# THE RIGHT TO LIVE IN HEALTH

# THE RIGHT TO

**ENVISIONING CUBA**
Louis A. Pérez Jr., *editor*

*Envisioning Cuba* publishes outstanding, innovative works in Cuban studies, drawn from diverse subjects and disciplines in the humanities and social sciences, from the colonial period through the post–Cold War era. Featuring innovative scholarship engaged with theoretical approaches and interpretive frameworks informed by social, cultural, and intellectual perspectives, the series highlights the exploration of historical and cultural circumstances and conditions related to the development of Cuban self-definition and national identity.

DANIEL A. RODRÍGUEZ

# LIVE IN HEALTH

*Medical Politics in Postindependence Havana*

The University of North Carolina Press  Chapel Hill

© 2020 The University of North Carolina Press
All rights reserved
Designed and set in Quadraat with Hypatia Sans by Rebecca Evans
Manufactured in the United States of America
The University of North Carolina Press has been a member of the Green Press Initiative since 2003.

A version of chapter 4 originally appeared as Daniel A. Rodríguez, "'The Dangers That Surround the Child': Race, Gender, and Infant Mortality in Post-Independence Havana," *Cuban Studies/Estudios Cubanos* 45 (2017): 297–318. Republished with permission.

A version of chapter 6 originally appeared as Daniel A. Rodríguez, "'To Fight These Powerful Trusts and Free the Medical Profession': Medicine, Class-Formation, and Revolution in Cuba, 1925–1935," *Hispanic American Historical Review* 95, no. 4 (November 2015): 595–629. Republished by permission of the copyright holder, Duke University Press.

Cover illustrations: photograph of doctor and patient by Julio Trigo, ca. 1920s–1930s (Fototeca, Caja 133, Sobre 117, registro. 4330, Archivo Nacional de Cuba); background, *Grunge Flag of Cuba* (© Fredex8, iStock).

Library of Congress Cataloging-in-Publication Data
Names: Rodríguez, Daniel A., 1976– author.
Title: The right to live in health : medical politics in postindependence Havana / Daniel A. Rodríguez.
Other titles: Envisioning Cuba.
Description: Chapel Hill : The University of North Carolina Press, 2020. | Series: Envisioning Cuba | Includes bibliographical references and index.
Identifiers: LCCN 2020004161 | ISBN 9781469659725 (cloth ; alk. paper) | ISBN 9781469659732 (paperback ; alk. paper) | ISBN 9781469659749 (ebook)
Subjects: LCSH: Cuba. Secretaría de Sanidad y Beneficencia—History. | Public health—Cuba—History—20th century. | Medical policy—Cuba—20th century. | Right to health—Cuba—History—20th century.
Classification: LCC RA395.C9 R63 2020 | DDC 362.1097291—dc23
LC record available at https://lccn.loc.gov/2020004161

**FOR SUSAN AND LOURDES**
*You make it worth it*

## CONTENTS

Acknowledgments xi

**Introduction** 1
The Meanings of Health in Postindependence Havana

ONE **A Nation of Spectres** 19
Reconcentration, U.S. Occupation, and the Modernization of the Public Health State

TWO **A Blessed Formula for Progress** 48
Medical Nationalism, U.S. Empire, and the Development of Public Health, 1899–1909

THREE **Salus Populi Suprema Lex** 86
Medical Modernity, Neocolonialism, and the 1914 Bubonic Plague Outbreak

FOUR **The Dangers That Surround the Child** 117
Gendered Poverty and the Fight against Infant Mortality

FIVE **With All, and for the Good of All** 146
Race, Poverty, and Tuberculosis

SIX **To Fight These Powerful Trusts and Free the Medical Profession** 176
Spanish Mutualism, Medicine, and Revolution, 1925–1935

**Conclusion** 201
The Right to Live in Health in Postcolonial Havana

Notes 209
Bibliography 241
Index 261

## FIGURES

Figure 1.1  Children dying on the palace porch  21

Figure 1.2  Los Fosos shelter, Havana  25

Figure 2.1  Postcard distributed by the Liga Contra la Tuberculosis en Cuba  61

Figure 2.2  Nursing students at Municipal Hospital No. 1  77

Figure 3.1  "War on the Rats!"  104

Figure 4.1  Advertisement for Maltina malted beer  136

Figure 4.2  Mothers and their babies attending the Consultorio de Higiene Infantil  143

Figure 5.1  Residents of the Solar Poloni  156

Figure 5.2  Residents of a tenement in Centro Habana  157

Figure 5.3  Tuberculosis consultation at La Esperanza  159

## ACKNOWLEDGMENTS

IT IS A TRUISM (that is nevertheless too often ignored outside "Acknowledgment" sections) that all academic work is a collective exercise, all books the product of countless influences and a lifetime of intellectual and personal debts. But it is without a doubt true.

The process of researching and writing this book coincided with a series of political and personal events that have profoundly shaped the writing process. Politically, the United States has been embroiled in over a decade of debate over the proper role of the government in ensuring that its population have access to affordable and quality health care. These debates, which often revolved around issues of the suitability of the capitalist market to meet the health needs of all, and the responsibility of the government in ensuring access, have informed the prism through which I have come to understand the health care debates of early-twentieth-century Cubans. Historical context, of course, matters, and the political culture of the early-twentieth-century United States is profoundly different from that of turn-of-the century Cuba; but I believe that by reflecting on the process through which Cubans came to take up health as a fundamental right rather than a privilege is indeed illuminating for those of us living today.

On a more personal note, as I was writing an early draft of this book, my wife, Susan—almost seven months pregnant with our first daughter—became acutely ill with preeclampsia and H.E.L.L.P. Syndrome. For the first time, I had to confront the real possibility that both my partner and my child could die. Thankfully, the doctors and nurses at Baystate Medical Center provided my family with the best care one could hope for. My wife made it through, and although our daughter, Lourdes, was born two months premature—weighing less than three pounds and fitting in the palm of our hands—she is now a thriving and creative first-grader. While these experiences profoundly affected me and my family, they also shaped this book. On an immediate level, they compelled me to research and write a chapter on infant mortality and child health. But they also brought me into deeper consideration of the possible meanings of illness and early death for the men and women who experienced these as a fact of life in Havana, in that period of history when a medical revolution was transforming our understanding of disease, but decades before antibiotics and new medical therapies would transform the ability of physicians to cure common illnesses. This book and my life have been informed by a new appreciation for the precariousness of health and the intertwining of family, medical, and community support that maintains us.

My research would not have been possible without the sponsorship of Cuban research institutions and the generous financial support of U.S. foundations. For sponsoring my research on the island and helping connect me to the vibrant research community there, I am indebted to the Instituto Cubano de Investigación Cultural "Juan Marinello" (and especially the ever-capable Henry Heredia), the Instituto de Historia de Cuba, Casa de las Americas, and the Fundación Antonio Núñez Jiménez de la Naturaleza y el Hombre. At different points, my research was made possible by the Tinker Foundation, the Torch Prize Fellowship, the Susan and George Field Summer Research Fellowship, and the Junior Faculty Development and Humanities Research Funds at Brown University. Invaluable time to write was made possible by the generous support of the Woodrow Wilson Foundation, the Mellon Foundation, and the Consortium for Faculty Diversity.

The support and warmth of Cuban archivists, librarians, and academics never ceases to amaze me. I am particularly thankful for the knowledge, patience, and support of the island's archivists and librarians, whose often thankless job is to preserve Cuba's cultural patrimony, despite the lack of state funding and the relentless attacks of the environment on archives and libraries full of crumbling paper and slowly deteriorating books. My special thanks go to wonderful staff at the Archivo Nacional de Cuba, especially Julio López Valdés, Silvio Santiago Facenda Castillo, Jorge Macle, and Olga Pedierro. This project literally could not have happened without the help of Graciela Guevara Benítez at the Museo Nacional de Historia de las Ciencias "Carlos J. Finlay," as well as the staff at the Biblioteca Nacional de Cuba "José Martí" and the Instituto de Literatura y Lingüística José Antonio Portuondo Valdor. My research was also pushed along by the wonderful community of open and generous Cuban historians, who gave me invaluable advice over cafecitos or amid piles of documents at the archive. Particular thanks go out to Enrique Beldarraín Chaple, Bárbara Danzie León, Victor Fowler, Tomás Fernández Robaina, Reinaldo Funes Monzote, Marial Iglesias Utset, Ricardo

Quiza Moreno, Alejandro Fernández, Pedro M. Pruna, Julio César González Laureiro, and Maikel Fariñas Borrego.

I am also indebted to the helpful and knowledgeable staffs at the U.S. National Archives at College Park, Maryland; the Library of Congress; the National Library of Medicine; Pennsylvania Historical Society; the Albert and Shirley Small Special Collections Library at the University of Virginia; the Rare Book and Manuscripts Library at Columbia University; Bobst Library at New York University; New York Public Library's Stephen A. Schwarzman Building and the Schomburg Center for Research in Black Culture; the Countway Library, Law School Library, and Lamont Library at Harvard University; and the staff at the Rockefeller and Hay Libraries at Brown University, especially librarians Holly Snyder, Patricia Figueroa, and Bart Hollingsworth for his patience with this inveterate Interlibrary Loan scofflaw.

My special thanks go out to those who generously read parts or all of this manuscript over the years and whose thoughtful commentary made it so much stronger. Ada Ferrer read many early drafts of this book, and her pushing, prodding, questioning, and support have made me a better writer, scholar, and teacher. Greg Grandin, Thomas Bender, Amy Chazkel, and Barbara Weinstein all provided important feedback at various stages of this book, and I'm grateful for their thoughtful comments and for showing me that excellent scholarship can be both politically relevant and rigorous. I was humbled when two of the historians I most respect—Alejandro de la Fuente and Eileen Findlay—took the time to read a draft of this book and come to Providence to spend the day workshopping it. And one of the joys of being faculty at Brown University has been the wonderfully generous and sharp colleagues who have taken the time to read drafts over the past few years, including Evelyn Hu-Dehart, the late Doug Cope, Naoko Shibusawa, Robert Self, Jeremy Mumford, Jennifer Lambe, Faiz Ahmed, Hal Cook, Debbie Weinstein, Lundy Braun and the members of the Race and Medicine Working Group, the History of Medicine Working Group, and the Legal History Workshop at Brown University. The fantastic group of students in my Race, Gender, and Medicine in the Americas seminar at Brown University provided the kind of useful feedback and support that one can only dream of, reinforcing my joy of teaching at Brown. The careful reading and comments of the two anonymous reviewers of the manuscript have without a doubt made this a stronger book, as has the phenomenal editing help of Rachel Kantrowitz. Finally, I would like to thank my editor Elaine Maisner at UNC Press for her support of this project and for her tireless support of now generations of scholars of Cuba.

Graduate school and post-Ph.D. academic life can be brutal, but survival is possible with the support of good friends and colleagues. At NYU, I had the pleasure of being part of a robust cohort of Latin Americanists and Caribbeanists, including Greg Childs, Anne Eller, Jennifer Adair, Ernesto Semán, Franny Sullivan, Jorge Silva, Michelle Chase, Justino Rodríguez, James Cantres, Christy Thornton, and Nathalie Pierre. Mike Bustamante, Brodwyn Fischer, Amy Offner, Jesse Horst, Kelly Urban, John Gutiérrez, and Ilan Erhlich have all helped shape this work through their own excellent research, as well as over shared meals and conversation. We would not have gotten through this past decade without the friendship and support of our now far-flung New York family, especially Greg Childs and Laura Cade Brown (and Carolina and Jamila, the best "sisters" we could ask for for our daughter), Samantha Seeley, Jen Wilson, Justino and Jared Rodríguez, Reynolds Richter, Geoff Traugh, Peter Wirzbicki, and Chester Soria. I am especially indebted to Linda Rodríguez and Mrinalini Tankha for their friendship, cooking skills, and research advice, and for getting me to the hospital when I fell into a pit in Havana. Linda Rodríguez died much too early, and her friends and loved ones feel her absence deeply. This book would not have been the same without her.

Since leaving New York, I have benefited from the personal, institutional, and intellectual support of many. The Smith College Program in Latin American and Latino/a Studies gave us a home and support as I finished my dissertation and welcomed the birth of our daughter, and Jeffrey Ahlman and Ann Zulawski extended much-needed support during our year in Northampton. And the Department of History at Kenyon College welcomed us during my postdoctoral fellowship there, while Ryan Phillips and Mollie Ring provided the friendship and delicious food that made that year much more pleasurable. At Brown University I've had the pleasure of being surrounded by a fantastic community of scholars that extended their friendship and ideas. I'm especially grateful to count among my colleagues Elena Shih, Emily Owens, Francoise Hamlin, Leticia Alvarado, Sarah Thomas, Iris Montero, Tara Nummedal, Seth Rockman, James N. Green, Ralph Rodriguez, Bathsheba Demuth, Jennifer Johnson, Ethan Pollock, Ken Sacks, Monica Martinez, and Daniel Vaca. And one of the pleasures of teaching at a place like Brown has been the amazing undergraduate and graduate students that have shaped my thinking, and special thanks go to the fantastic Ph.D. students Dan McDonald, René Cordero, and Thamyris Almeida, as well as undergraduates like Angelica Cotto, Brais Lamela, Camille Garnsey, Marga Kempner, Rachel Trafimow, Daniel Muller, Ella Satish, and Yilena Jimenez. All of these students have helped shape my thinking and sharpen my writing over the past few years.

My interest in the Cuban past was fostered over decades of stories of childhood, love, and family in small-town eastern Cuba, told and retold by my *abuela* Elvia Torrejón and by my *tía* Pilar Torrejón and *tío* Alfredo Torrejón, and especially by my mother, Silvia R. Torrejón. As an immigrant single mother struggling to raise three children and make ends meet in the increasingly expensive city of Boston, she imparted her love of family, history, and the deep joy of learning. Childhood stories about Havana from my *abuelo* José "Pepe" Rodríguez and my father, Joseph Arturo Rodríguez Armada, also stoked a deep interest in the Cuban capital that has yet to be quenched. My family in Vázquez, Cuba, has been a bottomless well of laughter, love, food, rum, and late-night chat fests in rocking chairs and terrifying motorcycle rides among the cane fields of eastern Cuba. While they are too many to list, my thanks particularly go out to Rosie and Elda, Bindo, Isis and Jorge, Lourdes, Omar, Javier, Pipito, Román, and Edelberto, all of whom have shown me the importance of family and have let me know that I will always have a home in Cuba. My extended family of *cubanos*, *puertoriqueños*, *dominicanos*, and *chilenos* always keep me grounded, and a special shout out goes to my wonderful siblings José Michael, Nicole, Giselle, Deandra, and Kathy, as well as my nieces Ava, Hannah, and Faye, and my cousins Christina, Jasmín, Natalia, Alisha, Mellissa, and Jessica.

But most of all, this project could never have been completed without the seemingly endless patience, support, wisdom, and sharp eye of my wife and partner, Susan Avalyn Rohwer. Our countless discussions on issues of health and politics, medicine and gender, childhood and state responsibility, shaped this project from beginning to end. Finally, to our daughter, Lourdes Avalyn Rodriguez Rohwer, whose joy and curiosity are infectious and who keeps us all grounded. Thank you. This is for you.

# THE RIGHT TO LIVE IN HEALTH

# Introduction
## The Meanings of Health in Postindependence Havana

ON APRIL 27, 1903, members of the Cuban House of Representatives met in Havana to discuss the creation of new government ministries to guide the work of the young republic, which had been inaugurated just one year earlier. During the meeting, José Ángel Malberty, a physician and legislator from the far-eastern town of Baracoa, surprised his colleagues by proposing the creation of a Secretaría de Sanidad y Beneficencia, a cabinet-level ministry centralizing in one body the administration of Cuban public health and welfare institutions.[1] The plan, however, proved controversial. As critics were quick to respond, no country in the world had a ministry dedicated specifically to matters of health, so why should Cuba?

But for Malberty, it was precisely the timing of Cuban independence that gave the new republic a unique opportunity and responsibility to make public health a matter of the highest state concern. As he told his fellow representatives, it made sense that none of the many nations "founded long before Sanitary Science was recognized as a Science" had established a Ministry of Health. After all, he explained, a nation's political and legal systems reflect the times in which they arise, and change thereafter only with some difficulty.[2] Indeed, as Malberty argued, reformers in England, France, Belgium, and the United States had in recent years pushed for the creation of ministries of health but had been stymied by inherited legal traditions that were resistant to change. But using this same historical reasoning, Malberty argued it was "logical and natural . . . that this Republic, born in this century," should establish a ministry dedicated to protecting the health of the Cuban people. The rupture of colonial ties, he believed, had created an opportunity to reimagine the essential duties of the state. As Malberty explained, "We must break with the past" and "take advantage of this constituent period to organize our government in accordance with the demands of modern Science."[3]

A second legislator, Pedro Albarrán Domínguez, rose to speak in support of the proposal. Like Malberty, Albarrán was also a practicing physician trained in Spanish medical schools and French hospitals during a period of unprecedented medical discovery, where he witnessed firsthand how bacteriology and new laboratory methods had fundamentally transformed both ideas of disease causation and the practice of medicine. But rather than see science and the state as separate spheres, Albarrán presented a forceful argument that as medical knowledge advanced, so too did the responsibility of the government to protect citizens' lives from diseases whose causes were finally known. Addressing his fellow legislators, Albarrán articulated this expansive theory of state responsibility: "The right to exist, the right to live," he argued, "necessarily comes before all other rights of man. The State has the obligation to guarantee these rights before all others. A considerable number of diseases that endanger man's existence can be avoided; therefore, each and every citizen has the right to demand that their government take the necessary measures to protect them."[4] The legislators were swayed by the words of Malberty and Albarrán, and they voted overwhelmingly in favor of the proposal. Although the bill initially failed to pass the Cuban Senate, six years later the government inaugurated the Secretaría de Sanidad y Beneficencia, or Ministry of Health and Public Charities, giving Cuba the distinction of having the world's first cabinet-level ministry dedicated to protecting the health of its people.

Though this debate took place over a century ago in the earliest months of the Cuban Republic, it nevertheless reveals an ambitious and far-reaching political project to join science and statecraft and secure health as a fundamental right of citizenship. For Malberty and Albarrán, protecting the health of the Cuban people was an essential task of government and the historical responsibility of the first independent nation of the twentieth century. But they were hardly alone. Indeed, for an entire generation of early-twentieth-century physicians, nurses, and public health officials, the political rupture of the end of colonial rule provided an unprecedented opportunity to use the tools of medical science to reshape Cuban society and create a modern and healthy republic. For these men and women, medical knowledge had profound political implications. Once the causes of diseases like yellow fever, tuberculosis, and infantile tetanus were known and practices to prevent them were established, Cuba's grim annual mortality rates were no longer inevitable facts, but a call to action. With the power to reduce or even in some cases eliminate certain disease threats, decisions over whether to extend public health services or expand access to public medical care became matters of deep political importance, reflecting the essential purpose of government and the most basic rights of citizens. But if medical science created new state responsibilities, these responsibilities were to be shared by citizens, who were increasingly called upon to adopt new hygienic practices to protect themselves and their fellow citizens from disease.

The Right to Live in Health explains how these ideas emerged during the transition from colony to republic, shaped the development of new health institutions and the lives of Havana's residents, and were contested, transformed, and taken up by ever-broader swaths of the urban population to make claims about citizenship and state responsibility. It examines the postcolonial history of Havana as urban residents confronted disease and early death during a period of dizzying political, economic, and scientific change. Between 1897 and 1935, Havana's residents experienced the devastating impact of Cuba's final War of Independence (1895–98), two U.S. occupations (1899–1902 and 1906–9), the birth of the republic, economic booms and collapses, the rise of a dictatorship, and a social revolution.

While these events were of profound importance to the men and women who lived and worked in the city, their lives were shaped in even more direct ways by events closer to home: the illness of a child or spouse or the untimely death of a loved one. Tuberculosis was an ever-present danger, disproportionately killing those in the prime of their lives, while gastroenteritis was especially deadly for the youngest, and yellow fever targeted primarily immigrants without the acquired immunity that protected native Cubans. These diseases, each targeting distinct populations and with distinct modes of transmission, transformed the lives of the families they touched. Each illness, each attempt to get care at a public hospital or dispensary, each interaction between medical workers and patients, was an occasion rife with personal, social, and political meaning. As Cubans of all classes negotiated these interactions and contested the meanings of disease and health in the postcolonial environment, they transformed the medical landscape. The central task of this book is to bring together these frames of analysis, highlighting the interdependence of the city's economic, ideological, and bacteriological environments, as the economy had profound epidemiological consequences and as disease and medicine came to take on profound political significance.

## MEDICAL NATIONALISM IN POSTCOLONIAL CUBA

In 1905, Carlos J. Finlay, the famed Cuban physician who discovered the cause of yellow fever transmission, wrote that "the young Republic of Cuba had the luck of being born at the dawn of an age of enlightenment, in the midst of a sparkling atmosphere of scientific discovery, so that its first breaths have been of progress and noble aspirations."[5] It is a truism of historical thinking that people interpret the world through the lens of their experiences, within specific cultural and material contexts. For figures like Finlay, Malberty, and the rest of the generation of medical nationalists that cohered during the transition from colony to republic, their linking of medicine and health to the promise of independence was firmly rooted in their experiences as practicing physicians deeply engaged in the rapid scientific and political change of their age. These turn-of-the-century medical reformers straddled two revolutionary currents. The recent "bacteriological revolution," set off by the research of Louis Pasteur and Robert Koch, and the revolution in surgery made possible by new antiseptic and aseptic techniques transformed the practice of medicine in the late nineteenth century.[6] The rapidly growing list of diseases whose cause and modes of transmission were finally known and the development of new hygienic practices to successfully ward off illness all led to a sense of rapid and inevitable medical progress. New procedures and better understandings of infection vastly improved surgical outcomes and postsurgical recovery. Public health practice was transformed, and officials increasingly claimed broad new powers to control disease in their jurisdictions. And physicians, health officials, and reformers increasingly preached the "gospel of hygiene," spreading practices like hand-washing, careful preparation and storage of food, and avoidance of the bodily fluids of others in order to prevent the spread of infection.

In Cuba, this period of scientific change coincided almost perfectly with the island's decades-long independence struggle. Cuban independence came long after the great Atlantic Age of Revolution, which rocked Europe and saw most of the Western Hemisphere shed colonial ties and embrace some form of republican governance. As Ada Ferrer and other historians have shown, as anticolonial rebellion spread across the hemisphere in the early nineteenth century, Cuban elites clung ever more closely to Spain, fearful of the racial implications of independence for the sugar colony whose wealth was based on the ever-expanding supply of enslaved African labor.[7] It was not until 1868 that the Cuban planter Carlos Manuel de Céspedes freed the enslaved men and women on his plantation and initiated what would be a decades-long struggle for independence that tied anticolonial rebellion to the process of abolition and, eventually, the ideal of a racially egalitarian nation.

Over the next thirty years and through three separate wars of independence, the protracted anticolonial struggle shaped the politics, practice, and meanings of Cuban medicine. Cuban physicians became central figures in urban underground revolutionary networks, were forced into exile where they gained valuable experience in cutting-edge clinics in Europe and North America, and practiced frontline medicine in the battlefields of the anticolonial wars. Cuba's final War of Independence (1895–98) provided a brutal denouement to colonial rule, as Spanish "reconcentration" policies displaced tens of thousands of rural Cubans, removing them from the countryside to prevent them from supporting the independence forces and pushing them into the cities where they had little access to food, shelter, or medical care. As a result of these policies, 150,000 to 170,000 civilians, close to 10 percent of the Cuban population, had died by the end of the war, mostly of disease and starvation. It was Cuba's worst demographic disaster since the Spanish conquest and became a grim symbol of the failures of colonial rule.[8] Immersed in an age of anticolonial ferment and scientific progress, and armed with new ideas and a desire to use their medical knowledge to benefit their people, Cuba's scattered nationalist physicians returned to the capital at the end of the war, ready to confront the health effects of the war and aid in the reconstruction of the island.

But while the end of one empire provided an opening, the emergence of a second cemented the role of medicine in Cuban national politics. After defeating Spanish forces in the "Spanish-American War" of 1898, Americans established the ostensibly provisional U.S. Military Government in Cuba (1899–1902). Hoping to finally eliminate yellow fever—the perennial threat to the southern U.S. coastline—from the Cuban capital, military officials immediately began tackling Havana's abominable health conditions. Officials organized a broad sanitary campaign to clean up the city, dredging the harbor, initiating round-the-clock street cleaning brigades, installing flush toilets, performing house-to-house health inspections, and eventually overseeing a massive campaign to root out the city's mosquitoes. As historians Nancy Stepan and Mariola Espinosa have noted, the military government's sanitary reforms amounted to a colonial public health program meant primarily to protect American lives and interests.[9] But, turning the lens slightly, we see that Cuban medical workers eagerly participated in this sanitary reorganization of the capital and were transformed by the process.

Cuban physicians took up administrative positions in new local and national boards of health, working as medical inspectors, hospital administrators, and government health advisors. From these positions they advanced their reform agenda, pushing back against the occupation government's singular focus on yellow fever and demanding increased funding for tuberculosis control and new clinics and hospitals to care for the sick. They saw in the military government's centralization of public health and medical services a model for postcolonial health work that reflected not the priorities of an occupying power but the health needs of the Cuban people. In short, they took advantage of American health concerns to assert their own priorities, in the process redefining a colonial public health agenda into a nationalist medical project that would reverberate in the coming decades.

For this generation of Cuban medical nationalists, disease itself was colonial, and medical science provided the blueprint for turning the broken former colony into a healthy and modern republic. Reformers saw biomedical science as an extension of the revolutionary anticolonial struggle, "a blessed formula for progress" for the Cuban nation. It would reshape the urban landscape of Havana and transform its inhabitants into healthy, modern citizens prepared for the responsibilities of independence. But while they were united in this broad medical nationalist vision for the republic, they differed quite a bit on the implications of this project on questions of race, the organization of the economy, and the contours of state versus individual responsibility for the health of the people. Indeed, they were largely middle-class white male professionals whose vision of modernity, hygiene, and the sanitary capacities of the Cuban people was shaped by long-standing racial, gendered, and class discourses that tied the capacity for "civilized" conduct to European norms. Many saw women and Cubans of color as disproportionately responsible for Havana's supposed sanitary backwardness. And some were explicit in their hope that sanitary reforms would, by reducing urban disease, attract European immigrants and help whiten the population into modernity. After independence, these differences came to take on much greater significance, leading to sometimes fierce disagreements over the appropriate amount of state intervention in the economy—over rents, food prices, and the size of the public medical sector—as well as whether the persistent health problems of the island resulted from fundamental flaws in its multiracial population or the failure of the government to fulfill its responsibility to protect the health of the people.

Like all nationalist discourse, Cuban medical nationalism emerged out of a complex interplay between external and internal pressures, and here, once again, the United States played a central role. When the Cuban Republic was inaugurated in May 1902, the city's health statistics had improved dramatically: yellow fever was all but eliminated, and sanitary improvements had helped lower the city's exorbitant mortality rates. But even as the U.S. occupation gave way to the republic, the United States forced upon the island the mechanism for continued sanitary oversight. The Platt Amendment, imposed on Cuba as a precondition for the withdrawal of U.S. forces, included as its fifth article the requirement that the Cuban government maintain acceptable sanitary conditions in its cities, in order that "a recurrence of epidemic and infectious diseases may be prevented, thereby assuring protection to the people and commerce of Cuba, as well as to the commerce of the southern ports of the United States and the people residing therein." Failure to do so risked additional American intervention. In a very real sense, then, Cuban sovereignty would be determined by the ability of health officials to control infectious disease. Cuban health officials and medical workers rejected the imperial pretensions that underlay the Platt Amendment's health clause, and they fumed at the lack of faith it showed for Cuban administrative ability and commitment to public health. But medical nationalists also used the clause to further their objectives, pressuring recalcitrant government officials to fund innovative health programs as the fulfillment of the nation's international obligations, thereby turning the central mechanism of neocolonial control into an essential tool for furthering a revolutionary health agenda.

Indeed, the early years of the republic were marked by an unprecedented expansion in medical work.[10] New state-run nursing schools—attached to newly nationalized hospitals across the island—produced Latin America's first professional nurses, who worked alongside hospital administrators to transform hospital care. In Havana, Cuban scientists convened at the National Academy of Science to share original medical research, while doctors and nurses worked to bring new medical knowledge and hygienic practices into the homes of city residents through an interconnected system of public dispensaries, home health education programs, and health journals aimed at popular audiences. Public health campaigns—by decade's end directed by the world's first Ministry of Health—extirpated yellow fever from the island and targeted infant mortality, tuberculosis, malaria, bubonic plague, and other diseases. While primarily felt in the capital, these new campaigns and institutions reached deep into the homes of urban residents, transformed the lives of citizens, and represented a vast expansion in state action. But urban residents experienced these changes differently, as both disease and medicine were shaped by class, race, gender, and national origin.

While illness spared no one, urban residents had differential access to the material conditions that could mean the difference between a long life and an early death. Economic inequality, race, and national origin structured uneven access to health care. While early-twentieth-century Havana could boast of having perhaps the highest per capita number of physicians anywhere in the world, it was the wealthy who had easiest access to quality private medical care, while Spanish immigrants and those who could claim Spanish descent—exclusively white Cubans in practice—had access to the city's system of low-cost private mutual aid hospitals and clinics established by Spanish immigrant workers. Disease also reflected and helped reinforce the city's gendered and racialized economy. Cubans of color and women were relegated to the lowest-paying jobs, which, in Havana's notoriously expensive housing market, meant that these families often lived in cramped and overcrowded *solares*, or tenements, and lacked regular access to healthy food. Economic insecurity forced poor mothers to wean their infants early, leaving them vulnerable to the gastrointestinal ailments that were the main cause of infant mortality, while the cramped living conditions, exhaustion, and insufficient nutrition of poor households made them ideal incubators for tuberculosis. In a grim cycle, the disproportionate disease burden of the poor often resulted in loss of household income, further impoverishment, and greater vulnerability to disease.

This book contends that, over time, the growing interactions between the urban poor and the agents of the expanding public health state were transformative for both. For the poor families who made up the majority of the city's population, vulnerable moments of illness and death were key points of interaction with new public medical institutions, as they competed for care in the city's chronically underfunded public hospitals, clinics, and dispensaries or welcomed into their homes public health nurses who sought to teach them how to avoid infection and care for sick children or family members stricken with tuberculosis. While these moments were always fraught with multiple meanings, over time they generated new expectations, as urban residents increasingly looked to public medical and welfare institutions to meet their health needs, eventually claiming access to these institutions and services as fundamental rights of citizenship.

But these interactions also transformed the medical workers who had the closest contact with the urban poor. Having worked under the medical nationalist belief that preventative health work, hygienic education, and new medical institutions would in themselves ensure the health of the Cuban people, medical workers were forced to confront the limits of this vision in light of a postcolonial economy that itself was responsible for so much disease and death. By the 1910s, it would be nurses, doctors, and public health officials that increasingly called attention to the limits of a medical nationalist vision that did not address the root causes of disease in the city's low wages and exorbitant rents. By the 1920s and 1930s, these insights facilitated a growing alliance between medical workers and labor unions, journalists of color, and radical intellectuals who called for more far-reaching medical and economic reforms that would finally meet the health needs of the Cuban people.

## DISEASE, DEATH, AND MEDICINE IN A CHANGING CITY

Essential for understanding how disease and health came to take on such political significance in early republican Cuba is the rapidly changing city of Havana itself. Rather than simply being set in the Cuban capital, this book takes as a starting point that Havana's urban environment was a profound epidemiological factor shaping the distribution of disease and mortality across an uneven field of race, gender, class, and national origin. Historians of the Caribbean have long characterized the region through its interconnections of trade, people, and ideas, and indeed Havana was a thriving port city whose trade and transportation networks connected it not just to the United States but to the broader Caribbean, Spain, and the rest of the Atlantic.[11] The epidemiological implications of these interconnections were clear to those Americans who imposed upon Cuba the requirement that urban centers be kept free from dangerous infectious diseases. In so doing, they hoped to protect southern U.S. ports from diseases like yellow fever, bubonic plague, or typhus, which were often spread by unseen microscopic hitchhikers on the bodies of the people, rats, and insects that journeyed across the Caribbean on ever-faster shipping networks.[12] As Cuban health officials emphasized, however, disease traveled in all directions, and at various points the Cuban port was closed to commerce from New Orleans, the Spanish Canary Islands, Puerto Rico, and Mexico, among others, as foreign port cities became sites of infection. Efforts to limit certain kinds of immigration were often couched in terms of the potential disease threat immigrant bodies might pose. Yet racial concerns often proved decisive for how these debates played out, as officials called for the barring of Chinese or black Antillean migrants while Spanish immigrants were welcomed as a "civilizing" influence on the young nation.

But beyond the microbial interchange that inevitably occurs through trade and travel, the social geography of the city was itself shaped in fundamental ways by these trade networks, in ways that had profound implications not just for the distribution of disease but also for how disease was interpreted in a city divided along lines of class, race, and national origin. A central, yet far too understudied, fact of urban life in Havana was the enormous influence that Spanish immigrants continued to exert over the postcolonial economy.[13] In the decades after the end of Spanish colonial rule, Spanish immigration to Cuba actually increased, with the capital being the main destination for most Iberian migrants. In the decades after independence, the Spanish-born consistently made up more than a fifth of the urban population. Yet their economic clout far outweighed their percentage of the population, as Spaniards came to dominate the urban banking sector as well as wholesale and retail commerce and many of the urban trades. This was evident to anyone walking along the city center. Spanish-owned warehouses—filled with imported potatoes, beans, and salted codfish—lined the blocks south of the city's docks, while Spanish immigrant workers delivered these wares across the urban core to Spanish *bodegueros* who sold them to city residents. By the 1910s, Spanish immigrant mutual aid associations—which banded together immigrants from specific regions of Spain such as Asturias or Galicia—had built imposing *centros*, or social clubs, in the city center, and low-cost monthly membership dues provided everything from entertainment and spaces to socialize to adult education and medical services.

The social and economic geography of Spanish commercial power profoundly shaped the medical landscape. It often pitted Cuban health officials and physicians against what they increasingly saw as the continued colonial influence of the former imperial power. One explosive moment occurred in 1914, with the arrival of bubonic plague in Havana. The disease likely arrived on the island as a microbial stowaway, traveling across the ocean within the bodies of the fleas attached to the rats that hid in the bowels of ships carrying food exports from the Spanish Canary Islands. The subsequent outbreak was centered in Havana's waterfront warehouse district. All of the initial victims were Spanish workers, but Spanish warehouse owners resisted public health orders, reluctant to have their goods ruined by antiplague fumigation measures. The ensuing conflict inflamed Cuban medical nationalist sentiment against Spanish merchants, culminating in the quarantine under military occupation of the entire commercial core of the city. But Spanish immigrant economic power shaped the medical history of the city in even more fundamental ways. With fully a quarter of the city's residents receiving low-cost private medical care through one of the city's Spanish immigrant mutual aid *centros*, Spanish institutions dominated the urban medical market. With many urban residents too poor to pay for medical services and reliant on underfunded public hospitals and clinics, Cuban physicians were forced to compete with private Spanish clinics for patients in a crowded medical market. Once again, anti-Spanish sentiment helped bring together Cuban physicians, whose professional organizing centered on opposition to Spanish *centros*. And once again, this came to an explosive end, with a 1934 medical strike, the bombings of Cuban pharmacies, and the assassination of a Cuban physician. In both of these cases, however, Spanish power pushed physicians to consider the economic limits of medical nationalist action and opened the way for more radical solutions to the problems of patients and physicians.

The very development of the city, its growth in population and land area, its property values and rental markets, its transportation networks, and its distribution of factories and workshops, hospitals and clinics—all of these had a profound effect on the health conditions of the people and the meanings they ascribed to them. Havana's postcolonial growth continued along the lines of its colonial development, lacking anything that could be described as intentional urban planning.[14] Between 1899 and 1931, the population more than tripled, while the boundaries of the city expanded far to the south and west, increasing the land area of the capital fourfold.[15] But even as the city expanded and incorporated new tony suburbs, real estate speculation kept urban property values extraordinarily high. Avaricious landlords took advantage of the tight housing market to charge exorbitant rents. This forced poor families to live in tight, overcrowded, and often poorly maintained tenements, where poverty and close proximity facilitated the spread of disease. The fluctuating urban job market shaped the fortunes of urban residents along lines of race and gender. Cubans of color and women occupied the lowest rungs of the economy, where low wages and high unemployment meant these households were often forced to live in the worst conditions, faced higher levels of malnutrition, and suffered from much higher rates of infant mortality and tuberculosis death. While census records show that less than a quarter of the city's population was of African descent, Cubans of color appeared at much higher rates in the annual mortality statistics. Over time, these facts took on sharp political meaning, as journalists of color, health officials, physicians, and nurses all called attention to the disproportionate rates at which Cubans of color were dying. In so doing, they highlighted the failure of the independence-era ideal of a racially egalitarian republic and called upon the government to fulfill its historical promise of a healthy Cuba for all.

## ARCHIVES, FIRES, AND FRAMEWORKS

Early in the pre-dawn hours of February 6, 1933, three decades after José Ángel Malberty first proposed the creation of a Secretaría de Sanidad y

Beneficencia, an incendiary device went off at the ministry's headquarters.[16] The ensuing fire engulfed the ministry's archives, finding ample fuel in the stacks of memos, reports, and missives that documented decades of funding requests and sanitary fines, hiring practices, and intra-agency conflicts. While no one was ever arrested for the arson, it came only months after a bomb destroyed a wing of the Ministry of Health. These were among a string of attacks during the violent final months of the dictatorship of General Gerardo Machado (1925–33), during which opponents of the regime often targeted government ministries that—like the Ministry of Health—were widely viewed as being especially corrupt.[17] One striking irony of the bombing, in fact, was its destruction of documentary evidence of the extent of corruption at the ministry, which had for years been plagued by accusations of graft and financial mismanagement. The destruction of the ministry's archive obviously poses certain challenges for historians, but it also forces us to cast a wider net across both state archives and a rich body of largely untapped sources for exploring new dimensions of early-twentieth-century Cuban life.

The bombing of the ministry's archive serves as a rather stark example of how power shapes knowledge production and a useful reminder that archives *always* reflect broader struggles. As Antoinette Burton reminds us, "Archives come into being in and as history as a result of specific political, cultural, and economic pressures—pressures which leave traces and which render archives themselves artifacts of history."[18] Like all archives, the Archivo Nacional de Cuba (the Cuban National Archive) reflects a long series of political decisions and encounters that work to shape the contours of the past. At the most basic level, by collecting material from various government ministries, the Archivo Nacional reflects historical struggles over the fundamental duties of the Cuban government. But the collections also reflect decisions over which specific documents are worth keeping and processing, choices over how to classify particular documents, national-level debates over how to fund the archives, and administrative decisions regarding who should be allowed access. Finding aids reflect the politicization of the past in post-1959 Cuba, with the period between the end of colonial rule and the 1959 Cuban Revolution officially classified as the *seudorepública*, or pseudo-republic, reflecting the official narrative of the republic as characterized by American neocolonial domination and fundamental continuity with Spanish colonial rule, only broken by the rupture of the 1959 triumph of the revolution.

Together, these forces have exerted a profound influence on historical scholarship, shaping the contours of historical research and our sense of the Cuban past. Indeed, while there has been much excellent scholarship on the republic, this work has tended to foreground themes of neocolonial dependency and political corruption, tracing broad lines of continuity between colonial and postcolonial forms of domination and social relations.[19] Undoubtedly, the effects of neocolonialism and corruption on Cuban life and politics are important themes, and indeed they are central to this book as well. But overall, this book takes a rather different approach. Inspired by a growing cohort of historians reexamining the republic on its own terms rather than simply as a "prelude to Revolution," and drawing lessons from postcolonial scholarship, recent work on nineteenth-century Latin America, and the rich literature on "everyday forms of state formation," *The Right to Live in Health* emphasizes rupture over continuity, highlights the contradictory effects of neocolonial influence, and sees public health as a central site of struggle and negotiation over the meanings of health, modernity, and independence in the decades after independence.[20]

Historians of twentieth-century Latin America have understandably emphasized the repressive aspects of governance in Latin America and the Caribbean. But "the state" was always more than its repressive function, and especially in the cities, where public services were much better developed, citizens experienced the state in a variety of ways beyond the coercive. Of course, medicine served an important disciplinary function, most obviously in the project to instill hygienic self-control, and public health is inseparable from the coercive power of the state to enforce the mandates of health officials, as became clear to all when the army was sent out to enforce the quarantine of the city's waterfront warehouse district during the 1914 bubonic plague outbreak.[21]

But power was not unidirectional. Even as new ideas and hygienic practices reshaped Cuban society, Cubans transformed the medical landscape, as they interpreted medicine through the lens of their own experiences and needs and, by claiming health rights, pushed physicians, nurses, health officials, and eventually lawmakers to recognize the right of all Cuban citizens to medical care. In narrating this story, this book highlights the postcolonial state as a key site of struggle, draws our attention to how rights are contested and developed at all levels of society before becoming officially articulated in constitutional law, and shows that Latin America was a center for the articulation of new social rights in the twentieth century. The history of social rights is usually told as a North Atlantic story, emerging out of the European Enlightenment and the French Revolution, and perhaps best represented by the 1793 Jacobin Declaration of the Rights of Man and Citizen, which articulated an expansive vision of rights, including the right to education and public relief.

But there is a long if underappreciated history of enshrining expansive collective rights in Latin American constitutional history, from the 1805 Haitian constitution and 1813 draft constitution of the Mexican revolutionary José María Morelos to the 1917 postrevolution Mexican constitution and postdictatorship Brazilian constitution, and scholars are increasingly turning their attention to Latin America's contributions to the history of social rights.[22]

THE RIGHT TO HEALTH is distinct from other rights, however, and emerges not in the eighteenth or early nineteenth century but only once medical science and public health practice had advanced to the point where they could generate new expectations and citizens began making novel claims on the state to protect the public health. This fact distinguishes the historical trajectory of health rights from other Enlightenment-era social rights. Cuba is at the center of this global story of health rights due to a confluence of factors: the timing of the independence struggle and its relationship to the transformation of medicine in the last third of the nineteenth century, the complex linkages between American empire and Cuban medical nationalism, and the decades of interactions between medical practitioners and patients in postindependence Cuba that led to new expectations and understandings of state and individual responsibility for health in the context of a postcolonial economy that precipitated so much suffering. By 1940, where this book ends, access to medical services was enshrined in the country's new social democratic constitution as one of the fundamental rights of all Cuban citizens.

This book is peopled with middle-class professionals: physicians, public health officials, nurses, journalists, writers, and politicians. These are the individuals whose perspectives, frustrations, actions, and ideas are most clearly preserved in the archival records and published materials of the time. As they lived through and struggled to make sense of this period of intense political, social, and scientific change, they debated the root causes of disease, the implications of the disproportionate mortality of the poor, and how to best improve the health conditions of their country. Some left especially prominent traces, allowing us to follow their shifting understanding of disease, health, poverty, and government responsibility, and these play an especially prominent role in this narrative. The physician and inveterate reformer Manuel Delfín, for example, founded a dispensary for poor children, wrote several books, and published the journal *La Higiene* with the goal of bringing the benefits of hygienic knowledge and practice to a literate middle-class readership, and he went on to found other organizations that sought to reduce disease by addressing the basic needs of the poor. The tireless nurse and educator Mary Eugénie Hibbard and health official José Antonio López del Valle would increasingly call attention to the role that housing conditions, poor wages, and malnutrition played in the city's terrible health conditions.

While the actions and ideas of these middle-class professionals are of profound importance to this story, just as important are the poor and working-class families who made up the majority of Havana's population. But the archive has left us few sources through which we can make sense of the meanings these women and men gave to disease and early death or to the health institutions created to improve the health of the Cuban people. Of course, from the end of colonial rule through the tumultuous decade of the 1930s, their habits, behaviors, forms of childrearing, and living conditions were the subject of much debate and analysis from reformers, medical professionals, journalists, and officials. So it is to the troves of paper that these debates generated that we must turn, carefully sifting through these documents to begin to access—however partially—the ideas, actions, and experiences of the urban poor. Perhaps the most important of these records were the health statistics published infrequently in the official Boletín of the Ministry of Health. These statistics give us a map of how the gendered and racialized postcolonial economy left its mark on the very bodies of the city's residents, marking certain groups for disease and early death while blessing others with relative health and long life. Disease reflected and reinforced racialized class disparities, but it also revealed them. Statistics give us a glimpse into the lived reality of Cubans who rarely appear in the written record except in the traces produced in their interactions with state and private medical institutions, as their births, deaths, and illnesses were fed into the city's mortality and morbidity reports.

Rather than simply reflecting on-the-ground health conditions, statistics themselves became powerful instruments, as health officials, reformers, journalists, and politicians read them as signs of modernity or backwardness, the collective ignorance of the poor, or the historic failures of the republic. The anthropologist Sean Brotherton has described the post-1959 Cuban government's fixation with specific public health markers as a form of "statistical fetishism," as certain health indices and Cuba's national ranking on World Health Organization lists came to symbolize the essential goodness of the revolutionary project.[23] But in the early twentieth century, it was Cuba's elevated infant mortality rate, especially in relation to the rate of other countries, that proved a profound source of embarrassment to medical nationalists and government officials alike. Later, activists of color and their allies saw in the disproportionate rates of black tuberculosis mortality the failure of the republic to live up to its ideals. These concerns generated public attention, which in turn generated more scientific studies and public and private health programs. These reports shine further light on the living conditions and mothering practices of the poor and tell of the complex and sometimes conflictual relationship between medical workers and urban residents.

## STRUCTURE OF THE BOOK

The structure of *The Right to Live in Health* reflects key moments, debates, and conflicts that were central to the transformation of Cuban medical politics through the early decades of the twentieth century. Chapter 1 explores the health crisis caused by Spanish reconcentration policies during the final War of Independence, tracing Cuban and U.S. efforts to provide relief to the city's *reconcentrados* as war gave way to the new U.S. military occupation, and as health and welfare work was systematized and centralized by the new Departamento de Beneficencia, or Department of Public Charities, which Cuban physicians and health workers saw as a model for the nationalization of health services in postcolonial Cuba. Chapter 2 traces the development of Cuban medical nationalism as both an anticolonial politics and an example of state formation as cultural revolution. During the period of the first U.S. occupation and first years of the republic, medical nationalism served as the organizing principle for the expansion of the postcolonial public health state, but it also required the transformation of Cuban habits in the service of a Eurocentric vision of national modernity.

The following four chapters explore different aspects of republican health work, focusing on how Cuban health politics emerged out of and in relation to the changing postcolonial economy. Chapter 3 explores the 1914 bubonic plague outbreak in Havana, examining the local, national, and international politics that shaped both state disease control efforts and popular responses to the outbreak, which was centered in the Spanish immigrant commercial enclave in the heart of Old Havana. In mid-April, public health authorities instituted a broad quarantine of seventeen city blocks in the heart of the commercial district, forcing 7,000 residents to leave the area, as the Cuban army was brought out to the streets of the capital to enforce the measures. Caught between international pressure to rapidly control the disease and Spanish resistance to public health measures, the bubonic plague outbreak highlights the economic processes that both justified and limited the power of medical nationalist health officials to act.

Chapters 4 and 5 expand on the relations between the postcolonial economy and public health, taking on the two central health concerns of the postindependence period: tuberculosis and infant mortality. These two chapters emphasize the limits of a medical nationalist vision that ignored the roots of disease in the neocolonial economy and show the growing demands for nationalist health policies that addressed poverty in addition to providing medical services and health education. Chapter 4 explores the expansion in child and maternal health work in early-twentieth-century Havana in the context of years of alarming infant mortality statistics. In response to the health crisis, and to accusations of government indifference, health officials organized the Children's Health Service. This new branch of the health ministry was responsible for the medical care of poor children and the creation of special sanatoriums for tubercular children, the supervision of midwives and wet nurses, the care and hygienic education of poor mothers and pregnant women, and other work, as part of a holistic effort to reduce the city's infant mortality rate. But while health reformers had advocated for a broad expansion in public medical care and free childcare options for poor mothers, the campaign against infant mortality focused primarily on educating poor women in modern childcare methods and urging them to breastfeed their children, and it would be up to private organizations to directly confront the economic bases of infant mortality.

Chapter 5 focuses on debates over poverty and tuberculosis in the context of the disproportionate rates at which Cubans of color died of the disease. This provides a view of the city's racial economy and the meanings that racialized disease took on in the context of a political system ostensibly based on racial egalitarianism. More than any other disease in the early twentieth century, tuberculosis highlights the broader social and economic dynamics that shaped the health conditions of the Cuban people. As journalists of color made clear, neither poverty nor disease were color-blind; rather, the disproportionate rates of black poverty and disease represented a failure of the Cuban state to fulfill its historical promise of a nation "with all, and for the good of all." Over the 1910s and 1920s, there began to emerge a growing sense of the need for deep structural reforms: new public medical institutions to address the immediate health care needs of the poor combined with broad economic reforms to increase wages and bring down rents and the cost of basic necessities. Through this process, urban residents, reformers, and black activists pushed for a medical nationalist project that secured health as a social right, combining access to health care with economic policies to eliminate the root causes of disease.

After my examination of the city's health politics from the perspectives of medical reformers, public health officials, and the residents of Havana, the last chapter explores the politics of medical practice and the medical market from the perspective of Cuban physicians. This chapter explores the radicalization of the Cuban medical class in the context of the political and economic crises of the early 1930s. I argue that a small group of physicians, in successfully pushing the broader medical class to broaden its sectoral demands to address wider problems in urban medical care, were able to take advantage of a revolutionary moment to benefit both doctors and patients.

The book's conclusion brings us to Cuba's 1940 social democratic constitution, which formally enshrined the right to health for all Cubans, and uses this historical moment to reflect on broader historical continuities and discontinuities during a century of profound political, social, and scientific change. Today, Cuba's association with medicine is well known, and perhaps the most enduring and transformative legacy of the 1959 revolution has been its formal commitment to providing quality medical care to all citizens. But, as this book shows, much of the medical nationalist discourse of the post-1959 period can be dated to this earlier period, which underscored the potential of an alliance between medicine and the state to transform Cuban society, even if that reality remained largely out of reach for most Cubans.

As this book goes to press, almost half of the world's population is under a "stay-at-home" order to prevent the spread of the novel coronavirus COVID-19. During times of crisis, it can be comforting to look to the past for guidance or understanding, but it gives me little comfort that so many of the dynamics present in early twentieth-century Cuban health politics are also shaping the current pandemic. As in Cuba a century ago, we see the health implications of a partisan media landscape, the medical scapegoating of the foreign-born, and hygienic education campaigns meant to change individual behavior and thereby reduce the spread of disease. As in Cuba before the creation of the national Ministry of Health, today in the United States we see the health consequences of a patchwork system of public health authority—with major public health decisions made at the local and state level and little national coordination and insufficient government funding. Most importantly, while disease spares no one, once again we see the health effects of global and national inequality, with the poor and those lacking social protections most at risk of dying in this new pandemic. But perhaps the current moment of crisis will jolt people to demand universal access to essential health services and an end to the entrenched inequalities that condemn so many to unnaturally short lives—just as a century ago, Cubans demanded health and medical care not as a privilege, but as an essential right for all.

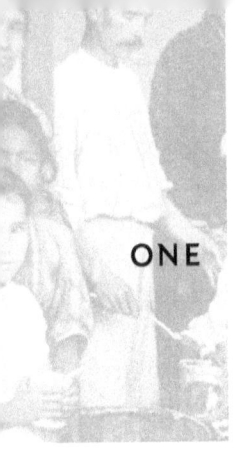

## ONE   A Nation of Spectres

Reconcentration, U.S. Occupation, and the Modernization of the Public Health State

RARE AMONG MAJOR FIGURES in turn-of-the-century Cuban medicine, Manuel Delfín did not come from an elite family. Born in 1849 in Baracoa, at the far eastern end of the island, Delfín had worked as a servant growing up. A promising student, he had earned a scholarship to study medicine in Madrid.[1] After returning to Cuba, he spent many years working as a small-town doctor, packing a medical bag onto his saddle and riding on horseback to attend to sick campesinos. It was here in rural Cuba in the final years of colonial rule that Delfín first confronted poverty the likes of which "he had never dreamed of in [his] life." Decades later, he recalled the sparse palm-thatched homes of households barely held together by single mothers, whose families would go days without food, resulting in malnutrition, disease, and early death for children and adults alike.[2] Delfín would go on to devote his career to addressing the relationship between gendered poverty and illness. Eventually moving to Havana, in the 1890s he founded the Hygiene Society and the journal *La Higiene*, both of which worked to advance the cause of public health and popularize scientific medical knowledge among the Cuban public. In 1896, Delfín was tapped by the bishop of Havana, Manuel Santander y Frutos, to run the Dispensario La Caridad, a free clinic for poor children that would be housed on the first floor of the bishop's residence on the outskirts of Old Havana. It was a natural fit for a physician-reformer dedicated to the health of the poor.

Within months, however, the little clinic was overwhelmed. Every day, hundreds, sometimes thousands, of starving and sick children and their mothers lined up along the streets of Old Havana, hoping to be attended by the clinic's all-volunteer staff. They were among the hundreds of thousands of Cubans displaced by the *reconcentración*, the infamous policy meant to extend Spanish rule in its last great American colony. Devised by the Spanish general Valeriano Weyler as a counterinsurgency strategy during

Cuba's final War of Independence, Spanish forces drove rural Cubans off their land and "reconcentrated" them in the towns and cities of western Cuba in order to deprive independence forces of much-needed support.[3] Within months, tens of thousands of *reconcentrados*—most of whom were women, children, and the elderly—were relocated to Havana and its surrounding towns, where they were forced to subsist on relief services. Little aid materialized. The *dispensario* began providing donated food in addition to free care and medicine, but as one of the few institutions in the city providing aid during reconcentration, the small clinic could not come close to meeting the overwhelming need. Delfín later described the clinic as filled with children crying, many suffering from fevers and the effects of starvation, their mothers curled up in the corners of the waiting room, frozen in fear and exhaustion. The eight to ten volunteer physicians and support staff provided what relief they could, but, he admitted, "almost all of those children later died."[4]

Cut off from food, shelter, or medical care, *reconcentrados* perished by the tens, or even hundreds, of thousands.[5] It was undoubtedly Cuba's greatest demographic disaster since the Spanish conquest, as some 155,000 to 170,000 civilians—close to 10 percent of the population—died of starvation and disease between 1897 and 1898.[6] But what would have been, in other times, a localized tragedy now became a global story. News of the plight of the *reconcentrados* reverberated widely across the Americas, sparking moral outrage at the Spanish counterinsurgency and spurring support for Cuban rebels. Aided by advances in photographic reproduction, images of the *reconcentrados* created a visual lexicon of Cuban suffering. In the United States, this was given new meaning by expansionist Protestant humanitarianism and turn-of-the-century "yellow journalism."[7] (See figure 1.1.) A flurry of U.S. newspaper and magazine articles described in lurid detail "children dying in the streets" of western Cuba and "babies found dead in the arms of their exhausted mothers."[8] In Havana, witnesses described hospitals lacking even basic resources and overflowing with the dying sick, while orphans begged for food at the city's train stations. "Everywhere," all agreed, "hunger, starvation, and illness reigned."[9] A potent symbol of Cuban helplessness and Spanish perfidy, these images galvanized American public opinion against Spain and helped build a compelling moral argument for American military intervention.

But once Spain was defeated and the U.S. Military Government in Cuba established, Americans inherited responsibility for the still-starving thousands too poor to return to their ruined farms. In Havana, the *reconcentrados*

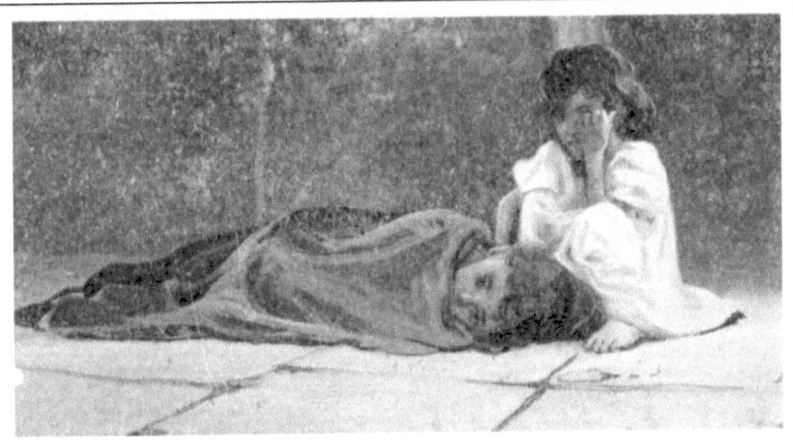

DYING ON A PALACE PORCH.

*The two little sisters lay dying on the stones in front of the Governor's Palace, Matanzas City  They lay for twelve hours untended  Died in hospital.*

Figure 1.1 Children dying on the palace porch. Images like this, reproduced in Columbia's War for Cuba in the summer of 1898, emphasized Spanish indifference to the suffering of Cuban children, women, and the elderly, highlighting American moral obligation to intervene. (Tupper, Columbia's War for Cuba, 170)

presented an obvious problem for U.S. officials: a desperately poor and highly visible population in the city that Americans were intent on using as a showcase for American-style modernization. Back home, the boosters of U.S. power hailed the military intervention and subsequent relief efforts as an unalloyed success, showcasing the United States as a progressive force for good on the world stage. But close attention to the on-the-ground interactions between Cubans and American relief workers and reformers reveals the profound ironies and unintended consequences of U.S. health and welfare policy, as racialized fears of Cubans "abusing American charity" hampered relief efforts, as Cubans' own priorities clashed with U.S. policy, and as new institutions meant to rein in public spending instead dramatically increased state health care expenditure.

This chapter explores how hunger, disease, and the various efforts to confront the effects of the reconcentration shaped the transition from Spanish to U.S. colonial rule and set the stage for debates over the rights of the poor and the sick. In the different Cuban and American responses to the reconcentration and its aftermath, we see a variety of ideas about state responsibility, as the crisis and the occupation created new opportunities to imagine what the state could—and should—do to address poverty, hunger, and disease. What was the responsibility of the state to provide shelter, medical assistance, or food to those suffering from the effects of the war? Once wartime conditions transitioned to something approaching normalcy, how did ideas about state responsibility change? Who was considered "deserving" of aid and who was not? In Cuba, as everywhere, these questions were profoundly gendered and inseparable from ideas about class, race, and the "burdens" of empire. At different moments, Cuban and American relief workers and officials ascribed different meanings to the suffering of Cuban women—especially poor mothers. Attention to these discourses provides insight into gendered political claims-making during this period of political transition.

Despite the extensive literature on the "Spanish-American War" and the subsequent military occupation of Cuba, little has been written on the development of social policy under U.S. rule.[10] But health and welfare policy were of deep concern to the architects of the occupation government. For American reformers and officials, social welfare not only provided aid to the sick and destitute and support and supervision to orphaned children; by delineating the proper spheres of government and private health and welfare work, occupation officials also hoped to instill in the Cuban people such ostensibly "American" values as self-sufficiency and charity, while avoiding the perennial problems of "dependency" and reliance on government. Occupation social policy, in other words, was meant to form a blueprint for both the postindependence Cuban state and a modern Cuban citizenry. But Cuban health and welfare reformers also saw the period of U.S. occupation as a "workshop" for social policy, and they had their own vision of how state power could be utilized to protect the health and well-being of the Cuban people. Through their often quarrelsome interactions with American social reformers and military officials, and through the process of helping shape new institutions, Cuban reformers grew increasingly convinced of the power and potential of a strong central authority governing public health and welfare. They would go on to apply these experiences to postindependence health and welfare work, becoming vocal advocates for strong government action on poverty, infant mortality, and disease and pushing the government for the expansion of state health and welfare institutions.

### RECONCENTRACIÓN AND SURVIVAL IN HAVANA

In February 1896, exactly one year after a series of uprisings across the island heralded the start of Cuba's third and final War of Independence, the Spanish general Valeriano Weyler issued his first order for the "reconcentration" of civilians in Cuba. Designed to deprive the insurgents of support in the countryside, reconcentration orders relocated rural campesino populations to towns and cities garrisoned by the Spanish. By moving civilians from the countryside and destroying their fields, the Spanish cut off the major food supply of the insurgency, which relied heavily on the crops, horses, and other materials it could glean from rural supporters and enemies alike. By preventing movement between the cities and the countryside, Weyler's policy blocked food, medicine, and information from passing between them. Initially applied only to the eastern Cuban provinces where insurgent forces were strongest, by January 1897 the reconcentration was extended westward to Santa Clara, Matanzas, and Havana provinces.[11] As many as 120,000 peasants were relocated in Havana province alone, with the majority sent to the capital, where most stayed in makeshift shelters hastily set up on the outskirts of the city.[12]

Weyler's counterinsurgency policies had a devastating impact on the economy, on urban residents, and especially on the reconcentrados themselves. By the summer of 1897, the colonial economy was at a standstill. Cuba's western provinces were littered with burnt crop and cane fields, as both the Spanish army and the Cuban insurgents set the countryside ablaze in order to keep the other side from having access to provisions. The combination of insurgent scorched-earth policies and Spanish counterinsurgency led to a collapse in sugar production, with exports reduced by 80 percent compared to just two years prior. Sugar's collapse hit the shipping, banking, and commercial sectors especially hard, but with so much of the urban economy either directly or indirectly dependent on sugar exports, urban unemployment skyrocketed. Those lucky enough to keep their jobs found their wages sharply reduced, but even then, the collapse in food production and distribution led to a sharp increase in the cost of food. Residents found the price of staples such as bread, milk, flour, yams, and plantains increasing as much as fivefold, and this combination of high prices and lower wages proved disastrous to the service sector. The city's bakers, restaurants, and food vendors, urban transportation workers, and repair shops were all affected as the economy ground to a halt.[13]

The rising cost of food affected everyone, but it was devastating to the urban poor, and especially the *reconcentrado* refugees, who lined up at the city's train stations begging for food or work.[14] Many who had the means fled the city. Those who remained were subject to new epidemics of disease and starvation. The final year of the war was the hardest for the capital, as, according to an American military official, "all general business, investments, imports, even that of food, had been impracticable for the greater portion of the year."[15] The city was left "bankrupt and prostrate" with an empty treasury and a population dying off in droves.[16]

Spanish officials were completely unprepared to care for the refugee population they had created. With the regular functions of civil government increasingly subordinated to the military effort, little care, it seems, was put into managing the capital's refugee problem. The *reconcentrados*, pushed into crowded, poorly constructed shelters, died by the tens of thousands of starvation and disease.[17] According to the Cuban physician Enrique López, many *reconcentrados*, weakened by starvation, simply "died in the thoroughfares without appearing to have anything more than anemia."[18] The numbers are astounding: in Havana alone, perhaps 42,000 *reconcentrados* died between 1897 and 1898.[19] Nevertheless, if these numbers are correct, then Havana's *reconcentrados* actually *survived* at a disproportionate rate compared with those "housed" in other towns, a fact perhaps explained by the relative availability of local and international relief aid in the capital that was unavailable to *reconcentrados* in the interior.

Thousands perished in a single shelter, Los Fosos, which became a grim symbol of the humanitarian disaster of the reconcentration (see figure 1.2). A little warehouse on the outskirts of the city originally built for storing carts, it was set aside by city officials for sheltering *reconcentrados*. But the numbers of *reconcentrados* quickly overwhelmed the small space. One U.S. military surgeon described the scene:

> There were 500 people found in and around this building, and of that number over 200 were found lying on the floor, sick and dying. I saw no child under ten years of age who could be considered in good health. . . . [A] conservative estimate of the death rate would be about 10 per day. The number is recruited by fresh accessions from the country. There were over 150 children below the age of ten years and I did not observe one whose chance for living thirty days, under the existing conditions, was good.[20]

The cramped quarters and inadequate food and medical attention of Los Fosos facilitated the rapid spread of disease, and thousands died there in the final year of the war. The *Minneapolis Journal* reported residents of the shelter falling in the streets, "where flocks of vultures, 'Weyler's chickens,' as they are termed in Havana, have feasted on the remains."[21] As Manuel Delfín remembered, "Those who did not get to see in those times the scene

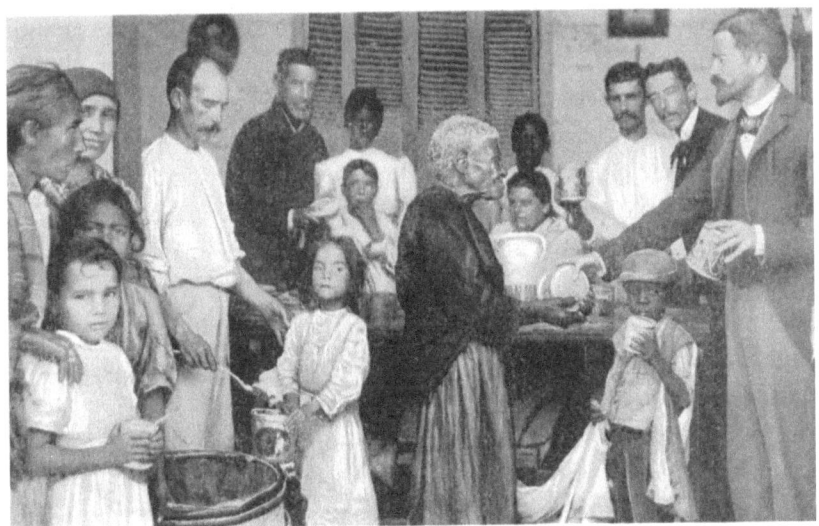

Figure 1.2 Los Fosos shelter, Havana. (Tupper, *Columbia's War for Cuba*, 184)

of our streets, the piling up [of bodies] in Los Fosos . . . have not been able to form an idea of the sacrifice made by the Cuban people. This was a nation of spectres (*era éste un pueblo de espectros*)."[22]

In the face of this crisis, *reconcentrados* used what survival strategies they could to keep themselves and their families alive. Some women and girls sold sex to support their families.[23] Others survived by begging. As Delfín later recalled, "Calle Obispo was difficult to traverse on the sidewalks, with innumerable women seated in the doorjambs with their almost moribund babies in their arms, demanding with their wails bread for their little ones, a coat for their flesh."[24] While most of the *reconcentrados* came into the city without the familial networks that sustained most poor Cuban families in hard times, many found some sources of aid. In the months after Weyler's reconcentration orders took effect, the poor extended their solidarity to the displaced and the sick, sharing what resources they had, and taking in children whose parents had died of starvation or at the hands of the armed forces. While few sources describe the experience of the reconcentration from the perspective of those expelled from their rural communities and herded into cities like Havana, many observers remarked on the local webs of solidarity that kept the death toll from being much higher than it otherwise would certainly have been. American military officials such as Jefferson Randolph Kean noted the "native kindness and generosity of the Cuban people, who showed such a willingness to share their little with those who had nothing."[25]

Such spontaneous, popular forms of support were essential to the survival of most *reconcentrados*, as the capital's hospital and asylum system, already taxed by years of official neglect, was completely overwhelmed by the health crisis of the reconcentration. The capital had a long history of charitable *beneficencia* institutions funded by religious organizations and the elite, but these were of little help during the war. With their endowments drying up in the economic crisis, rents unpaid, and rural properties unable to produce, many of Havana's hospitals and other charitable institutions were unable to continue their normal functions, let alone support the influx of refugees. At the Mazorra hospital, the insane asylum on the outskirts of the city, almost 50 percent of the inmates died from diseases facilitated by their slow starvation from insufficient rations.[26] Making the situation more dire, many institutions and all of the city's principal hospitals were commandeered by the Spanish for military use.[27] For example, the Casa de Beneficencia y Maternidad was the city's most important charity institution, an enormous structure overlooking the ocean on the outskirts of the city that functioned as an orphanage, a foundling home, and a residence for the aged destitute, with a capacity to accommodate more than 800 residents.[28] But even as the war increased the need for its services, General Weyler ordered the building emptied, its residents transferred to other city institutions so the building could be used as a military hospital.[29]

The influx of poor and sick *reconcentrados* would have been a challenge for the city's medical system during "normal" times, but the war left institutions like Manuel Delfín's Dispensario La Caridad doubly under pressure. Havana had always been the medical center of the island, but during the war, physicians fled the city into exile abroad or to the countryside to avoid the diseases ravaging the capital, leaving few doctors to address the growing health crisis.[30] Although Delfín had practiced medicine for decades, the reconcentration "produced medical disorders [he] had never before seen." As is common in situations of acute malnutrition, gastroenteritis—the inflammation of the intestines, usually accompanied by severe diarrhea—was responsible for "countless victims."[31] But many also died of illness related to consumption of contaminated foods, as sick animals were sold for food in the city's markets. To address these needs, Delfín turned the dispensary into an important food distribution center, giving out free rations of corn, flour, rice, and "a bit of condensed milk" to the city's poor. Especially during the American blockade in the spring of 1898, food was difficult to procure, and provisions often ran out. But the need remained high, as "the number coming to Dispensary never fell below two to three thousand."[32]

All of Havana's residents were affected by the reconcentration, the American blockade, and the war in general, but each according to their social position and economic resources. The wealthy, as always, were better able to ride out the food crisis, but institutions like Delfín's dispensary and the *cocinas gratuitas*—soup kitchens organized by the city's civil government—provided some limited relief to the poor.[33] While the lack of reliable statistics makes a precise demographic breakdown impossible, it is clear that white Cubans and Spanish immigrants had greater access to the economic and organizational means to survive. During the crisis, a little bit of economic security could mean the difference between life and death. But Cubans of color were already overrepresented among the city's poor and disproportionately lived in the rural areas where the reconcentration was deadliest, so they almost certainly died at greater rates.[34] Further, whites benefited from segregated health institutions, like the well-funded Spanish mutual aid hospitals and clinics, which remained an important source for medical services to those Spanish immigrants and white Cubans who could afford the low-cost membership fees.[35] Finally, some *beneficencia* institutions, reflecting the racial caste system of colonial society, limited care to white children.[36] Overall, it is clear that the city's racialized class system and segregated colonial institutions facilitated the disproportionate mortality of Cubans of color. But, as we will see, while the suffering of Cubans of color was obscured by a visual discourse that emphasized the suffering of white women and children, the prevalence of Cubans of color among the *reconcentrados* shaped subsequent U.S. relief efforts as Americans sought to prevent what they saw as the "abuse of American charity."

## THE LIMITS OF AMERICAN AID

Back in the United States, the American public was riveted by the crisis in Cuba. Newspaper sales exploded as reporters described in lurid detail the suffering of reconcentrados. A constant flow of reports presented stark depictions of Spanish cruelty toward Cuban civilians, echoing and amplifying calls for humanitarian aid to Cuba, as gendered images of Cuban helplessness framed arguments for American humanitarian and, later, military action. As Kristin Hoganson has argued, proponents of American intervention successfully marshaled gendered imagery of feminized Cuban helplessness and American masculinity to press for a chivalric intervention on behalf of the *reconcentrados*.[37] But the meanings Americans ascribed to Cuban suffering were also profoundly racialized. Before the U.S. intervention, newspaper articles, along with accompanying lithographs and cartoons, almost always emphasized the plight of white women and girls. These discourses implicitly framed American aid as a masculine nationalist imperative to save helpless white Cuban women and children. Ultimately, however, relief efforts were hamstrung by military priorities, logistical problems, and an increasingly racialized distrust of those forced to rely on aid for survival.

In his 1897 Christmas appeal, President William McKinley called on Americans to donate "money, provisions, clothing, medicines and the like articles of prime necessity" to alleviate the *reconcentrado* crisis.[38] The public response was resounding. The U.S. State Department organized a Central Cuban Relief Committee to coordinate efforts and process donations from the local relief committees that sprang up across the country. In Philadelphia, for example, wealthy and poor alike sent donations of clothing, food, and money to the local relief committee, sometimes attaching hand-scrawled notes indicating their support of "the suffering Concentrados [sic] of Cuba."[39] Support for "the suffering Cubans" came from groups like the National Society of Patriotic Workers and the Philadelphia Daughters of St. Paul's Church.[40] But others were more circumspect, highlighting the growing popular belief that what Cubans needed was not just charity but an end to Spanish colonial rule. One Philadelphia woman donated $2 to the cause, even as she criticized the U.S. government for its official policy of neutrality in the Cuban conflict, writing that "it is rather unusual for a government to insist its citizens shall relieve the oppressed while it is engaged in upholding the crime of the oppressor." She asked for assurance that her donation not be used "to help purchase Spanish bullets to be used against the unfortunate Cubans."[41] Similarly, if less eloquently, the Philadelphia-based Cuban exile physician Juan Guiteras responded to the call for donations with a terse "I regret to have to differ with the aims of the Committee and cannot, therefore, contribute," reflecting frustration with any solution to the *reconcentrado* crisis that left unresolved the fundamental political question of Cuban independence.[42]

By February 1898, the American Red Cross had arrived in Havana to coordinate the distribution of food and clothing from the United States and began building makeshift hospitals to care for the sick and asylums for children orphaned by the reconcentration.[43] This work was invaluable; but even with this infusion of relief, thousands in the city continued to die of starvation, and many more succumbed in the surrounding towns and villages.[44] American involvement escalated quickly when, following the mysterious explosion of the U.S. battleship *Maine* docked outside Havana, the U.S. Congress formally declared war on Spain on April 25. Although the war was ostensibly a humanitarian effort in support of suffering Cubans, the U.S. naval blockade actually prevented even the most needed supplies from reaching the island—including food shipments—and therefore exacerbated the humanitarian crisis. Some Americans had anticipated the effects of a war on the *reconcentrados*, for whom it was ostensibly fought. As *Harper's Weekly* warned, "If it is really our aim promptly to relieve the *reconcentrados* of their present misery, we should jump at the chance of doing this peaceably, for the very simple reason that armed interference . . . would forcibly separate us from the objects of our benevolence and doom them to further sufferings."[45] Indeed, the naval blockade and ensuing war made an already critical situation significantly worse. With war declared, even the Red Cross fled the island, leaving tens of thousands of starving and sick *reconcentrados* with few sources of aid.

Vastly outgunned, Spain was defeated in a short series of naval battles and land skirmishes and sued for surrender on July 26, but the formal transfer of power to the United States did not occur until January 1, 1899. In the intervening months, American news reports of the *reconcentrados* practically disappeared, and U.S. relief committees began redirecting their efforts away from *reconcentrados* and toward supporting American soldiers occupying the island. Even the American Red Cross began preparations to close down operations on the island.[46] But even as war gave way to an uncertain peace, conditions for the *reconcentrados* continued to deteriorate, and the death rate for Havana in the fall of 1898 was actually *higher* than at any point during the reconcentration.[47]

The relief work of George W. Hyatt during the summer and fall of 1898 highlights both the limits of U.S. relief efforts and the continued humanitarian crisis under conditions of "peace." Hyatt was an American businessman who had spent decades living in the small town of Guanabacoa, across the bay from Havana. During the height of the reconcentration, as his adopted town was inundated with *reconcentrado* refugees, Hyatt became a local agent of the Red Cross and helped distribute food aid across the greater Havana region. But while the American Red Cross abandoned relief efforts during the U.S. naval blockade, Hyatt repeatedly broke the blockade with small ships loaded with relief supplies from Key West, smuggling needed food and medical aid to the island.[48]

Even after the short war was over, Hyatt found that supplies were difficult to come by. In a series of increasingly desperate letters, Hyatt struggled to convince Red Cross leadership that even months after Spain's defeat, and despite the imminent transfer of power, "Weyler's design of general starvation" remained intact, as *reconcentrados* continued to die in the streets of Havana and surrounding towns.⁴⁹ As he explained in October, "The stage of misery and starvation and sickness is *more than ever, and on the increase.*"⁵⁰ Indeed, refugees from smaller towns where relief had long since vanished continued to make the journey to Havana in search of food, exacerbating pressures on the insufficient relief system.⁵¹ Even those "of the once reputable and self-supporting class" were dying of starvation, including "American citizens of the once-fashionable and well-to-do society of Habana," for, as he added, since pride prevented many elites from begging in the streets for food, they "could only live in despair until death came."⁵² But despite this continuing starvation, Hyatt had to plead continually for food supplies to be sent to the island, peppering his letters with personal appeals. Using the gendered language of suffering women and children that had proved so effective one year before, he urged Clara Barton, the aging founder of the American Red Cross, to "remember the starving women and babes you saw in Cuba, and not forget the thousands of those since dead and dying."⁵³ By the end of 1898, however, this discourse was not nearly as powerful as it had been one year before. American attention had turned elsewhere, to the problems of governing the new island territories that had come under U.S. control.

With the termination of Spanish sovereignty on January 1, 1899, the United States officially inherited the problem of feeding and sheltering the *reconcentrados*. The task was daunting: according to the Cuban relief worker Miguel R. Suárez, at the beginning of the year, "some 17,000 to 20,000 persons, of both sexes and of all ages and conditions in life, roamed around the city, either destitute, sick, or starving."⁵⁴ But military relief efforts were hampered by an uncooperative military bureaucracy, and the military government's own policies reflected both the general elitist bent of welfare thinking in the United States and a rapidly developing distrust of the Cubans themselves. Given few resources, and with U.S. officials increasingly distrustful of recipients of aid, the military relief effort ultimately proved insufficient and contradictory.

Problems with the U.S. military relief effort emerged immediately, as the food distribution system was hamstrung by a time-consuming inspection system to prevent "fraud" and "abuse."⁵⁵ With the numbers of the destitute overwhelming the paltry six officers assigned to investigate all pending cases, General William Ludlow turned to the elite Junta Patriótica, whose leadership was composed of "Cuban gentlemen of standing," to sort through the cases and recommend those "worthy" of government food and medical aid. Reflecting broader American concerns over the issuance of state support to the "undeserving poor," a thorough investigatory regime was instituted even as Havana residents continued to die of starvation and malnutrition.

Surprisingly, Ludlow's reports are remarkably candid about the failures of the military government to provide aid to the sick and starving. Repeatedly, Ludlow found, the needs of Cubans were subordinated to those of the invading army. Mirroring Spanish military policies during the War of Independence, American officials commandeered local hospitals for U.S. military use.[56] Unable to secure additional resources, Ludlow was forced to rely on the already overburdened system of local and private asylums and hospitals to aid the thousands of sick and starving Cubans perishing on the streets of the capital.[57] While noting that medical and relief work "was done as effectively as practicable," Ludlow lamented that "a large number must have perished who could have been saved if proper provision could have been made for them."[58]

Back in the United States, concern for the *reconcentrados*, which had done so much to fuel the push for war against Spain, began to shift as worries over the "abuse of American charity" and the rise of Cuban "pauperism" tempered earlier charitable concerns. The *Brooklyn Eagle*, for example, warned of a "permanent pauper class" emerging as the "shiftless, dishonest and incapable have gathered in and around Havana and Santiago to be fed, clothed, and supported by the United States government."[59] These sentiments went against the thinking of those military officials now responsible for the island. General John R. Brooke, the new military governor of Cuba, reminded a subordinate that "we are feeding a great many men, women, and children who otherwise would starve," adding, "It will not do to restrict the issue of food too much at this time, as men who might work if they had the opportunity are often too much reduced physically to do so."[60] Nevertheless, the idea that "shiftless" Cubans were "taking advantage" of American charity found wide purchase. The *Chicago Daily Tribune* wrote that "unlimited almsgiving" was turning Cubans into "chronic paupers." According to the *Tribune*, these "pauper reconcentrados ... would all prefer to sit down and be fed by Uncle Sam, and not a few already consider such to be their just right."[61] A reporter for the *Washington Post* concurred, arguing that "undeserving persons" were taking advantage of American charity and that many Cubans would rather collect rations than work. Nevertheless, the correspondent begrudgingly conceded that "there is no work for most of [the *reconcentrados*] at present."[62]

The shifting American discourse on the *reconcentrados* reflected a broader shift in how Cubans were perceived after the advent of the American occupation. Over the course of 1898, American perceptions of Cubans underwent a dramatic shift, as Americans came face to face with a racially heterogeneous population at odds with the sanitized image of white Cubans in need that had fed the rush to war.⁶³ In the months after the landing of U.S. troops in Eastern Cuba, Louis A. Pérez Jr. writes, "a new American consensus took shape," as Cubans came to be seen as "unworthy of further American sympathy and undeserving of continued American support."⁶⁴ As Ada Ferrer has shown, Americans marshaled racial knowledge formed in the United States in their attempts to make sense of the Cuban people and their "capacity for self-rule," but in dialogue with their day-to-day experiences with Cubans themselves.⁶⁵ Given the fraught history Americans had with questions of relief and dependency, as well as charity and poverty, it is not surprising that what began as humanitarian concern for the *reconcentrados* would quickly turn into a racialized suspicion of the recipients of "American charity."⁶⁶ In the United States, anti-Catholic sentiment and racialized assumptions of the propensity of the African American and immigrant poor for "pauperization," and fears that "hand-outs" would erode the will to work, surely shaped Americans' perceptions of the Cuban poor. Indeed, even at the height of the reconcentration crisis in early 1898, the Red Cross worried about the potential long-term impacts of "indiscriminate" medical aid, convening a group of Cuban physicians to devise a "plan for avoiding the creation of a pauper element, through the abuse of out-patient clinics."⁶⁷

By the summer of 1899, officials at the Havana Relief Department, worried about fostering dependency, began cutting off recipients from government aid. In order to prevent the "able-bodied poor" from continuing to receive aid, relief agents were ordered to investigate further each individual or family seeking continued food aid, so that "only the extremely destitute ones are attended to, and all possibility of misplaced charity is carefully avoided."⁶⁸ In effect, resources were shifted away from aid and toward the investigation of the poor, to "oblige [the poor] to seek some means of self-support" within a still-fragile economy.⁶⁹ Yet work was difficult to find, especially for women. Wages were depressed all around, and women's paid labor, when available, was particularly poorly remunerated. As Miguel R. Suárez—the Cuban superintendent of the Relief Department—noted in 1900, making ends meet was particularly difficult for the poor women of Havana, who, after years of war and disease, often found themselves the heads of their households. Suárez described women who were "able-bodied and skilled in various domestic arts, such as sewing, embroidering, cigarette making, etc., [but who] on account of the scarcity of work, are unable to earn a subsistence, and consequently find the struggle beyond their resources."⁷⁰ Labor supply greatly outmatched demand, he noted, so the poor women of the city would "have to drift along for a time until the condition of the country so adjusts itself as to offer a more profitable field for their labor."[71] Nevertheless, fearing "dependency," the military government discontinued food aid for these women.

Miguel R. Suárez's reports to the military government are striking for their attention to this gendered urban economy and the problems poor women faced in supporting their families. As superintendent of the Relief Department, he envisioned a more expansive role for government action. Suárez hoped that "some sort of co-operative workshop might be established with the government support, and some well-organized system of labor exchange for women, which would be the means of helping the willing class to get work."[72] In April 1900, he oversaw the creation of "working exchanges and shops . . . to enable destitute women to become self-supporting by means of their own labor."[73] These workshops employed women in making clothing for children, providing needed training for women unaccustomed to wage labor. Funds previously allocated for rations were used to purchase materials and to pay these women a wage of 50 cents per day.

While these workshops surely helped many women, scarcity of work was not the only problem poor mothers faced. Those lucky enough to have found employment still needed some form of childcare. Suárez noted in a report that "the establishment of the Habana Industrial School for Girls at Compostela Barracks [a shelter for destitute children created by the military government] has been the means of aiding a great many destitute mothers, who, by being relieved of the care of their children, are enabled to earn their own living."[74] Unfortunately, these measures were temporary; despite Suárez's advocacy, no government-organized cooperatives were formed and no permanent workshops were created to continue training or employing women. Over the course of the occupation, tensions persisted over the appropriate limits of government aid to the poor beyond feeding the starving, and efforts to directly employ poor women, or provide training, loans, or any form of industrial relief, were rejected by military officials as "paternalist." The gendered urban economy would remain skewed, to the detriment of women seeking employment, for years to come, and the city's poorest women and their children would continue to face higher rates of disease and early death.[75]

#### FROM COLONIAL *BENEFICENCIA* TO SCIENTIFIC CHARITY

Having reined in expenditures on rations for the *reconcentrados*, American officials soon turned to the *beneficencia* (public welfare) system as a whole. In late 1899, the U.S. Military Government's Division Headquarters ordered the inspection of all hospitals, asylums, and other institutions supported by insular funds. Finding these institutions in "a most lamentable condition of disorganization, want and neglect," military officials decided that in addition to immediate repairs of individual institutions, "a more centralized and uniform system of administration was necessary."[76] The legal framework that governed charitable institutions, dating from the late colonial period, was deemed backward and inadequate for modern conditions. According to General Leonard Wood, the Cubans in charge of the island's charities "were entirely unfamiliar with the work at hand." Endowments were poorly managed, he argued, while the lack of modern scientific administration led to the proliferation of preventable disease. "In short," he concluded, "the whole system was unqualifiedly bad."[77]

What was needed, then, was the thorough revamping of the colonial *beneficencia* system. Mirroring earlier efforts to force Cubans off public rations, officials hoped that by instituting a modern centralized system of administration for the island's *beneficencia* system, government expenditures would be reduced and "institutional dependency" prevented. But reshaping the island's fractured social welfare system required new legal frameworks and a new government body to oversee this work, so General Wood turned to a young reformer named Homer Folks. Steeped in American "scientific charity" thinking, Folks would oversee the creation of the Departamento de Beneficencia—the first national body with broad authority over the island's entire health and welfare system.

On February 9, 1900, Laura Drake Gill, from the New York–based Cuban Orphan Society, wrote to Homer Folks, then secretary of the New York State Charities Aid Association, a leading American social reform advocacy organization. Writing at the behest of Military Governor Leonard Wood, Gill solicited Folks's aid in organizing a Departamento de Beneficencia, or Department of Public Charities, for the island, appealing to his expertise in the "scientific classification of such matters."[78] Two months later, thirty-two-year-old Folks boarded a Ward Line steamer for Havana, where, during a six-week stay and after touring the island's hospitals, orphanages, and other charitable institutions, he drafted the military order that would form the basis of Cuban welfare law for the next forty years. Homer Folks would go on to become a major public health and welfare reformer in the United States, helping found the National Child Labor Committee and serving as an advisor to Franklin D. Roosevelt on welfare issues in the 1930s. In 1900, he was already well known for his advocacy of state oversight over private charities and as a prominent advocate of adoption (called "placing-out" at the time) over the "institutionalization" of children in orphanages.

Like many welfare reformers at the time (and still), Folks believed that "indiscriminate" direct aid led to dependency and pauperization. This was, in fact, the central tenet of the Scientific Charity Movement closely identified with his New York State Charities Aid Association. The most prominent theory in welfare reform in the late nineteenth century, scientific charity posited allegedly universal truths around poverty, relief, and charity that could be condensed into well-defined principles. Advocates believed that any form of "out-door relief" only bred dependency, and they strongly opposed state charity. Instead, private charity based on personal relationships between the donor and the recipient, with strict supervision and "moral encouragement," would instill self-respect in the poor, building character and self-sufficiency.[79] As Jefferson Randolph Kean, the future head of the Cuban Department of Public Charities, would describe it, "Modern scientific charity, which is a branch of political economy . . . while relieving distress, strives to prevent pauperism and to build up character."[80] Folks's desire to streamline public health and charities administration found a receptive ear in Leonard Wood, whose own vision of government activism was based on the belief that organization and efficiency, a "business-like way of doing things," were essential to progress and civilization. And Folks's Progressive Era understanding of the importance of state action meshed well with Wood's own authoritarian centralism. Finally, American racial understandings of Cubans, who they already believed were predisposed to pauperism and "abuse of charity," certainly lent support to the idea of reorganizing Cuban *beneficencia* along the lines of American scientific charity.

Cuban Civil Order 271, drafted by Homer Folks and signed July 7, 1900, transformed the organization of health and welfare services in Cuba. It created a national Department of Public Charities with broad powers to inspect and oversee all private and public charitable institutions on the island, including hospitals, orphanages, and asylums, and defined the lines of division between state, municipal, and private charities, clarifying what the proper domains and responsibilities of each would be.[81] The state was charged with the care of all destitute children, rather broadly defined, and new institutions for the care of delinquent or destitute children were to be created and placed under the authority of the department.[82] A new Bureau for Placing Children in Families was also created to organize the shift from the institutionalization of orphans to their legal adoption by Cuban families.

The law also nationalized the Mazorra insane asylum, making the inmates legal wards of the state, and, finally, tasked the Department of Public Charities with creating schools for training nurses.[83]

According to Folks, many of the major provisions of the new law were based on the most "advanced" laws in the United States, reflecting social welfare innovations from Minnesota, Wisconsin, Massachusetts, and New York, among other states.[84] The military government gave Folks the power to organize and regulate a national public welfare system with a freedom that would have been unthinkable in the United States. A *Chicago Daily Tribune* correspondent was correct in noting, "There was one advantage Mr. Folks had. He was able to steer for his port without having to reckon with the crosscurrents of State Legislature politics. He made his law and General Wood issued it." Indeed, the reporter added, "This was tyranny, [but the Cubans were] well-pleased with being treated tyrannically."[85]

As this reporter suggested, this system would have been impossible in the United States, where decentralization was the norm and public welfare varied tremendously from state to state. Designed to impose administrative order over an unruly national public and private social welfare system, the Department of Public Charities centralized in one body the administration, regulation, and oversight of all of the island's hospitals, asylums, orphanages, nursing schools, reformatories, and training schools. It was enormous centralized power, and despite the intentions of individuals like Folks and Wood, who envisioned a clear delineation between state and private responsibility for the sick and the poor, in the coming years the work of the department would inspire greater and greater public investment in the health and welfare of the Cuban people. But in 1900, American observers saw this colonial experiment in social policy as an opportunity to test the principles of scientific charity on an entire nation.[86] Replacing "backwards" colonial administrative methods with "efficient and modern" American methods, the new *beneficencia* system was designed as a testament to the superiority of American administrative know-how. By delineating the proper roles for public and private charity, the new law sought to shape both the nascent Cuban state and its people, fostering "enlightened" statecraft informed by Progressive Era American legislation and a modern, self-sufficient Cuban citizenry in the (self-) image of East Coast, urban, middle-class reformers. But despite the enthusiasm of officials and reformers, this American experiment in colonial social policy came up against the ideas and actions of Cubans who had their own visions for how the state should intervene in dealing with hunger, poverty, and disease.

## SCIENTIFIC CHARITY IN PRACTICE: GENDER, CLASS, AND THE DISMANTLING OF THE RELIEF SYSTEM

The goals of the Scientific Charity Movement—reducing poverty by limiting direct support to the poor, thereby compelling them to find employment and learn "self-sufficiency"—dovetailed perfectly with Military Governor Leonard Wood's vision for limiting the size and expense of the colonial (and, he hoped, postindependence) government. But in 1900 Cuba was in the midst of the colonial transition, with hundreds of thousands of Cubans still displaced and the economy barely recovering from decades of war. In this context, the goals of scientific charity and Wood's vision for limited government represented a kind of colonial "shock doctrine" for the Cuban poor who relied on public support for food, medicine, and shelter.[87] For the many women whose husbands had left or died during the war, these plans to curtail government support represented an existential threat to their families. With the gendered economy providing few employment opportunities for women, they relied on whatever relief services they could find to feed and house their families. But as archival records for the dismantling of children's asylums and the infamous Los Fosos shelter show, these women did not take lightly state efforts to dismantle the haphazard relief system upon which they depended.

In the occupation government's focus on orphans, we see clearly the interconnected goals of reducing state expenditures and using social policy to foster the creation of "modern" Cuban citizens. One key innovation of the 1900 *beneficencia* law was that it sought to do away with the institution of the orphanage, which was seen both as costly to the state and as having negative effects on children. According to the director of the Department of Public Charities, U.S. Army surgeon Jefferson Randolph Kean, orphanages inhibited independence and self-sufficiency. A child raised in an orphanage, he argued, with its "affections atrofied [sic], its will undeveloped, and its entire ignorance of the economies and mutual sacrifices of family life, cannot make a good citizen."[88] Municipal and private orphanages supported by the state were therefore phased out, and a broad experiment in state-supervised adoption began. Already by April 1900, officials began dismantling the system of emergency children's asylums set up in 1898–99 by the Red Cross and other organizations. These asylums housed thousands of *reconcentrado* children—most of whom were orphans who had lost one or both parents during the war—and employed hundreds of *reconcentrado* women to cook, clean, and help care for the children. But by 1899 these small emergency asylums relied largely on the military government for financial support, which officials were increasingly unwilling to provide.

Debates over children's asylums exposed tensions between relief advocates and occupation officials over the proper sphere of government aid. Citing the burden they placed on the occupation government's finances, military officials called for their immediate closure.[89] But Clara Barton herself vigorously defended these asylums while arguing that supporting orphans was actually the proper responsibility of the occupation government, not private charity. In a sharply worded letter to Leonard Wood, she argued that Red Cross emergency shelters were meant to complement and facilitate—rather than replace—government relief work. The organization's "gathering of [orphaned children and] cleansing them of filth and disease, by no means released them from the care of the government or from the distribution of the food which it was there to administer." "I might say," she added, "that we had taken them in like lambs from the storms, provided them a fold and a litter, and arranged a rack for the government to fill with its rations of food—that food for the starving, *for which we had raised an army, fought a war, and buried our dead.*"[90] As Barton reminded General Wood, if aiding the *reconcentrados* was the entire point of the war with Spain, then why was the occupation government so determined to limit relief services when they were still needed? Interestingly, the decision to close these asylums was a matter of some debate within the government. According to Homer Folks, who was present for these discussions, many, "including a large number of prominent Americans," argued that these shelters should continue to receive government support for as long as the need existed. But concern over the imputed social effects of these asylums won the day. Articulating the colonial scientific charity discourse at the heart of U.S. social policy in Cuba, Folks argued that "every unnecessary institution was sure to undermine the independence of the Cuban and to teach him to rely upon government aid." Leonard Wood concurred, and "keenly alive to the temptations which [these institutions] offered to weak parents," he ordered the dismantling of the emergency orphanages.[91]

Ironically, rather than teaching them to "rely on government aid," orphanages and asylums provided the means for some Cuban women to support their families by supplying much-needed employment and facilitating women's search for work. The Habana Industrial School for Girls—an asylum and training school on Compostela Street—provided many poor women with a place to care for their children while they worked or searched for employment.[92] Sometimes these asylums were a needed source of employment for *reconcentrado* women. As Homer Folks himself admitted, "Widows and other homeless women were glad to [work in these asylums] as matrons, cooks, seamstresses, etc., without salary, themselves and their children being cared for."[93] While they were always insufficient to meet the needs of the *reconcentrado* women as a whole, these institutions provided vital support to those able to access them. And while the archive is mostly silent regarding how those affected by these closures felt about them, a couple of sources provide tantalizing glimpses into the responses of the women who depended on these asylums to support their children. One telegram to Governor Wood, signed simply "Mothers," pleaded for an asylum in Sancti Spiritus to remain open, but this petition was rejected. In his comment on the request, Captain K. P. Fremont argued that the asylum closure would create no hardship for these families, but "if the mother is unsuitable . . . the child should be removed for its own good."[94] Blind to the effects these closures would have on the women who relied on them, and ignorant of the lack of opportunities available to poor mothers in the postwar economy, officials soon shuttered the emergency asylums. The American scientific charity experiment would continue.

By the middle of 1900, U.S. officials were also anxious to close the infamous Los Fosos shelter that had roused such interest and sympathy among Americans in the months before the U.S. invasion. For American relief workers like Folks, steeped in the theories of scientific charity, the continuing presence of *reconcentrados* at Los Fosos was proof that relief bred dependency, laziness, and mendicancy. Of course, neither Folks nor the American officials in charge of relief examined the gendered economy of urban employment in Havana, nor could they grasp how the reconcentration had severed many of the social ties that the popular classes relied on in difficult times. While in many ways the urban economy was improving by 1900, the situation continued to be especially difficult for women. As Miguel R. Suárez noted, in Havana "the field for women's work [remained] . . . quite limited," with the few jobs available to women among the poorest-paid.[95] Women therefore struggled to find work capable of supporting their families in an expensive city. Nevertheless, from Folks's limited vantage, the "free shelter and free food [at Los Fosos] had begun to reap their natural result, and able-bodied people for whom work could easily be [found] shrugged their shoulders and trumped up some excuse for remaining."[96]

The case of Hermenegilda Fernández provides another glimpse into the experiences of *reconcentrado* women as they struggled to simultaneously navigate the government bureaucracy and the tenuous urban economy. In 1900,

Hermenegilda Fernández was a thirty-seven-year-old widow from Luyanó who had come to Los Fosos during the reconcentration. She had a thirteen-year-old son learning cigar making in the city and a twelve-year-old daughter whom she hoped to be able to send to school. Her husband, a foreman of public works, had died four months before. Most of her friends were also dead. According to notes from Elsa Trotzig and Homer Folks, who interviewed each of the remaining inmates at Los Fosos, Fernández hoped to find work during the day and "have her [daughter] come to her side at night." She "did not know what she could do," but she was "willing to do any kind of house work."[97]

Four months later, Fernández reappears in the archival record, in a report from Knowllys E. Nevins, a young American woman employed by the Department of Public Charities and charged with closing Los Fosos. Nevins naturally encountered broad resistance to the closing of the shelter, but mothers with young children gave her the most trouble. One particular woman had made the eviction work especially difficult, and Nevins found it necessary to "write a letter to the mayor complaining of Hermenegilda Fernández, who became not only impertinent, but abusive, writing anonymous letters and causing mutiny among the women, which again gave trouble."[98] If in the earlier report the description of Fernández seems sympathetic, especially in contrast to the reports on other inmates at the shelter, four months later the demure, hardworking mother appears to become an impertinent mutineer, organizing other women out of desperation that the only source of support she has is being taken away by an American bureaucrat. Rather than being the passive recipients of elite charity, as the Americans hoped they would be and as they seemed in newspaper reports in 1898, the women of Los Fosos fought against the difficult situation the military government put them in and used what resources they could muster to try to remain in the shelter. Nevertheless, by the fall of 1900, the shelter was shuttered, and Hermenegilda Fernández and the other residents of Los Fosos disappear from the archival record.

These on-the-ground conflicts reflect the inability of many *beneficencia* workers to understand the dynamics of Cuban poverty in the wake of the crisis of the reconcentration. The nascent Department of Public Charities was staffed by a mix of U.S. military officers, Cuban aid workers, and idealistic young American reformers. Some Cuban *beneficencia* workers, like Miguel R. Suárez, understood the gendered dimensions of Cuban poverty and became strong advocates for continued state support for shelters, orphanages, and programs to employ poor women such as government-organized cooperative workshops or labor exchanges for women.[99] But while the American employees of the Department of Public Charities came to Cuba out of a missionary zeal to alleviate the effects of the reconcentration and confront Cuban poverty and disease, their methods for addressing complex social problems were rooted in an often disdainful ignorance of the actual lives of the poor. In Cuba, they lived far removed from the objects of their work, immersed in a social world of North American expatriates and Cuban elites. They viewed the Cuban poor through an elitist lens developed through their immersion in Progressive Era scientific charity work in places like Philadelphia, Boston, and New York City.[100] These Americans came to Cuba confident in the superiority of North American methods for addressing poverty and sickness. They firmly believed that any form of state support would wreak havoc on the Cuban people. By forcing the poor to fend for themselves in an unstable postwar economy, they thought they would help foster a nation of hardworking independent citizens. But, unsurprisingly, by imposing a foreign theoretical understanding of poverty and dependence on a Cuban people still suffering from decades of war, they simply left the poor, especially poor women and their families, with fewer means to survive.

## HOSPITAL ADMINISTRATION, STATE SUBSIDIES, AND THE DANGER OF MEDICAL PAUPERIZATION

Despite the protests of affected families, the military government quickly closed emergency shelters and cut direct aid to the families still experiencing the effects of the reconcentration. Similar efforts to cut state funding for the hospital system, however, would not be so easy. The central goal of the Department of Public Charities was administrative reform for all the institutions under its purview, which included the nation's entire *beneficencia* system of hospitals, dispensaries, orphanages, and shelters. As with the Cuban poor, the goal was to wean institutions from government support, and American officials hoped that by improving the accounting methods and administration of the island's *beneficencia* institutions, the government could end the system of state subsidies upon which most institutions relied. The department therefore began exerting strict administrative oversight over the island's charities, requiring them to submit regular reports detailing expenses, properties, and sources of income, as well as the purposes for which the funds were expended. The department would then send out teams of investigators to promote the "vigorous, economical and systematized administration" of these institutions.[101] Efforts to eliminate subsidies for local health institutions, however, were hobbled by on-the-ground health and economic conditions that demanded continued government support. Despite American concerns over the "medical pauperization" of the Cuban people—the idea that Cubans would come to see health care as a right rather than a charity—the still-recovering postwar economy and local health conditions forced officials to continue the system of government subsidies they found so dangerous.

Early on during the occupation, few argued that Cuban hospitals did not require extensive government support. Years of wartime neglect left the city's public and private hospital system in tatters: many were left without essential medicines, bedding, or functioning disinfection plants and were unable to safely perform surgeries or prevent the spread of infection among patients.[102] It took many months of sanitary and institutional reform—discussed in the following chapter—for the city's hospitals to regain a semblance of normalcy. Just as hospital conditions had begun to improve, the 1900 *beneficencia* law reaffirmed local rather than state responsibility over municipal hospitals, dispensaries, and homes for the aged destitute. Given the collapse of municipal finances during the war, however, most cities and towns could not afford to support these institutions. Further, although many private charities owned a very large amount of property upon which they could, in normal times, draw rents to support their finances, the "unproductiveness of investments incident to the war" meant that even the institutions with the largest endowments, such as the Casa de Beneficencia y Maternidad in Havana, were still dependent on state funds.[103] According to Major Jefferson Randolph Kean, the superintendent of the Department of Charities, the department was "well aware of the evils and dangers inherent in so extensive a system of subsidy-granting," even as it was understood to be a temporary "necessary evil owing to the utter destitution of these institutions."[104]

Beyond the occupation government's goal of reducing state expenditures, these reforms once again used social policy to reshape the habits and customs of the Cuban people. Institutional subsidies, officials believed, had a deleterious effect not just on the poor who relied on these institutions but on the entire Cuban people, who, officials believed, would come to accept state support for hospitals, shelters, and other charities as a natural duty of government. Kean, like other U.S. officials and American scientific charity reformers, worried that if the system of state subsidies was not soon ended, "the charitable instincts of the Cuban people [would] suffer serious deterioration."[105] Similar to the belief that relief aid would eventually make the poor dependent on charity, officials asserted that aid to private institutions would "dry up the sources of private charity," as wealthy citizens would come to expect the state to cover the costs of the institutions.[106] Ending state subsidies to municipal and private charities was so important to the occupation government that an early pamphlet listed this as one of the department's two primary goals.[107] As with relief to the *reconcentrados*, the answer to this municipal and private institutional dependence on state aid was a shifting of state resources from monetary support to inspection, with the Department of Public Charities overseeing the finances of all institutions receiving state subsidies, even going so far as to shut down some institutions incapable of self-support and redistributing their assets to other *beneficencia* institutions.

Hospitals, however, were not like other *beneficencia* institutions. Unlike orphanages and homes for widows or the elderly, Havana's hospital system was a key node in the urban medical landscape, vital to the occupation government's central goal of controlling infectious disease. U.S. officials hoped to quickly end state subsidies to municipal hospitals, but this proved impossible. As J. R. Kean explained, although the Beneficencia Law of 1900 required municipal governments to fund local hospitals, the lingering economic effects of the war left municipalities across the country far too broke to do so, so that even by 1902, "no city in the Island" was able to support its municipal hospital.[108] Over the course of the occupation, in fact, this de facto state support for local hospitals became official policy, as eight of the larger municipal hospitals were made state institutions under the direct authority of the Department of Public Charities, where they served as both training schools for Cuban nurses and frontline health care institutions serving the needs of the Cuban poor. Ironically, therefore, even as department officials sought to reduce national involvement in the provision of local health services, the department's responsibility over local health care expanded dramatically during the course of the occupation. As the next chapter will demonstrate, rather than see this as a problem, Cuban health officials embraced this expanded state responsibility over the island's municipal medical system, turning this unintentional dynamic into an argument in favor of the nationalization of the island's health services.

But with the state now funding all municipal hospitals, the question of who gained admittance became a charged issue. Like most hospitals in turn-of-the-century Latin America, United States, and Europe, municipal hospitals in Cuba were public charities, providing free medical care to those too poor to pay for private medical services. Kean worried that public hospitals were too freely admitting sick people without making sure they were truly poor, as hospital administrators were compelled by politicians to admit patients without verifying their poverty.¹⁰⁹ Indeed, in keeping with colonial practice, Havana's municipal officials did attempt to exert control over hospital admissions, forcing department officials in 1901 to send letters reminding municipal hospital directors that city officials had "no authority whatsoever to issue orders governing the administration of institutions maintained by the State."¹¹⁰ But the issue was broader than political influence. According to Kean, not only were hospital administrators generally unwilling to investigate the economic circumstances of patients to ensure that only the "truly poor" gained admission, but "hospital authorities [were] also, as a rule, timid about discharging patients until they are willing to leave on their own accord." For Kean and other American officials, this amounted to a shameful waste of government funds and led to the overcrowding of Cuban hospitals. Even more troubling for Kean, however, this situation was leading to the "medical pauperization of the people," with the poor coming to see admission to public hospitals as a *right* rather than a charity. Until the state stopped funding municipal hospitals, Kean alleged, this situation "injur[ious] to public morals" would continue.¹¹¹

As these debates make clear, at issue was more than a question of state finances, but the kinds of claims citizens could make upon the state. Was medical care a right or a privilege? For Kean, schooled in American scientific charity thought, the availability of state-funded medical services for the poor would inevitably result in Cubans claiming health care as a right of citizenship. The only remedy was to quickly end state subsidies to municipal hospitals and institute strict income requirements to ensure that only the truly poor could access services. But while many Cuban *beneficencia* workers, physicians, and officials also worried about the negative fiscal and social effects of too-easy access to public medical services, some were equally vocal in their advocacy of expanded public medical services to those in need. Indeed, for Jorge Dehogues, a physician in Havana's Hospital No. 1, the state had the "obligation to give aid to all citizens in poor health who cannot through their own resources get medical assistance," and "all poor patients have the right to occupy a hospital bed" without undergoing onerous inspections to prove their poverty.¹¹² But for Emilio Martínez, the director of Havana's Tamayo Dispensary, the fact that medical services were paid for by the state was indeed the central problem. Describing the claims Havana's residents were making on the public medical system, Martínez complained that "every citizen believes they have this right because they believe that what pertains to the State pertains to them and it is not a charity but rather a right that they exercise without thinking that others are working to underwrite the costs which it occasions."[113]

## RELIEF, BENEFICENCIA, AND THE MEANINGS OF CHARITY IN POSTCOLONIAL CUBA

For both Cubans and Americans, relief was never only a state or a private function. Both complemented each other, even when both proved woefully inadequate. U.S. relief work in Cuba was informed by Protestant missionary idealism, humanitarian solidarity, and a colonial belief in the fundamental superiority of American methods. It was the product of an emerging expansionist American sense of purpose, as Americans increasingly looked beyond their borders to help make sense of their role in the world. Informed by both American and recent international relief efforts, U.S. relief organizations articulated different ideas of American responsibility, predicated on assumptions of shared humanity but also embedded within an emerging imperial relationship between Cuba and the United States.

The United States entered the twentieth century as the world's newest imperial power. For those who embraced this new reality, the United States represented a fundamentally different kind of global power, distinct from the "old" empires of its European rivals; it was a self-styled progressive force for good in the world. Many pointed to American relief work in Cuba—and the successful transformation of the island's colonial *beneficencia* system into a modern and efficient system of health and charities administration—as the clearest evidence of the benefits of American power abroad and an implicit refutation of both Cuban and American anti-imperialist sentiment. As John Kendrick Bangs wrote in his 1902 *Uncle Sam Trustee*, "What has American imperialism—this terrible bogey . . . done for these suffering people? It is a very simple story, yet one which should give to every American a thrill of joy that he may account himself such, and of pride that the army which represents him, under such difficult conditions has produced men capable of achieving such marvelous results."[114] In this narrative, the U.S. occupation had rescued a starving people and bestowed American expertise upon a passive and grateful Cuban people: "In charities, as in sanitation and in education, Cuba has sat at the feet of the United States," noted the *Chicago Daily Tribune* shortly after the inauguration of the Cuban republic. "As far as the apparatus of charitable work goes, no other country is now better off than the little republic just set up by the army and the Congress of America."[115]

That the results of the U.S. occupation of Cuba were never as marvelous as these boosters proclaimed should not surprise us, but neither should we assume that American philanthropic concern was merely a cover for imperial aggression. Rather, the history of food and medical relief and *beneficencia* in Cuba presents a complex fabric of conflicting motivations, actions, and institutions.

For the Americans in charge of the transformation of the Cuban social welfare system between 1899 and 1902, poverty was first and foremost a behavioral rather than a structural issue. As such, the methods employed to alleviate suffering on the island often seem contradictory: military officials rejected plans to offer inexpensive loans to impoverished farmers as "paternalistic" and shuttered state-supported women's cooperatives in the capital, but they invested a great deal of money into building up an inspections regime to prevent Cubans from receiving food or medical aid. Worried that Cubans would fall too easily into expecting support from their government, U.S. officials worked tirelessly to build a legal and institutional social welfare system based on *limiting* aid. In the process, however, they created a centralized body with broad authority that would serve as the institutional basis for further experimentation in social policy during the Cuban Republic.

For the Cubans who staffed and led these *beneficencia* institutions or sought aid for themselves or their families, this work took often profoundly different meanings. Embedded in debates over whether the poor and sick should be cared for by the state or by private charity were competing notions over whether the model of private charity in the United States fit the cultural and economic realities of postindependence Cuba. In the decade after independence, scores of physicians, public officials, journalists, reformers, and public and private *beneficencia* workers met for the annual Conference on Beneficencia and Corrections. Each multiday conference met in a different city across the island, and sessions were held on topics ranging from how to support the island's fledgling nursing schools to how best to care for orphans, the blind, the elderly, and the sick. Together, the published speeches and debates allow us to see not only the breadth of private organizing and state action during a time of rapid political and cultural change but also how Cubans made sense of this work and the meanings they attached to it.

According to the physician Carlos E. Finlay, son of the famous bacteriologist Carlos Juan Finlay and member of the Central Committee of the Department of Public Charities, the purpose of these conferences was to popularize scientific charity in Cuba and reinforce the idea that private charity, not the state, should primarily be responsible for caring for the sick. But, he argued, these ideas had found little purchase in Cuba, whose people and institutions reflected the "eminently centralizing regime of the Colony" and who, as he put it, "looked to the State" to address local needs.[116] As Finlay understood, despite his best efforts, it would be difficult for scientific charity to gain a foothold in postcolonial Cuba, for the island's *beneficencia* traditions reflected centuries of centralized Spanish colonial governance and its emerging political culture embraced a strong role for the state and a nationalist responsibility for those at the margins. As we will see, the emerging Cuban health and social welfare system—whose embryonic form was already apparent in 1901—reflected both the centralizing push of the occupation government and the medical nationalist politics of this generation of Cuban physicians, nurses, and *beneficencia* workers.

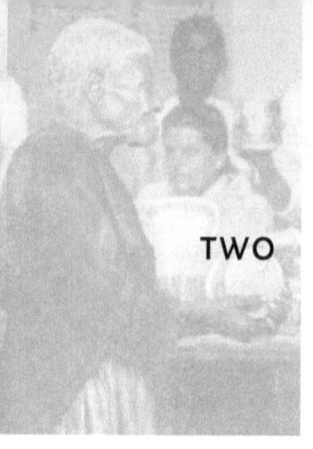

## TWO  A Blessed Formula for Progress
### Medical Nationalism, U.S. Empire, and the Development of Public Health, 1899–1909

ON MAY 15, 1902, just days before the Cuban Republic was formally inaugurated, the social, political, and scientific elite of Havana gathered to celebrate the new home of the Cuban Academy of Science. That evening, many "elegant ladies and distinguished men of science" crowded into the academy's stately dark wood lecture hall illuminated by the warm glow of electric lights.[1] At the front of the room sat the guests of honor, including the military governor of Cuba Leonard Wood and president-elect Tomás Estrada Palma, alongside two of the evening's invited speakers: the noted bacteriologists and physicians Juan Santos Fernández and Enrique Barnet. They came together that evening to celebrate the recent renovations that transformed the former San Agustín convent into this "new temple of science" for the Cuban people.[2] The timing of the event and the symbolism of its location seemed to suggest that an age of rationalism and national science had eclipsed colonial superstition and empiricism. Science and medicine would no longer be relegated to the margins of public consciousness or the nation's political priorities. Indeed, they could no longer be ignored, for the reality of tropical disease and Cuba's uneasy relationship to the United States required that the Cuban people embrace science, modernity, and the responsibilities of hygienic self-discipline. At the cusp of independence and the dawn of a new century, medicine represented more than a set of healing practices and technologies: it was a blueprint for a modern and healthy republic, a "blessed formula for progress" for the Cuban nation.

For the men and women gathered that evening, medical science and a government committed to public health action were the keys to the redemption of a tropical island long known as a hotbed of disease and death. As Juan Santos Fernández reminded his audience, "Our country, until yesterday, was considered on par with others in the tropical Americas, as poisoned ground that made civilized men pay with their lives for daring tread" upon

Cuban soil.³ Just months before, a joint effort of Cuban and U.S. scientists and health officials had finally managed to rid the island of yellow fever, the disease that targeted the foreign-born and had since the eighteenth century done profound damage to Cuba's economy and international reputation. The extirpation of yellow fever proved that environment was not destiny, that the tropics were not necessarily coterminous with disease, death, and backwardness.

For Cuban health advocates, the success of the yellow fever campaign was vivid proof that once the cause of disease was determined, concerted state action could reduce or even eliminate infectious disease. For Enrique Barnet, this meant that governments had a responsibility to do everything in their power to protect their citizens from disease, for "society has the right not to have . . . disease in their midst."⁴ But this right came with its own responsibilities, for Cuban citizens would have to assimilate the new lessons of the laboratory and adopt the hygienic bodily practices that would protect them and one another from infection. Barnet warned that citizens would have to be led, by force if necessary, into this hygienic modernity, for "the neglect of personal habits, [and] lack of cleanliness and personal hygiene are very common among the ignorant classes."⁵ He therefore urged his audience to embrace the task of popular health education, likening it to a religious calling, "so that science comes to be like the priesthood" for those that preached the life-saving "good news" of modern hygiene.⁶

If medicine was to have a privileged place in postcolonial Cuban life, however, it was not just because it could help Cuba achieve health and national modernity. Not far from the surface of this discussion was the pervasive threat that disease could pose to Cuban independence under the provisions of the Platt Amendment, imposed on Cuba as a precondition for the withdrawal of U.S. forces. Its fifth article required the Cuban government to maintain "acceptable" health conditions in its cities in order to prevent the spread of disease to southern U.S. ports. Failure to do so risked another military intervention. With the Cuban president-elect standing before him, Santos Fernández demanded that the new political leadership "turn their attention even more than they have to the importance of our health problems," for with the loss of sovereignty hanging over the island, "one would have to close their eyes to reason to not grasp that we will not have a country if we cannot maintain our public health."⁷

This evening, on the cusp of Cuban independence over a century ago, gives us a clear picture of the excitement, hopes, and anxieties of an entire generation of Cuban physicians, nurses, and public health officials. Coming of age at the apex of a period of scientific change, they hoped to use their knowledge to shape the coming republic. Engaging with and at times vigorously condemning the U.S. occupation government, Cuban medical nationalists worked to shape the contours of the postcolonial health landscape. They participated in institutional health reform and spearheaded public health campaigns, but just as important to these reformers was the transformation of the Cuban people into a modern and healthy population, prepared for the responsibilities of independence. For Cuban medical nationalists, independence represented a sharp break with the past, a political and social rupture that allowed them to insert their own visions of a healthy and modern Cuba into the very DNA of republican life and government. This chapter focuses on the ideas and experiences of these Cubans, as they responded in unexpected ways to American public health priorities, made sense of the transition from colony to republic, and created new institutions that would transform Havana's postcolonial health landscape.

While historians have rightly emphasized the colonial self-interests that shaped U.S. health policy in Cuba, far less has been said about the Cuban physicians and nurses who carried out these policies, whose actions and ideas helped shape U.S. policy, and whose work redefined this colonial health agenda into a nationalist medical project.[8] This medical nationalist project was a cultural revolution with implications for all aspects of Cuban society: from how Cubans ate, fed their children, interacted on the street, and went to church, to the basic functions of the Cuban government. Nowhere did this cause more conflict than with the establishment of Cuba's first nursing schools during the U.S. occupation, which elites and the Catholic hierarchy fiercely opposed as a violation of gendered and religious norms. Like other modernizing discourses, medical nationalist discourse served multiple, sometimes competing purposes as it was taken up by different groups to make claims about the proper ordering of postindependence society. For some elites, the failure of the poor—especially poor women and Cubans of color—to live up to elite standards of hygienic conduct served to justify class hierarchies and naturalize social segregation. But in the hands of the working-class women who became the first generation of Cuban nurses, this discourse allowed them to make forceful claims for inclusion while providing them with a means to support themselves and their families. During this period of political, social, and scientific change, matters of health became deeply politicized and took on outsized importance. The hospital, the home, the street, and the state all became battlegrounds in a cultural and medical struggle whose implications spread far from personal or national health, taking on international dimensions with the Platt Amendment's imposition of American sanitary oversight. This dynamic among personal habits, national politics, transnational science, and international relations is the subject of this chapter.

## "CLEANSING THE AUGEAN STABLES": COLONIAL PUBLIC HEALTH UNDER U.S. OCCUPATION

On New Year's morning 1899, the U.S. flag was hoisted high above El Morro castle at the entrance to Havana Bay, signaling the formal transfer of sovereignty and the end of four centuries of Spanish rule in the Americas. For the New York Times, Spain's "Bourbon incapacity for modern progress" was at the heart of its many failures, and its failures were no more apparent than in the abominable health conditions of the Cuban capital. Indeed, the Times alleged, with the threat of yellow fever emanating from Havana, the most important duty of the new Military Government in Cuba, after establishing order, was "the sanitary purification of that unspeakable town." But this sanitary campaign would require more than brooms and shovels. For the Times editors and U.S. military officials alike, 400 years of Spanish rule had left an indelible mark on the sanitary habits of the Cuban people. For it was precisely "the barbarous avoidance of all the decencies and conveniences of modern city life" of Havana's residents that allowed "the germs of yellow fever to find a permanent breeding-place in that city." As the New York Times warned, "Driving out the hydra [of Spain] from Cuba was the easiest of our Herculean tasks. The army and the navy did that in a few months. The cleansing of the Augean stables will be a longer and more arduous task. We can build sewers and close cesspools. But after that we must begin the sanitary education of a people sunk deep in ignorance and notably impervious to new ideas."[9]

It is impossible to overstate how important the sanitary reformation of Havana was for Americans at the onset of the occupation. For over 200 years, yellow fever had been the perennial scourge of the American South, costing untold damage to U.S. commerce and claiming as many as 150,000 American lives.[10] Recurrent outbreaks in southern U.S. port cities had been traced to Havana, where the disease had been endemic since the eighteenth century.[11] For foreigners in Havana as well as those in the path of periodic outbreaks in the U.S. South, the disease—with its high mortality rate and grisly symptoms—was a terrifying spectre. Most people infected with the virus experience only the initial stage of fever, chills, muscle pains, headaches, and vomiting. But for roughly 15 percent of cases, a brief remission is followed by a second toxic and highly dangerous phase of the disease, with delirium, seizures, severe abdominal pain, and kidney and liver damage—the latter resulting in the telltale jaundice that gives yellow fever its name. Bleeding from the eyes, nose, and mouth can follow, with some victims vomiting coagulated black blood due to gastrointestinal hemorrhaging—leading to its grim nickname of *vomito negro* or "black vomit." Up to half of those who experience the second phase of the illness die. A painful and gruesome disease, it almost exclusively afflicted the foreign-born, due to the lifelong immunity granted by a relatively mild childhood infection in places, like Havana, where the disease was endemic.

The carefully organized collection of yellow fever case files compiled by William Crawford Gorgas, the chief sanitary officer of Havana, gives us a sense of those whose lives were impacted, and sometimes ended, by this dread disease during the early years of the U.S. occupation. They were disproportionately male and working class, reflecting the fact that most foreigners that came to the island to work were men. Most were young and most came from Spain, like nineteen-year-old Angel Menéndez García, who had been on the island for ten months. Menéndez Garcia had been taking bookkeeping lessons at night in the hopes of moving up from his position as a clerk in a Spanish-run wholesale grocery store, but in late August 1899, he came down with the fever and chills of yellow fever. Although he was quickly admitted to the Spanish immigrant Quinta de Dependientes hospital, there was little doctors could do. Within a week, he was dead. Others that fell ill included a Dutchman employed as a painter in the lieutenant governor's palace, a Spanish tailor who took night classes, a forty-year-old American acrobat named Archie, several former American soldiers who returned to the island after their tours of duty were complete, a Spanish barber who enjoyed gin and his evening walks along Central Park, and a sixty-five-year-old French housekeeper who liked to watch her daughter perform at the Tacon Theater.[12] These brief files give us the smallest glimpse into the lives, hopes, and social networks of the foreigners who came to Havana seeking work. These men and women lived and worked alongside Cubans and often socialized with them, but unlike the native-born, they were vulnerable to this often-fatal disease. For those who succumbed to yellow fever, news of their deaths reverberated along both sides of the Atlantic, providing yet more evidence that the city of Havana was a diseased and dangerous place for foreigners.

For American officials, then, the military occupation was a long-awaited opportunity to finally tackle the disease at its source. And tackle it they tried, expending tremendous effort to effect a sanitary transformation of every aspect of the postwar urban environment. By day, Cuban workers busily repaved the city streets, while teams of white-uniformed street cleaners scoured the capital every night and mule-drawn wagons traversed the city sprinkling electrozone, a mild disinfectant, onto the streets. Hospitals were cleaned, disinfected, and given new medical supplies, and efforts were begun to dredge up Havana harbor, the foul-smelling depository of the city's raw sewage. Meanwhile, 114 Cuban physicians hired by the occupation government as medical inspectors fanned out across Havana, performing what was essentially a sanitary census of the city.[13] If conditions were found wanting, building owners were ordered to complete required sanitary work, such as painting, removing rubbish, and cleaning out cesspools, in a timely manner or be subject to fines.[14] For "unusually dirty" houses that were deemed to present a disease threat, the Health Department sent teams to clean out, remove clutter from, scrub, and whitewash these homes.[15]

This sanitary campaign represented a tremendous undertaking. Yet although it took place well into the bacteriological revolution of the late nineteenth century, it was based largely on pre-bacteriological disease theories that focused on filth as the source of contagion. As historians of science have long pointed out, scientific change is a slow and messy process, and for Americans entering Havana in late 1898 or early 1899, there seemed to be an obvious relationship between the city's state of sanitary abandon and yellow fever. Indeed, American newspaper articles, commercial advertisements, and political cartoons reflected and reinforced the idea that American responsibility on the island required, in the words of one letter to the editor, "a thorough and unrelenting crusade against filth."[16]

But in 1899, the method of yellow fever transmission was still in dispute: although the Cuban scientist and physician Carlos J. Finlay had published a study in 1881 proposing that yellow fever was spread through the bite of the *Stegomyia* mosquito, his research had been widely dismissed outside Cuba.[17] In the absence of a widely accepted understanding of yellow fever transmission, Americans directed their efforts to the kinds of sanitary reforms that were the hallmark of nineteenth-century public health work: street cleaning, garbage collection, and to a lesser degree, sewer construction and improving the city's water supply. But the focus was really on the "filth" of the city, the garbage, human waste, and dead animals that American visitors invariably commented on when they visited the city.[18] Of course, as Cuban physicians often noted, these conditions were the result of years of colonial neglect of public services, but for Americans they were simply proof of the "filthy habits" of the city's residents, as the *Times* alleged.[19]

In the occupation government's urban sanitary campaign, we see the overlapping goals of U.S. colonial health work. At once a plan to protect American lives and interests, reduce Cuban mortality, and highlight the superiority of American methods, the sanitary campaign became a powerful argument for the benefits of U.S. rule. For American officials, hygiene was more than a set of tools for combating disease; it was, as Marial Iglesias Utset has argued, a discourse on civilization and modernity, counterposing the alleged backwardness and disregard for hygiene of the Cuban people to the sanitary know-how and attention to personal cleanliness of the occupation forces.[20] It was a central part of a broader racial discourse that legitimated American control over the island, that tied hygienic discipline to capacity for self-rule. For William Crawford Gorgas, chief sanitary officer for Havana, hygienic tutelage was but part of the project of cultural and political Americanization that would counteract Cubans' "Latin" predisposition to disorder and conflict and prevent the island from becoming "a Hayti No. 2."[21] For Gorgas, the home inspections regime was the centerpiece of the entire sanitary campaign, "in all probability, the most prominent work the department is doing," for by forcing people to "clean their own houses" under threat of fines, they "thus get into the habit of cleanliness."[22] That Cubans would only learn these habits under pressure and guidance from the United States seemed obvious to some American observers. As the American correspondent Franklin Matthews asserted, the city would only be healthful once Cubans "learned something of sanitation and have educated themselves into abhorring bad smells."[23]

Already by April 1899, just a few short months into the sanitary campaign, the *Washington Post* marveled that "Havana, once remarkable for its filth, is being transformed. . . . There is no accumulation of dirt in the gutters, no litter of paper, no refuse of any character."[24] Even Manuel Delfín, often a critic of U.S. health policy, admitted that the daily sweeping of the city's streets produced "a truly notable difference in their appearance today, from that of before."[25] As with all aspects of the military government's work, however, this urban sanitary project took on multiple meanings, as Cubans and Americans, military officials and city residents, and reporters and physicians interpreted the campaign through the lens of their own experiences and within their own cultural and political frameworks. Havana's clean streets and improving health statistics contrasted sharply with the chaos, filth, and want of the final years of Spanish colonial rule. For Americans this represented the superiority of American scientific capacity and administrative know-how. But the sanitary transformation of Havana—itself more partial than its boosters admitted—was largely dependent on the work and leadership of Cuban physicians, who staffed reorganized hospitals, performed home inspections, and took up administrative positions in local and national boards of health and the new Departamento de Beneficencia. Indeed, while the occupation government's sanitary project was meant primarily to protect American lives and interests, the Cuban medical workers who carried out this project redefined it, asserted their own public health priorities, and in the process transformed a colonial public health program into a medical nationalist project.

## "TO PROMOTE THE HEALTH OF THE PEOPLE IS TO PREPARE IT FOR ITS FREEDOM": MEDICAL NATIONALISM UNDER U.S. OCCUPATION

For Cuban physicians, the end of Spanish colonial rule represented an opportunity to use their professional expertise to free the island and its people from the disease, death, and backwardness they associated with the recent colonial past. Poised at the cusp of independence and at the height of a period of rapid medical and scientific advancement, this generation of Cuban doctors articulated a medical nationalist vision for Cuba that would reverberate in the coming decades. Based on the idea that science was the key to transforming the former colony into a prosperous, modern, and healthy republic, and that both individual citizens and the state had a central role to play in its creation, this medical nationalist vision for Cuba overlapped in some important ways with that of U.S. military officials. For Cuban doctors, however, this amounted to an explicit program for the decolonization of Cuban society and, eventually, ensuring Cuban independence in the face of American neocolonial intentions.

Cuban physicians at the turn of the century were well positioned to engage in an expansive health reform project. Far from being a medical backwater, late-nineteenth-century Havana had perhaps the highest number of physicians per capita of any city in the world.[26] In addition to their daily work of attending to patients, these physicians organized a vibrant intellectual community, conducting original research and participating in transnational scientific debates. The last third of the nineteenth century was a period of intense scientific research and organizing in Havana, starting with the 1861 founding of the Royal Academy of Medical, Physical, and Natural Sciences of Havana, which brought together Cuban medical researchers, botanists, zoologists, physicists, chemists, and other scientists to share their research and discuss new scientific and medical discoveries.[27] It was at the academy in 1881 that Carlos J. Finlay presented his groundbreaking paper asserting that yellow fever was transmitted through the bite of the *Stegomyia* mosquito (later renamed *Aedes aegypti*). Another important institution, the Instituto Histo-Bacteriológico de la Habana, a bacteriological laboratory founded in the mid-1880s, provided a cutting edge space for collaborative scientific research and produced a rabies vaccine for the island.[28] New journals published original medical and scientific research; became spaces for debating recent scientific discoveries from Europe, North America, and Latin America; and became venues for the dissemination of public health and medical knowledge.[29]

Through their scientific journals and professional organizations, laboratory work, correspondence, and travel and study abroad, this generation of Cuban physicians engaged with and helped shape the most dynamic period of medical change in the history of the world. The "bacteriological revolution" set off by the research of Pasteur and Koch in the 1870s and 1880s and the revolution in surgical techniques made possible by antiseptic and aseptic surgical reforms transformed the practice of medicine. The final decades of the nineteenth century were an unprecedented period of global medical ferment. In a span of just a few years, the microbial cause and mode of transmission of some of the world's most notorious diseases were discovered, including tuberculosis, rabies, diphtheria, leprosy, anthrax, cholera, typhoid fever, and the bubonic plague. While truly effective therapeutic responses to many of these diseases would have to wait decades, vaccines were rapidly developed conferring varying degrees of protection for many of them. Meanwhile, new hygienic practices—like hand-washing and avoiding contact with bodily excreta—allowed the healthy to successfully ward off diseases like tuberculosis, typhoid, and cholera, which were among the greatest scourges of the nineteenth century. All of these discoveries and new practices led to a sense of rapid—even inevitable—medical progress. For Cuban physicians, however, this period of scientific progress coincided with and bled into the decades-long independence struggle, which upended the lives of Cuban doctors and transformed the practice of Cuban medicine.

While Cuban physicians had always held a variety of political positions, perhaps more than any other profession they were associated with the anticolonial struggle—as martyrs, political exiles, and frontline doctors on the battlefields of the Wars of Independence. In 1871, three years into the first War of Independence (1868–78), a group of eight medical students in Havana were executed for allegedly defacing the tomb of a renowned Spanish veteran. The unusually harsh sentence helped galvanize nationalist sentiment, and the students were hailed as martyrs to the independence cause. In the coming years, many physicians were among those exiled for their support for independence, including figures such as José Ángel Malberty, who, as a physician in the urban underground, had helped organize Cuba's short-lived Guerra Chiquita war against Spanish colonial rule (1879–80) and was later forced into exile in New York and Mexico.[30] Another was the future bacteriologist, internist, and secretary of state, Diego Tamayo y Figueredo, who joined the insurgent army during the Ten Years War, but was wounded, captured, and later exiled to the United States.[31] For many of these doctors, political exile provided the opportunity to practice and study abroad. They gained valuable experience working in centers of scientific research and surgical innovation like Paris, Philadelphia, and New York City.[32]

It was Cuba's final War of Independence (1895–98) that would be most closely associated with physicians. For José Martí, the revolutionary thinker and architect of the final War of Independence, Cuban physicians were ideal conspirators: they were professional men with the broad respect of the community, and their movements day or night would not attract attention, as they were expected to make house calls at all hours. For these reasons, Martí once said, the final war would be "the revolution of the doctors."[33] Indeed, they were central to urban revolutionary networks. At the beginning of the war, the surgeon and future founder of Cuba's first school of nursing, Raimundo Menocal, was named the first *delegado de la revolución*, or revolutionary delegate, in Havana, responsible for smuggling arms and medical supplies and conveying correspondences between insurgent leadership in the field and political leaders and supporters abroad.[34] Although forced into exile, he continued this anticolonial work in New York City, forming with the sanitarian and future secretary of health Enrique Barnet an organization of exiled Cuban medical professionals that helped provide "the revolutionary armies of Cuba and Porto-Rico" with surgical and medical supplies.[35] According to Manuel Delfín, this was an especially dangerous period for Cuban physicians, who were often put on government lists as suspected conspirators, "because it was said that this Revolution was the work of doctors."[36] Some were imprisoned for suspected anticolonial activities, like Emiliano Nuñez, the medical director of Havana's Mercedes Hospital, who was sent to a Spanish penal colony off the west coast of Africa.[37] But many of those who fled the cities joined the revolutionary army itself, practicing frontline medicine under extremely difficult circumstances, like the obstetrician Eusebio Hernández and the surgeon Enrique Nuñez de Villavicenio.

With the cessation of the war, these geographically dispersed anticolonial physicians converged on the Cuban capital. Armed with their experiences abroad and immersed in this era of scientific innovation, they imbued their own ideas of nationalism with a fervent belief in the promises of scientific reform. They saw the end of Spanish colonial rule as an opportunity to use the new tools of biomedical science to create the institutions that would ensure the health of the Cuban people and shape the coming republic. For this generation of early-twentieth-century medical nationalists—many of whom saw firsthand the death and destruction of Spanish reconcentration policies—disease represented the colonial past. Biomedical science, by contrast, was the key to an independent and prosperous Cuban Republic, "a blessed formula for progress," in the words of the physician Ramón María Alfonso y García.[38]

Physicians from this period often commented on what they saw as the nationalist significance of hygiene, science, and sanitary reform. For Ernesto Edelmann, who participated in the early government sanitary inspections, it was "just and logical [to] desire to banish from Cuba the germs of avoidable diseases, making our homeland an enviable country from the hygienic point of view," for all "health work is eminently patriotic."[39] In January 1900, the medical journal La Habana Médica proclaimed a "new age of hope" in the wake of Spanish colonial rule and urged Cuban physicians to take up the task of "making this country healthy," for "our sanitary state [is] the basis of all progress."[40] These sentiments represented a kind of nationalist inversion of the colonial health project of the U.S. occupation. For both Cuban medical nationalists and American officials, hygiene was as much a technology for improving health statistics as a discourse on modernity and civilization. But while Americans saw Cubans as hopelessly mired in backward habits, medical nationalists believed that promoting hygienic consciousness would lead the Cuban people to modernity and health.

Of course, the capaciousness of this project was the key to its strength. Medical nationalists were divided by class origin and party affiliation. Some medical nationalists emphasized the responsibility of individuals for their own health, while others looked more to the state; for some medical nationalists, a "modern and prosperous" Cuba depended on the whitening of the island through greater European immigration, while others directed their health work to the problems most affecting poor Cubans, black or white. Nevertheless, medical nationalists were united in their belief that medicine and science were the keys to national progress, and that a combination of popular hygienic education and strong state action was essential for achieving hygienic modernity. And they agreed that Cuban physicians themselves would help guide Cuban society to health and modernity.

Strikingly, the U.S. sanitary campaign, conceived as a means to protect American lives and interests, helped shape this emerging medical nationalist project. As Manuel Delfín writes in his memoir Thirty Years a Doctor, the scores of Cuban physicians who participated in the American health campaign were transformed by the experience. While colonial sanitary neglect had left the city, in the words of Gastón Cuadrado, "an immense trash heap," the American sanitary campaign presented the stunning contrast of military officials who were eager to improve the health conditions of the city, who followed the counsel of Cuban physicians, and who were "obedient to the dictates of science."[41] Despite their sometimes fierce criticism of the occupation, Cuban physicians seem to have been overwhelmingly supportive of the sanitary campaign and saw the military government's exercise of authority over health matters as a model for future action. But the work itself, of inspecting the homes of the city's poor, was also transformative. While most had experience tending to the medical needs of the poor in the city's public hospitals and free dispensaries, few physicians had confronted the terrible living conditions of the city's poorest residents. "We saw things we would never have dreamed of," Delfín wrote in his memoir. Although some received the medical inspectors with suspicion or anger, "the majority of residents blessed the moment in which something good would be done for those who suffered the horrors of a home without hygiene, true sources of disease."[42]

These experiences underscored the reality that medical nationalists wanted to change: replacing squalid living conditions with healthy homes and educating the poor in proper hygiene. As their published articles, personal letters, and meeting minutes from this period highlight, turn-of-the-century physicians consistently grappled with the question of changing popular habits in the service of health and national modernity. Speaking to his colleagues at the National Academy of Science, the physician Julio San Martín admitted that Havana's residents were "not yet sufficiently enlightened" to understand the new hygienic measures passed by the intervention government.[43] This sentiment was widely shared among Cuban physicians, nurses, and public health officials and surely reflected the reality—common across all urban centers at the turn of the twentieth century—that only a small if growing subset of urban residents understood and practiced the new hygienic precepts that allowed for the control of infection. Old theories of disease causation were only slowly eclipsed by the new lessons of bacteriology.⁴⁴ The behaviors that gave people some modicum of control over the spread of illness—actions such as hand-washing, avoiding contact with bodily secretions, not sharing objects such as spoons and cups, and preparing and storing food so as to avoid the growth of dangerous bacteria—were slow to seep into daily consciousness.⁴⁵

But for some turn-of-the-century physicians, this hygienic divide only reinforced their elitist conceptions of the backwardness of the Cuban poor, for medical nationalism was still deeply embedded in colonial structures that helped legitimize racial and gender hierarchies. With their understandings of hygiene, modernity, and the sanitary capacities of the poor shaped by long-standing class, gender, and race discourses, some found women and Cubans of color to be disproportionately responsible for Havana's supposed sanitary backwardness. Manuel Delfín was a complex figure in this regard. He was proud that his Dispensario La Caridad served the Cuban poor "without distinction by race, nationality or place of origin" and was often quite astute about the effects of the gendered urban economy on women's poverty.⁴⁶ And yet he lamented "the heterogeneity of this population, so influenced by the inferior races," which he believed "contributes to [a] criminal disdain" for hygiene among the Cuban people.⁴⁷ He also decried the "lethal ignorance of mothers" and saw their "truly criminal indifference" to the health of their children as a primary cause of Havana's high infant mortality rate.⁴⁸ Still others blamed Chinese or Antillean immigrants for disease outbreaks or expressed the hope that sanitary reforms would facilitate greater European immigration, leading to the progressive whitening of the island.⁴⁹

In many ways, this anticolonial medical vision itself was a kind of colonizing project: the poor were expected to conform to the enlightened vision of elite medical experts who often viewed the cultural practices of Cubans of color as an impediment to national progress and who often barely hid their disdain for the Cuban poor. Nevertheless, medical nationalists expressed confidence that proper training could extirpate colonial habits, instill in the Cuban population the habits of hygienic discipline, and transform the Cuban people into a modern and prosperous polity.⁵⁰ For the medical statistician Jorge Le-Roy y Cassá, a cultural education in hygienic modernity was an essential step on the path to decolonization, for to "promote the health of the people [was] to prepare it for its freedom."⁵¹ Implicit in this discourse was the idea that the Cuban people were not yet ready for independence, but with time and the proper education, they could be.

Medical nationalists therefore worked to popularize the new medical knowledge through public health poster campaigns, new journals aimed

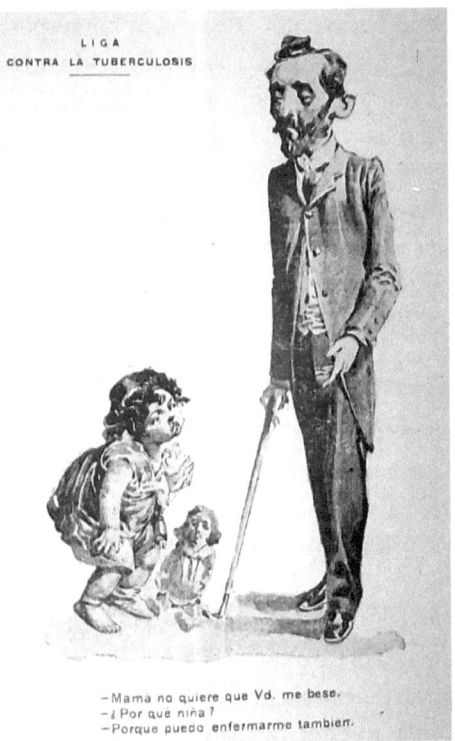

*Figure 2.1* Postcard distributed by the Liga Contra la Tuberculosis en Cuba: "Mother doesn't want you to kiss me." "Why, little girl?" "Because I could get sick also." (*Boletín Mensual de la Liga Contra la Tuberculosis de Cuba*, January 1903, 98)

at popular audiences, pamphlets, public lectures, and articles in the local press. With an evangelical fervor, they spread the lifesaving "gospel of hygiene" to all who would listen.[52] They tried to get Cubans out of the habit of kissing each other in greeting, encouraged priests to sanitize holy water basins to prevent the spread of disease, urged mothers to breastfeed their newborns, and entered factories to teach workers about disease prevention. They pushed for laws to protect women and children factory workers, establish tuberculosis insurance for the poor, and institute high taxes on alcohol, under the belief that alcohol was a major factor in reducing the body's immunological protection against tuberculosis.[53] They preached the practical benefits of hand-washing and regular bathing, urged Cubans not to spit (or if they had to, to use spittoons), and taught mothers how to properly disinfect baby bottles. All aspects of everyday life, in short, were subject to the hygienic cultural revolution that these physicians hoped to inspire.

It was precisely to transform the hygienic habits of urban residents and curb the city's exorbitant tuberculosis mortality that two prominent medical figures, Joaquín Jacobsen and Juan Santos Fernández, founded the Cuban Anti-Tuberculosis League in 1901.[54] In order to fulfill their mission, the league opened a small and perpetually underfunded dispensary for the poor, where its volunteer physicians diagnosed the disease, provided healthy meals for a small number of patients (as funding allowed), and worked tirelessly to spread popular awareness of the measures needed to prevent the spread of the disease. Indeed, in the decades before antibiotics finally provided a medical cure for the disease, antituberculosis work was largely educational, teaching the sick and their families how to avoid infection and promoting the rest and proper nutrition that were essential to recovery. In order to spread their message to as many Cubans as possible, the league got creative, distributing postcards with pithy lessons on tuberculosis prevention and even getting local manufacturers to print the league's "twenty prophylactic tips" for avoiding the disease on matchboxes and the backs of the colorful fans that so many Cuban women used to cool themselves in the hot tropical weather.[55] And they started a monthly journal, the *Boletín Mensual de la Liga Contra la Tuberculosis en Cuba*, which was distributed for free to city residents.

As historians such as Louis A. Pérez and Marial Iglesias Utset have shown, turn-of-the-century Cuba was a place of deep cultural struggle over the meanings of *cubanidad*, of political independence, and of modernity and democracy. The creative adaptation of foreign models to suit Cuban needs was at the core of this dynamic.[56] Nowhere was this more evident than in medical nationalism. Cuban medical journals constantly reported on health programs in other countries and reprinted articles from Latin American, European, and North American medical journals. This catholic interest in foreign health news reflected the excitement and sense of possibility of the age, the hope that innovative health and social policies from across the world could be fruitfully adopted on the island but reshaped to meet local health conditions and cultural dynamics.[57] But it also reflected the transnational medical education many physicians of this period received, the experiences they had studying and practicing medicine in places like New York, Paris, Madrid, Mexico City, and Costa Rica, where they were able to see firsthand how health and welfare services were organized in other countries.[58] Especially during the early years of the republic, when the possibilities for change seemed so much greater, these foreign experiences and foreign models provided the inspiration for a wave of innovative health programs designed to address local health concerns.[59]

Perhaps nowhere was the struggle between foreign and local, traditional and "modern" more fraught than with issues of gender. Medical nationalist physicians and nurses were careful to articulate a vision of modern Cuban womanhood that was traditional and "Cuban" while also scientifically informed. Indeed, as we will see, nursing was a central battleground over the meanings of Cuban womanhood during this period of political, social, and scientific change. But this delicate balancing act was evident in much of the writings of medical nationalists of the period and was especially so in the pages of Manuel Delfín's La Higiene. Perhaps the clearest articulation of Cuban medical nationalism, La Higiene was written for a popular audience and seems to have been widely read, with a print run reaching 10,000 copies. In the pages of La Higiene, Delfín and other medical nationalists vigorously criticized the health policies of the occupation government, advocated for stronger health reforms, and worked to popularize new medical discoveries and hygienic practices among the city's residents.[60]

More than any other medical publication of the period, the journal sought to develop a female readership, reflecting the idea common among turn-of-the-century sanitarians that women were the key to the widespread dissemination of hygienic principles within the home. La Higiene therefore regularly published practical tips on hygienic childcare practices, such as detailed instructions on how to properly bathe children, instructions on proper infant nutrition, and advice on how to pick a sanitary wet nurse.[61] In an effort to make hygienic precepts and bacteriological concepts accessible to a broad readership, almost every issue had a section called "Mañanas científicas," or "Scientific Mornings," which consisted of quippy dialogues between "the doctor" and his nosy maid "Filomena" where they discussed various topics related to health and science, delivered in a humorous and simple language.[62] For Delfín, Cuban women were expected to be modern, but only insofar as it reinforced their traditional roles. They were to incorporate the lessons of the laboratory into their daily feminine labors of keeping healthy homes and raising healthy children. Women who did not heed the new hygienic precepts, however, were therefore to blame for the deaths of their children, while those who took the wrong lessons from the island's exposure to American cultural influences—who, for example, sought a greater public role for women or engaged with political issues—were decried as rejecting the ideals of Cuban womanhood, "running in the streets like men with skirts."[63]

Turn-of-the-century medical nationalists embraced the hope that the end of colonial rule meant the beginning of a new era, a rupture with the past and the disease, death, and ignorance they associated with Spanish rule. Their speeches and writings, their new private organizations, and their medical institutions all reflected this moment of hope and possibility. They believed that as medical professionals they were uniquely positioned to take advantage of this historical moment; they would transform Cuban culture and habits, as well as build the institutions that would ensure the health of the Cuban people, serve as a testament to Cuban scientific knowledge, and prove Cuban capacity for self-rule. For the remainder of the U.S. military occupation, however, they had to work under American officials whose goals were often at odds with their own. They were locked, therefore, in a set of nesting power relations, subordinate to U.S. power but using their access to the levers of public health authority and moral suasion to transform the Cuban people, whom they saw as mired in backward colonial habits. But over time, their relationship with U.S. officials grew increasingly fraught, as cooperation increasingly turned to frustration and resentment.

## "THE SAME UNDER THE AMERICANS AS WITH THE SPANISH": COOPERATION AND CONFLICT

During the three and a half years of the first U.S. occupation, the military government relied on the labor and expertise of Cuban physicians in numerous ways. In performing home health inspections, they helped train Cubans in disease prevention while also assessing the urban living conditions that exacerbated the city's high mortality rates. When diagnosing their patients at home, in public dispensaries, or in the hospital, they were relied upon to quickly report cases of infectious disease to the Department of Health, allowing the government to track outbreaks, quarantine the sick, and maintain accurate health statistics. They managed the island's hospital system, worked closely with the Department of Public Charities, were appointed to local and national public health advisory boards, and were key figures in the new Yellow Fever Commission. In short, Cuban physicians—and increasingly, Cuban nurses—formed the backbone of the island's public health system and were indispensable for meeting the sanitary goals of the occupation government. But while Cuban physicians strongly supported the occupation government's overall focus on matters of health, they were also often its most vocal critics. Cuban doctors clashed regularly with U.S. officials over which disease threats should be prioritized and the level of attention given to issues like sanitary housing, sewer construction, and health education. While Americans remained fixated on yellow fever, a disease that primarily affected Americans and other foreigners, Cuban physicians demanded the occupation government address the health problems that most affected the native-born.

In their publications and public meetings, Cuban scientists and physicians expressed their growing dismay with the pace and priorities of the military government's health work. Vicente de la Guardia lambasted the American sanitary campaign for focusing on "palliative measures" such as street cleaning and home inspections while neglecting essential infrastructural reforms like modernizing the city's decrepit sewer system and ensuring urban residents had access to clean water.[64] Others echoed this call for greater attention to urban health infrastructure, expressing frustration that despite the clean streets, "the city continues to be as infected as before."[65] Part of the problem, according to a debate that broke out at the Cuban Academy of Science, was that American officials were not enforcing basic sanitary ordinances. While the Department of Health plastered the city with notices prohibiting spitting in public establishments like restaurants, streetcars, and government buildings, these measures were roundly ignored by urban residents and were rarely, if ever, enforced. Despite laws meant to protect the health of urban residents, Rafael Montalvo told his fellow academicians, "nothing practical or true can be accomplished if the Authorities do not know how to enforce their health regulations."[66]

Over the course of the occupation, there was a growing disconnect between the priorities of U.S. officials and those of Cuban doctors and scientists. Initial enthusiasm slowly turned to frustration and even anger as Cubans felt their expertise ignored or disparaged and their criticisms met with silence or even punishment. In many ways, Manuel Delfín's shifting relationship with the occupation government on health matters mirrored that of other reformers. Delfín, who was among the scores of physicians who volunteered to inspect the homes and factories of the city early in 1899, was initially very pleased by the effects of American health policies. He wrote to American officials congratulating them for the "better sanitary condition of the City," which, he added, in his slightly awkward English, "demonstrates a progress for the good of all."[67] Over the following year, however, Delfín's initial enthusiasm waned, as American officials ignored the counsel of Cuban doctors and remained frustratingly fixated on yellow fever alone. In 1899, a commission of Cuban doctors and veterinarians was sent to inspect all of the city's stables to investigate their conditions and make recommendations for government regulations that could reduce the spread of glanders in Havana.[68] The commission found them in filthy condition, with many obvious cases of glanderous horses, along with many suspected cases. According to Manuel Delfín, however, the commission's proposals were never carried out, and "glanders continues on its path, the same under the Americans as with the Spanish."[69]

Conflicts also emerged over military officials' treatment of Cuban doctors and critics of U.S. health work. In 1900, with yellow fever coming back after the seeming success of initial sanitary policy, military health authorities asked the newly organized Yellow Fever Commission to verify all yellow fever diagnoses.[70] While this was based on the sound idea that health officials needed the most accurate health statistics in order to assess the impact of their sanitary efforts, this apparent lack of faith in the diagnostic capabilities of Cuban physicians annoyed many. As Vicente de la Guardia asked, "Do we, the rest of the physicians of Havana, do we not understand or know how to diagnose the yellow typhus? Do we have some interest in raising the number of cases?"[71] For de la Guardia, this was but part of a broader pattern of American heavy-handedness and disrespect for Cuban doctors.[72] But American military heavy-handedness was sometimes even more punitive, as some officials sought to punish those who openly criticized occupation policy. For example, in 1900, U.S. officials in the town of Trinidad sought to arrest a newspaper publisher and suppress his newspaper *Los Cubanos en Campaña* for publishing an article critical of U.S. health policy.[73] And according to de la Guardia, a Cuban physician was fired from his post at the Aldecoa Hospital after his article criticizing American health policy published in *Progreso Médico* was translated and reprinted in the *New York Sun*.[74] While this doesn't seem to have been official policy, it highlights the tensions that arose between military officials seeking to impose hygienic order on the island and the Cubans who felt their interests were being trampled by occupation officials.

But by far the greatest source of conflict between Cuban physicians and American officials was over which diseases to prioritize. The central focus of American health policy was always eliminating the threat that yellow fever posed to Americans on the island and to southern U.S. ports. It was, as Luis de Abrisqueta put it, "the pimple on the tip of the nose of the North American continent," the singular obsession of a scared people.[75] Of course, yellow fever was certainly an important cause of death in Havana, but those afflicted were overwhelmingly the foreign-born.[76] As Cubans increasingly pointed out, diseases like tuberculosis, enteritis, malaria, and typhoid were far more dangerous to native-born Cubans, but they received very little of the military government's attention.[77] Cuban physicians and scientists regularly pushed the occupation government to make tuberculosis a priority, to redouble health education, fund the construction of sanatoriums, and address the crisis of poor urban housing conditions that made the disease the scourge of the urban poor. But these calls largely went unheeded. For Manuel Delfín, this dynamic spoke volumes, laying bare the colonial pretensions that privileged the lives of Americans and foreigners on Cuban soil over the lives of the Cuban people. "It is true," he wrote, "that the intervention government is only concerned with yellow fever, as if Cuba would always be the exclusive patrimony on the unclimatized: neither the tuberculosis that destroys our youth nor the glanders which humiliates us in the eyes of the civilized nations enter into the calculations of our non-Cuban governors."[78]

## TOO EASY A JOB: YELLOW FEVER AND THE IMPOSITION OF IMPERIAL SANITARY OVERSIGHT

By the summer of 1900, the occupation government's yellow fever campaign was floundering amid a new outbreak, demonstrating the failure of a purely sanitary response to the disease. As the *Washington Post* chided, health officials had "made the mistake of assuming that yellow fever can be suppressed by means of brooms and dustpans," but sanitation efforts alone had no effect on the disease.[79] Given the spike in infections, military health officials began exploring different theories of yellow fever transmission, and with the British scientists Patrick Manson and Ronald Ross having recently published their research proving the transmission of malaria through the mosquito vector, it was time to reassess Carlos J. Finlay's twenty-year-old mosquito theory. Through a series of experiments, U.S. army medical researchers Jesse Lazear and Walter Reed confirmed Finlay's theory that the only method of yellow fever transmission was that of human-to-human infection through the intermediary of the female *Stegomyia* mosquito.[80]

The confirmation of Finlay's theory transformed the military government's anti–yellow fever campaign. Armed with this new understanding of the mosquito's role in yellow fever transmission, the occupation government completely restructured the health campaign in early 1901. While earlier efforts revolved around keeping the city's streets and buildings free from filth, isolating the sick, and disinfecting their clothes and homes, going forward the campaign focused almost exclusively on destroying the eggs and larvae of the *Stegomyia* mosquito. Health Department resources were shifted away from street cleaning, with new work crews organized into "Stegomyia Brigades" that were tasked with finding and destroying mosquito breeding areas across the city.[81] All residents were ordered to mosquito-proof their cisterns, wells, water tanks, or other areas of standing water, either through mosquito netting or by applying crude coal oil to the water, which would float to the top and kill any mosquito larvae.[82] To enforce these orders, the Health Department levied fines against residents who did not comply. If inspectors found water barrels that were not oiled or mosquito-proofed, they would dump them out and smash them.[83]

The results of the yellow fever campaign were rapid and startling. Year after year, the summer months always saw the highest number of yellow fever cases. But after four cases were diagnosed in early May 1901, the rest of May and the entire month of June passed without another incidence of yellow fever in the Cuban capital. As Mariola Espinosa notes, "This was truly an accomplishment; since at least 1761 no June in Havana had ever been free of yellow fever."[84] While a few isolated cases occurred in the following months, their number was minuscule in comparison with earlier years. After early October, Gorgas would not find another case of yellow fever in Havana for the remainder of the U.S. occupation. Writing that autumn, Gorgas described his shock at the rapid success of the campaign: "I, myself, am so entirely taken aback at the result of our mosquito work, that I hardly know what to think. It can't be chance, and yet it seems too much to expect that we could have controlled yellow fever as we have this year. We seem to be able to stamp out the foci wherever established."[85] With the Cuban campaign a phenomenal success, Gorgas looked ahead to new tasks. "My ambition is soaring. What I want to tackle now is New Orleans, after she had been well infected. Havana, and the little towns about, is too easy a job."

With the success of the yellow fever campaign in the fall of 1901, and with only months left before the occupation government ceded power to the new republic, military health authorities finally began paying attention to other health concerns. By November, the military government began tackling Havana's glanders problem, putting more medical inspectors to work examining the city's stables.[86] Smallpox began receiving more government attention as well, with additional resources dedicated to vaccinating and revaccinating the population of Havana. And after years of prodding from Cuban medical reformers, the military government established a dispensary dedicated to caring for the city's poor tuberculosis patients—named the Dispensario Furbush in honor of the military surgeon who provided vital support for the project—and began the process of building a small sanatorium in the former yellow fever pavilions of Hospital No. 1. But much more was needed, so in March 1902, Juan Santos Fernández and Joaquín Jacobsen wrote to Military Governor Leonard Wood on behalf of the Academy of Science, asking the military government to put further resources into efforts to control tuberculosis. Noting the great success of the yellow fever campaign, they added that nevertheless, "this work will be incomplete" without addressing tuberculosis, which was responsible for a sixth of Cuba's annual deaths.

They continued: "This hidden plague, responsible for so many deaths, is nevertheless easy to control if the Government were to decide to make even half the monetary sacrifice so wisely used to extinguish yellow fever."[87] But that was asking too much, according to military officials. Although the new dispensary and sanatorium were important steps in addressing the city's tuberculosis crisis, the military government did not expand this work further.

With the success of the yellow fever campaign, the sanitary pacification of Havana seemed complete. But with independence looming, American officials worried about the long-term ability of Cubans to maintain acceptable sanitary standards in their major ports and thereby prevent future outbreaks that could pose a threat to the United States. As Military Governor Leonard Wood admitted, "The purpose of the war was not only to assist the Cubans, but, in a general sense, to abate a nuisance. It is probable that if we leave the island . . . we shall soon find Havana and all other large cities in practically the same conditions as during the Spanish War and a menace to our Southern seaports."[88] While Wood supported Cuban scientists and other elite professionals, he was deeply distrustful of most Cuban politicians, as well as the Cuban electorate as a whole, and insisted that some mechanism be put in place requiring Cubans to control infectious disease in their ports.[89] "This question of control of sanitation in Cuban ports is, in my opinion, of vital importance to the United States," he declared.[90]

The answer was the Platt Amendment, a series of articles that the United States required Cuban legislators to append to the constitution as a precondition for the U.S. withdrawal from the island. The Platt Amendment would structure U.S.-Cuba relations for decades, severely limiting Cuban sovereignty by laying out specific conditions under which the United States could unilaterally intervene in the internal political affairs of the republic. While an early draft of the proposed amendment made no mention of public health, in response to Wood's concerns, a new fifth article was added, holding the Cuban government responsible "for the sanitation of the cities of the island, to the end that a recurrence of epidemic and infectious diseases may be prevented, thereby assuring protection to the people and commerce of Cuba, as well as to the commerce of the southern ports of the United States and the people residing therein."[91] In December 1901, after fierce debates in Congress, Cuban legislators approved the amendment. As Cuban health officials understood, infectious disease now threatened not only the lives of Cubans but the very independence of the republic.

While the Platt Amendment infuriated many Cubans, some medical nationalists were particularly incensed with the fifth article. Having worked closely with the intervention government on health matters, having demonstrated their administrative and scientific capabilities, and having proven their zeal for the sanitary reform, they found the Platt's sanitary scrutiny galling. As Matías Duque later proclaimed, Cubans were committed to public health work "not in obedience to the provisions of Article V of the Platt Amendment attached to our Constitution, but because we labor for dignity, patriotism and for our welfare, because we do not ignore what public health signifies to a people. To affirm that we are obliged to maintain a good sanitary condition because the United States of America so demands, is to lay an anathema on our nation, which degrades and dishonors us."[92] Indeed, Manuel Delfín fumed, there "was absolutely no health measure enacted during the Intervention that was not asked for a thousand times" by Cuban physicians, both under colonial rule and during the U.S. occupation.[93] For Delfín the fifth article "confirms the lack of faith that our neighboring government has in our desire for sanitation: American legislators believe that the Cuban people will stumble when we are without the wise direction that we have had during the years of the Intervention. They believe that our neglect will be certain because Latin blood runs through our veins; and because of this, they put this clause in the Platt law, sure that in this way we will fall straight into their hands."[94] Delfín was not mistaken, for in the coming years Cubans would have to respond to a steady stream of often racialized accusations of Cuban sanitary "backsliding" from American newspapers, medical journals, and politicians.[95]

The Cuban journalist Julio César Gandarilla would later write, "Spain and the United States have two distinct systems of governing and administering: the first master turns the colony into a latrine; and the second, into a lustrous warehouse, into a factory and a tin workshop, with plenty of Sanitation. One does not use bathrooms; the other is more hygienic and endeavors to sanitize the colony for his recreation."[96] While Gandarilla was certainly correct in pointing to the colonial interests underlying the occupation government's public health work, this discourse obscures as much as it reveals. As we have seen, Cuban physicians did not engage with and help shape the military government's health campaign to further American interests but to transform Cuban society. Cuban medical nationalism emerged during the U.S. occupation as a complex response to the starvation, disease, and death of the final years of colonial rule; the hopes Cuban physicians had in medical science to reshape Cuban society; and the sanitary campaigns and institution building of the U.S. occupation. It was, at its heart, a cultural revolution meant to reshape Cuban ideas and habits, transform the Cuban state, and build lasting health institutions.

But only by turning to these institutions can we see how the Cuban people responded to and engaged with this project during the transition from colony to republic. The hospital was perhaps the central site of this institutional and cultural struggle over the meanings of modern medicine for Cuban society, and the new career of professional nursing was at the heart of these debates. At stake were questions posed across the world at this moment, such as who was the hospital for and was it an appropriate space for "respectable" women to work? However, with the transformation of the hospital and the establishment of professional nursing occurring during the U.S. occupation and the transition from colony to republic, these issues became fraught with even greater significance. Was nursing a foreign imposition ill-suited to Cuban culture and needs? Did contact between these young women and a multiracial body of patients represent a threat to Cuban morals and racial hierarchy? Far from being simply a medical issue, the development of professional nursing in early-twentieth-century Cuba provides a fascinating perspective on how gender, race, class, and science were implicated in the transition from colony to republic.

## A CIVILIZING ELEMENT IN CUBAN SOCIETY: GENDER, PROFESSIONAL NURSING, AND THE DECOLONIZATION OF THE HOSPITAL

On the evening of November 8, 1902, Trinidad Cantero joined six other young women in the lecture hall of the recently inaugurated General Wood Laboratory in Havana to celebrate their graduation from Cuba's new national Schools of Nursing. As evidenced by the attendance of some of the country's leading political figures, scientists, and members of elite society, this was no ordinary graduation. Not only were these seven women the first Cubans to receive the title of professional nurse: they were the first women from anywhere in Latin America, Spain, France, and Italy to have earned that title.[97] Resplendent in their crisp blue uniforms and beaming with pride, they stepped forward one by one as the Cuban secretary of state Diego Tamayo called their names to receive their diploma and a pin from President Estrada Palma.[98] For those in attendance, the event was a turning point for Cuban women and for the history of Cuban medicine. The graduation of these first seven Cuban nurses represented, in the words of Carlos E. Finlay, "a new stage along the path to professional and scientific advancement, a new stage along the path of social progress."[99] It was, according to La Lucha, a "new triumph" for the young republic, representing "the national pride." They would be, it seemed, the face of modern scientific Cuban femininity, on the front lines of the transformation of the hospital, the fulfillment of Cuba's medical nationalist promise.

Despite this broad show of support, however, the emergence of professional nursing in Cuba was fraught with controversy. As Trinidad Cantero had recently asserted, "The truth is that the woman that dedicates herself to the profession of Nurse has to possess a special character."[100] Barely out of their teens, Cantero and her fellow nurses had already overcome a great deal. They were all from humble backgrounds, and most had suffered greatly during the war and reconcentration. Then came three exhausting years of difficult study and long hours at Mercedes Hospital training under the strict supervision of Mary Agnes O'Donnell, a veteran nurse from New York City. But in some ways, their real difficulties would only now begin. They would have to confront a host of obstacles, from the opposition of patients to the indifference or outright hostility of much of Cuban society, who believed professional nursing to represent an antireligious institution and an immoral occupation unfit for Cuban women. As we have seen, turn-of-the-century Cuba was a time of rapid cultural, political, and scientific change. But nowhere was the struggle between medical modernity and entrenched social values more fraught than with the advent of professional nursing. Although supported at the highest levels of the occupation and republican governments, professional nursing seemed to many a violation of gendered norms, a foreign imposition ill-suited to Cuban values, and a rejection of religious tradition. In short, it became a lightning rod, pitting medical nationalist nurses and their physician allies against much of the island's social and religious elite.

Beyond the meanings ascribed to secular nursing, the emergence and growth of the profession provided young women with the means to financially support themselves and their families while also being central figures in Cuba's turn-of-the-century medical revolution. Perhaps more than any other group, professional nurses were the on-the-ground figures responsible for the modernization of the Cuban hospital system and the transformation of popular hygienic habits. They administered anesthesia and assisted in surgeries, and they took meticulous care of patients in their wards, ensuring that medications were taken at the correct time and wounds were properly cleaned and dressed and patients were fed nutritious food. And they were on the front line of teaching their patients and their families—and therefore Cuban society as a whole—the practical basics of bacteriology, showing them how to prevent infection and support healing through the new rituals of cleanliness and germ avoidance. The development of professional nursing in Cuba therefore represented more than the opening of a new occupation for Cuban women; it was a central site of struggle over the gendered meanings of medical modernity, the changing nature of the hospital, and the role of scientific knowledge during Cuba's transition from colony to republic.

The founding of the first Cuban nursing schools in 1899 reflected the idea—shared by both Cuban physicians and American officials—that the island's crumbling hospital system needed radical transformation and that trained nurses would be an indispensable part of this process. Cuban hospitals had suffered greatly during the final War of Independence and were pushed to the point of collapse by the reconcentration and U.S. blockade in the spring of 1898. With the partial exception of Havana's private mutual aid clinics for Spanish immigrants, which fared better than most, the city's hospitals were prostrate at the end of the war: overcrowded, lacking medicine, and often without the proper facilities for disinfecting surgical equipment and bedding. In a 1901 report, Lucy Quintard, one of the American nurses employed by the Department of Public Charities to inspect Cuban hospitals, was blunt in her assessment of the "appalling condition" of Cuban hospitals at the onset of the occupation, writing that they "were dens of immorality and uncleanliness in every form" that did as much to spread disease as they did to cure it.[101] But while exacerbated by the war, substandard conditions predated the final War of Independence, for Cuban hospitals had long had a reputation of being "only places to die in," providing little more than "shelter, food, and a canvas-bottom cot, where [patients] lay in their rags and received the doctor's visit."[102] For many Cubans, they were an option of last resort. Emiliano Nuñez described the "true horror that the Cuban people felt when going to the hospitals," noting that Cubans would generally avoid them at all costs, only seeking admission after exhausting all other options and usually "when the illness had reached such proportions that medical assistance would turn out to be useless."[103]

Improving their physical condition was relatively easy. Military officials ordered hospitals cleaned, painted, and reorganized. New disinfection facilities were installed, and they were stocked with new surgical equipment and medical supplies donated by American hospitals. But improving hospital administration and patient care would prove more complicated, for while physicians were, on the whole, highly trained and competent, all of the hospital's nursing was done by untrained *enfermeros* and Sisters of Charity. The work of cleaning patients and attending to their basic physical needs was delegated to *enfermeros*, who held the lowest position in the hospital hierarchy and were decried as "slovenly," "vulgar" men, "the lowest type of humanity."[104] But if the "very name of *enfermero* . . . was a term of degradation," in contrast Cubans were loath to speak ill of the Sisters of Charity, who were universally praised for their "abnegation, Christian charity, and valor" and for the "enormous benefits [they] offered to a suffering humanity."[105]

Yet these benefits were largely spiritual, not medical. Cuban physicians, especially surgeons and others who worked primarily within the hospital system, found Sisters of Charity to be wholly inadequate to the needs of the modern hospital. With their religious order being "resistant to all advances and progress," they necessarily lacked "the most elemental understandings of medical science" and put "their religious practices . . . before the scientific needs of the patient."[106] And indeed, with their religious vows preventing them from seeing their patients' naked bodies, they refused to perform many of the tasks professional nursing required, such as bathing their patients and cleaning and dressing their wounds.[107] For Enrique Nuñez, this "absolute lack of subaltern staff accustomed to the antiseptic methods of contemporary surgery" had devastating effects on patient care in Cuban hospitals, creating the conditions for an "era of surgical infections that devastated hospital wards from one side to the other."[108]

These conditions surely fed into the negative assessment many Cubans had of the hospital, but elite antipathy to the institution also reflected long-standing cultural norms that justified class hierarchy through rigid social separation. In much of Europe, Latin America, and the United States, the late-nineteenth-century revolution in antiseptic and aseptic surgical techniques that dramatically reduced hospital infection dovetailed with and fed a growing acceptance of hospitals as medical treatment centers among the middle and elite classes.[109] But in Cuba this process was interrupted by the upheavals of war. Cuban hospitals continued to be largely places for the poor and the chronically sick, especially single male immigrants without families to help care for them. They were avoided at all costs by the privileged, who could pay for a visit from their family physician and preferred to receive care at home or in a private medical clinic. During the occupation, this elite aversion to the hospital precipitated conflicts with military authorities when individuals with infectious diseases were ordered to be isolated in local hospitals. One such clash occurred in the town of Trinidad in 1900, after the editor of a local newspaper, *Los Cubanos en Campaña*, wrote a scathing critique of the military authorities for forcing "honorable and order abiding citizens of this town" to enter the hospital during a smallpox outbreak. The gendered authority of the father over the family was central to his argument. Addressing his readers as fellow "fathers of families," he called on the local authorities not to allow health officials to force families, especially "pubescent and modest young ladies," into the heterogeneous social space of the hospital. For this newspaper editor, this amounted to "an assault to their humanity" and a dangerous usurpation of patriarchal authority.[110]

This picture of hospitals as dangerous, immoral, and largely male spaces that rather than curing diseases were responsible for their spread is precisely what Cuban physicians and American health officials hoped to change with the introduction of professional nursing to the island. The first attempt to establish schools of nursing began in early 1899, when the noted surgeon Raimundo Menocal organized a nursing school with twenty-two students. During the final War of Independence, Menocal, like so many other pro-independence physicians, went into exile in New York, where he raised funds for the revolutionary struggle and worked as a practicing surgeon. During his time in exile he experienced the benefits of working alongside trained nurses, and shortly after returning to the island, he organized a small school of nursing attached to the Sanatorio Habana.[111] The sanatorium, along with its fledgling nursing school, closed just months later; but the idea was taken up by the military government, and in the summer of 1899 a new, more permanent school was established at the Hospital Mercedes. This school, like the others that would be formed in its wake, was run by American nurse superintendents—dubbed the "Americanas" by their Cuban students—who were given significant authority "to organize the school for Cuban nurses, equip the hospitals, modernize the system, and make necessary changes in the domestic departments" of Cuban hospitals. For Mary Eugénie Hibbard, an American nurse whose career in Cuba would span decades, the break from colonial rule and the broad mandate to transform Cuban hospitals and create from scratch the new institution of professional nursing on the island meant that nursing schools "could work unhampered by dictate or tradition."[112] But tradition did, in fact, provide a significant obstacle to the success of the nursing program.

The new nursing schools were of paramount importance to both medical nationalist physicians and American officials. But the schools received unexpectedly virulent opposition from elites, the conservative press, the church, and prospective students' own families, all of which hampered their ability to recruit young women. By the summer of 1901, eight nursing schools had been authorized by the military government, attached to hospitals in all of the provincial capitals. But of these, complained J. R. Kean, "only two have obtained the desired number of pupils, and four are partial or total failures on account of the difficulty in procuring pupils." For Kean, the source of this failure was the "systematic opposition on the part of priests of the Roman Catholic church" who "lose no opportunity of speaking ill of trained nurses as a class, and of prejudicing the women and young girls of their congregations against professional nursing." Indeed, in a country whose elite was deeply Catholic, the wholesale replacement of revered Sisters of Charity with secular women gave the schools the reputation of being "antireligious institutions."[113] According to Mary O'Donnell, the superintendent of the nursing school at Mercedes Hospital, this "opposition, sometimes active, sometimes passive, came from all parts" and also reflected deep-set elite beliefs about the impropriety of young women working outside the home. With such opposition from family members and the church, it is no surprise that many of the early students in the training programs were young women who had been orphaned during the War of Independence and the reconcentration.[114]

Central to elite and familial opposition was how they interpreted the cross-class, cross-gender physical contact between nurse and patient that professional nursing required. For both nurses and their supporters, the daily physical labor of bathing patients, cleansing wounds, and changing bedpans could be "unpleasant" or even "repugnant."[115] This was, of course, precisely the kind of gendered care work that was regularly expected of women when family members fell ill, but this level of intimate physical contact with nonfamily members, especially men, was seen by elites as inherently dishonorable.[116] As Mary O'Donnell explained, many Cubans believed that it was impossible for women to "carry out the specific duties of the nurse without losing the propriety and respect of those with whom they had contact . . . [and] this being the general opinion, naturally prevented many young women who would have been good nurses from entering the training schools."[117] Racism was at the heart of this dynamic. Carlos E. Finlay admitted that "opposition from family and friends to their entry into this profession" was due, in part, "to racial prejudice."[118] As American nurse and hospital inspector Lucy Quintard explained, while all of the schools initially found it difficult to recruit students, the school in the eastern city of Santiago de Cuba was "one of the most difficult to establish, owing to the fact that the population of Santiago de Cuba is fully two-thirds negro."[119] With nursing students generally drawn from "honorable" nonblack families, the

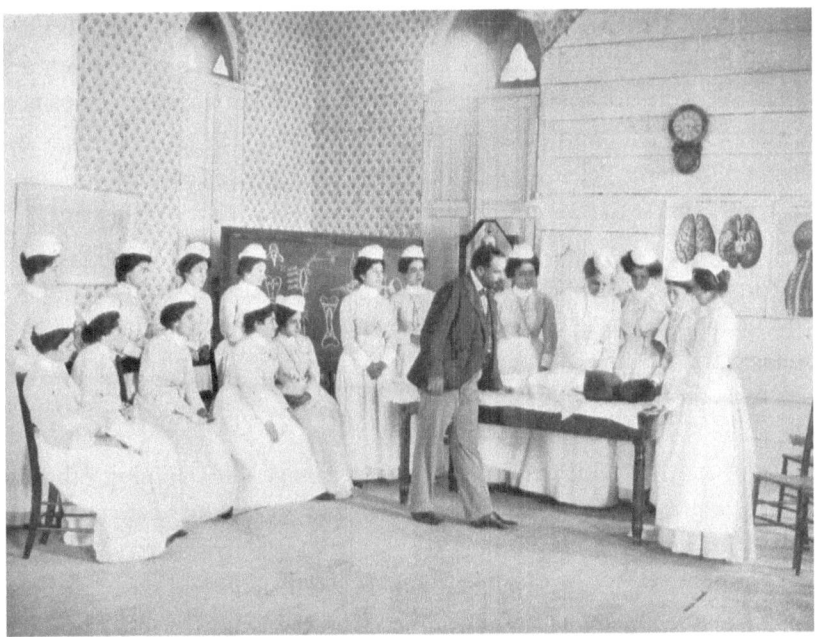

Figure 2.2 Nursing students at Municipal Hospital No. 1. (Biblioteca Nacional de Cuba José Martí, Fotos Cuba, Sala Cubana, album 146)

cross-racial, cross-gender physical contact that would be required especially of nurses in Santiago created particular recruitment difficulties. In light of this "race difficulty," Quintard added, officials had to resort to financial "inducements" to get students to enter the schools.[120]

American and Cuban officials did what they could to change public opinion, but Cuban nurses were perhaps the strongest advocates for their profession. Speaking at the 1902 National Conference of Beneficencia and Corrections, nurses Verena Jover and Trinidad Cantero directly confronted antinursing sentiment. Confronting accusations of immorality and lack of femininity, Jover asserted that nursing was actually a decent and honorable way to earn her subsistence in an independent manner and in harmony with her sex.[121] Cantero addressed the "frequently heard" belief that "the nursing profession is incompatible with religious principles." But she flipped this idea on its head, arguing that "on the contrary, they could not be more intimately united," for nursing itself represented the ideals of mercy and charity at the heart of Catholic social practice.[122] Jover echoed this idea, emphasizing that nursing required sacrifice, humanitarianism, and "the greatest abnegation." It is no coincidence that Cuban nurses and their allies defended their work using precisely the language others used to describe the Sisters of Charity: abnegation, tact, duty, love, and charity. But this new sisterhood was secular, scientific, and dedicated not to spiritual salvation but to saving lives. For nurses and their allies, professional nursing was not dishonorable, a foreign model ill-suited for Cuban women, but rather the height of modern, scientific Cuban womanhood. It allowed Cuban women to "contribute, with their own effort and intelligence, to the prosperity and good fortune . . . of the country."[123] Nurses spoke of the nationalist desire to help "fulfill the aspirations of our beloved Nation," asserted the patriotic duty of nursing, linked their work to the revolutionary anticolonial struggle, and declared the first Cuban nurse to be "she who treated the first wounded soldier in the camp of the Revolution."[124]

BUT WHILE NURSES and their allies sought to change public opinion, officials moved to prevent scandal. In 1901, J. R. Kean, desperate to stem church opposition, asked for help from the military government, requesting "that such steps be taken as may put a stop to this systematic opposition" to professional nursing, an institution "upon which the well-being of the sick in Cuba so largely depends."[125] Officials struggled to gain the support of elite Cubans but worked to ensure that they avoid additional stigma, by preventing, for example, registered prostitutes from being admitted to hospitals with nursing schools and through the strict moral regulation of nursing students.[126] Even as the schools struggled to find students, prospective candidates were forced to undergo strict background checks, providing references attesting to their moral character. During their three years of study, "their conduct is carefully observed . . . to filter out all students whose morals are not irreproachable."[127] As Finlay argued, it was vitally important to "not in any way tolerate the smallest transgression," as this would be "a most powerful weapon in the hands of the enemies of the institution" of professional nursing.[128] Soon, however, one important enemy of the institution raised a very public alarm.

In 1904 the conservative *Diario de la Marina* published a pair of articles railing against secular nursing in Cuba, making clear what had been a regular criticism of Cuban nursing: that it was an immoral foreign implantation ill-suited to Cuban culture and temperament. For the Havana daily, recent "scandalous events" at the hospital in the city of Cienfuegos were proof of the mistake American and Cuban officials had made in adopting the institution of secular nursing, as they were but "a natural consequence, fatal in a way, of the substitution of Hermanas de la Caridad with lay nurses in the hospitals."[129] For the editors of *Diario de la Marina*, no amount of moral supervision would suffice, for only religious sisters, with their "heroic virtues," could surmount the temptation and degradation of the hospital ward. Those who sought out this career "implanted in Cuba" by the United States were inherently morally suspect, for the "intellectually and morally well-educated woman . . . has other careers available, and they as well as their families prefer these to that of nurse."[130] It was, of course, precisely this continued stigma against professional nursing that prevented more young women from choosing the career early in the republic. But this was the bind nurses faced. By definition, those forced by economic circumstances to seek employment outside the home were not considered the most "honorable" members of society.

According to Trinidad Cantero, many Cubans continued to believe, like the *Diario de la Marina*, that "only people of low class dedicate themselves to this profession," people who "are incapable of representing in society the role that has been entrusted to them." Speaking at the Third National Conference of Beneficencia and Corrections, she expressed a frustration surely shared by fellow Cuban nurses: "The truth is that the public should already be persuaded about what our profession is, of the benefits that result for a humanity that suffers and recognize also the abnegation and spontaneous sacrifices that we impose upon ourselves . . . in order to dedicate all of our care, all our eagerness to comfort the poor soul who suffers."[131] But culture changes slowly, and it would be the greater part of a decade before nursing began to achieve widespread support.

As they struggled for acceptance, they confronted these restrictive notions of femininity and articulated their own brand of medical nationalism that allowed them to redefine the boundaries of honorable womanhood. Nurses argued for acceptance on the basis of the results of their work, and in so doing, claimed a new understanding of honorable womanhood, based not on their families' class position but on the social value of nurses' medical labor. While long-standing colonial class discourse held that women's paid labor was inherently dishonorable, Cuban nurses turned this formulation on its head, arguing that it was precisely their labor—useful, scientific, and beneficial to humanity—that proved their worth. For Edelmira Fernández, "our professional existence should not rest solely on elevated philanthropic sentiments in favor of the weak sex" but, rather, "on the benefits we can bring to the sick."[132] For this first generation of Cuban nurses, their own actions and perseverance showed professional nursing to be both "honorable and worthy of approbation," in the words of Trinidad Cantero, representing not only a means to gain subsistence but also duty to nation and "a suffering humanity."[133] Fernández was confident that as Cubans came to experience the benefits of professional nursing—as did Cuban physicians—"the rich patient as well as the poor will demand our service."[134] And indeed, over time and through both their speeches and their writings, but especially in their everyday ministrations—tending to the sick, assisting in surgeries, and counseling patients and their families in how to avoid infection—nurses slowly changed public opinion, eroding elite opposition and winning the support of patients, physicians, the clergy, and the press.

For medical nationalists like Edelmira Fernández, Trinidad Cantero, and Verena Jover, the growing acceptance of nursing was just one aspect of the medical cultural revolution that was reshaping Cuban society during the transition from colony to republic. "The ideas and habits brought by modern civilization," Fernández asserted, were beginning to eclipse old ideas about Cuban women that, "like a fruit of colonial life," held that women without the "strong arm of the father to protect his family" were destined for "either the washing trough or the sewing machine" or to selling "their flesh for a crust of bread."[135] For Fernández, the "common success" of Cuban nurses was "an object lesson in just how capable" Cuban women were. In the coming years, as more women graduated and the corps of Cuban nurses grew, these women increasingly became the backbone of the Cuban health system. With the creation of the Ministry of Health's Section on Tuberculosis Nursing, they entered the homes of the city's poor and taught families how to best care for the sick, while avoiding further infection. They taught mothers to care hygienically for their children, to feed them nutritious foods appropriate to their age. They were increasingly hired by private clinics and Spanish-run hospitals and soon became an indispensable part of the private medical system, assisting in surgeries, caring for patients, and educating the sick. As they reflected on their work and experiences, however, these women became among the most vocal advocates for the expansion of health services to the poor and for government policies that might address the structural causes that led to the disproportionate mortality of those on the margins of Cuban society.

## PATRONAGE, POLITICS, AND THE WORLD'S FIRST MINISTRY OF HEALTH

On May 20, 1902, as the U.S. military occupation gave way to the new Republic of Cuba, Cuban officials assumed—for the first time—full responsibility over the country's health landscape. The challenges they faced were daunting, but with key medical nationalist figures now at the helm of the Department of Public Charities and the new Junta Superior de Sanidad, or Superior Board of Health, they hoped to be able to build on the public health successes of the occupation while directing these new national institutions toward health concerns that most directly affected the Cuban people. Continuing their educational mission, health officials published books and pamphlets and distributed leaflets to spread scientific and medical knowledge and train the new citizens to control the spread of diseases like tuberculosis, scarlet fever, diphtheria, and yellow fever.[136] The main thrust of their reforms, however, was institutional. While the Department of Public Charities and its growing corps of Cuban nurses helped transform the nation's hospitals, the Superior Board of Health was tasked with coordinating the island's entire public health system, ensuring that local health officials performed inspections, enforced health regulations, and carried out the sanitary work that would prevent future outbreaks of infectious disease. This important work was stymied, however, by a legal landscape that granted extensive autonomy to cities and towns and left local governments with the responsibility to fund and carry out public health work. To the growing dismay of medical nationalists in Havana, municipal autonomy led to chronic underfunding and facilitated the subordination of public health to local political influence. These conditions led to the breakdown of local public health services, setting the stage for new disease outbreaks, and, as we'll see, creating precisely the conditions that led to the adoption of the world's first Ministry of Health.

In the early years of the republic, national health officials struggled to exert control over the island's decentralized public health landscape, but patronage politics and the limitations of municipal finances proved to be insurmountable barriers. Local health officials were appointed by mayors or municipal councils, a fact not forgotten by health inspectors tasked with the sometimes delicate work of issuing fines for noncompliance with sanitary regulations. Charles Magoon astutely described this dynamic in 1907, noting that local health officials sometimes "were unable to enforce the sanitary requirements because an attempt at enforcement usually produced a rebuke, and not infrequently removal from office. The sanitary inspectors and other officials were subject to the Municipal authorities and very soon learned the personal advantages of moving along the line of least resistance."[137] Further, on the rare occasions when local health officials had employees assigned to them as assistants, the power to hire or fire them was the purview of local politicians alone. Reluctant to issue sanitary fines, powerless to hire competent technical staff, and unwilling to criticize the politicians upon whose favor they relied for continued employment, local health officials were left without the independence of action their work required. In the words of the Havana's director of public health José Antonio López del Valle, political influences "shackled" local health officials "in bonds as pernicious as powerful, and swamped all their energies, and in many cases broke the willpower of the best prepared and most generous minds."[138]

Conditions were not much better in the country's public hospitals. After independence, the Department of Charities lost much of its autonomy after it was placed under the Ministry of the Interior, where, over time, it was "reduced to a sort of Consulting or Advisory Board" with little authority to ensure that the island's hospitals, dispensaries, and other public medical charities were run and managed by competent technical personnel, rather than those with the best political connections. According to Juan Manuel Plá, the physician and longtime Beneficencia official, when officials at the Department of Charities resisted political pressure to appoint well-connected candidates to cushy or prestigious positions such as hospital directorships, "the consequence of this friction has been the above-mentioned curtailing of our executive powers." As Plá explained in 1906, political influence eventually "extend[ed] so far that the presidential approval is required for the appointment of even the most insignificant employee of any of the hospitals or asylums," resulting in the "most baneful influence . . . of politics into the solution of Charity problems."[139]

But if patronage politics limited the independence of health officials, a chronic lack of funds left them "tied hand and foot," completely unable to perform their duties.[140] According to existing law, municipalities were responsible for funding local health work, but, as J. R. Kean reported, "the municipalities upon which local sanitary organizations depended were as a rule in financial difficulties, and not greatly concerned with sanitary matters."[141] Health officials were paid such "shameful" and "ridiculous" salaries that they were forced to pick up better-paying work that took time away from their official duties.[142] Worse still, low salaries served as an inducement for less-scrupulous inspectors to take bribes in exchange for not reporting health violations.[143] But the ultimate effect of insufficient municipal funding, low-level corruption, and political influence over the hiring of inspectors was that important preventative work, such as mosquito control, was not performed.[144] The results of this situation became painfully clear when in late 1905 yellow fever once again appeared in Havana and quickly spread to smaller towns outside the capital, where the disease "adopted revolutionary tactics," attacking small villages and settlements along the railroad lines and proving difficult to extirpate.[145] Using what little authority it had, the Superior Board of Health ordered local health officials to confront the outbreak by enacting thorough mosquito control measures, but, as Kean noted, these orders "were met with the inevitable reply, 'No hay de que,' and for even the smallest operations against yellow fever . . . the National Government had to furnish the money and the personnel."[146] The lingering yellow fever outbreak proved a profound embarrassment to Cuban health officials, who were anxiously aware that the U.S. press was blaming it on the sanitary "indifference of natives and officials" and that U.S. State Department officials were considering invoking the Platt Amendment against Cuba if officials could not quickly get the outbreak under control.[147]

For the Cuban legislator José Angel Malberty, the yellow fever crisis of 1905–6 must have seemed especially tragic. If the outbreak was at least partly the result of insufficient public health funding, local political influencing, and a lack of coordination between national and local health officials, each of these problems could have been prevented had the Cuban Senate approved his 1903 proposal to create in Cuba a Ministry of Health. As he had argued before his fellow representatives, health officials should be afforded the highest level of independence, free from political influence, and the island's public health apparatus should function as a single coordinated body. In the words of Pedro Albarrán, public health must be guided by "scientific criteria," not political meddling, and "perfect unity of action among those charged with enforcing sanitary laws, without which the necessary results will never be achieved."[148] The proposed ministry would have granted national health officials direct authority over the island's local health offices, ostensibly eliminating the influence of party politics on hiring practices, ensuring the proper distribution of funds for preventative health work like mosquito mitigation efforts, and quickly directing emergency resources to confront new outbreaks whenever they arose. While neither Malberty nor Albarrán mentioned the Platt Amendment in their speeches in favor of the proposal, it was clearly in the minds of legislators, who saw in the proposed ministry an institution capable of safeguarding Cuban independence. As the legislator Pedro Cué admitted, the "Platt Law obligates us to dedicate profound attention to public health," and failure to do so risked "through an unpleasant intervention, the independence and sovereignty of our nation."[149]

But although the disease still popped up with frustrating regularity in the towns and villages outside Havana, it was not yellow fever that precipitated another U.S. intervention in 1906. That summer, a different crisis hit the island, as Liberals, angry at what they saw as a rigged election ensuring a second term for President Tomás Estrada Palma, staged what became known as the August Revolution. In the mounting political crisis, Estrada Palma was forced to resign in early September, and American officials invoked the Platt Amendment, landed troops in Havana, and initiated the Second Occupation of Cuba. Like its predecessor, the new Provisional Government of Cuba (1906–9) was profoundly concerned with the public health landscape of the island, and especially with yellow fever. But while Cuban medical nationalists had a sometimes contentious relationship with American officials during the prior intervention, this time their interests aligned, and U.S. officials became vocal advocates for the nationalization of public health and the establishment of the Ministry of Health. As Jefferson Randolph Kean, who returned to Cuba as advisor to the Sanitary Department, put it, "A sanitary service to be able to act with promptness, vigor, and effectiveness in the face of epidemics and to be able to withstand when necessary popular opposition, must have autonomy and large discretionary powers."[150] He therefore persuaded provisional governor Charles Magoon to sign Decree 894, nationalizing the administration of public health in Cuba and putting all municipal health work under the direct control of the central government, and then pushed to make these changes permanent by adopting Malberty's proposal for a Ministry of Health.[151]

On January 19, 1909, the leaders of new Secretaría de Sanidad y Beneficencia were sworn in. For Cuban medical nationalists, this was a crowning achievement. With the world's first ministry of health now established and staffed by the island's leading medical nationalist scientists and health officials, they believed they would finally have the resources and authority to fulfill their dream of a healthy and modern republic that would be the envy of its neighbors. Together with the confirmation of Finlay's theory of yellow fever transmission, this moment seemed to cement Cuba's place at the forefront of global medicine.[152] For the new secretary of health Matías Duque, it "signified a great step forward in the progress of public health" for the entire world."[153] Indeed, the creation of the Ministry of Health was a world-historical event of profound significance; it was, as J. R. Kean proclaimed, "an important step forward in the history of State medicine" throughout the world and "an epoch-making incident in the advance of the Science of Sanitation." As a student of international public health legislation, Kean was correct in noting that by the beginning of the twentieth century, the "trend of public opinion in all progressive countries" was "constantly increasing importance of the agencies which have to deal with Public Health, and the tendency is to enlarge the powers and jurisdiction of the National Sanitary authorities which alone can deal satisfactorily with such great questions as water pollution, pure food, control of epidemic diseases, vital statistics, etc." But Cuba was far ahead of the curve in this growing global trend toward the centralization of public health work and would therefore "exercise a marked influence on future legislation of this character in the Spanish American Republics and perhaps also in the United States."[154] Indeed, in the coming years more and more countries would follow Cuba's lead and create national-level ministries to coordinate and oversee public health work.

For Duque and many other medical nationalists, the ministry was a tremendous achievement, heralding a bright future. But for others, this hopefulness was tempered by a lingering pessimism about Cuban politics or the capacities of the Cuban people to meet these expectations. To the young intellectual Emilio Teuma, in light of the Republic's endemic corruption and political subordination to the United States, the ministry was perhaps "the only thing, really, that [Cuba] can offer as an example to the world."[155] For the editors of the new medical nationalist journal *Vida Nueva*, however, the meaning of this moment was yet to be written. "If success crowns this effort," they wrote, "then it will be the greatest mark of glory of the Republic." But, they added, "if this effort . . . sinks into failure, then we will recoil into the dark shadows where dwell those who are incapable of entering that luminous atmosphere that encircles the great membership of civilized nations."[156] This mix of hopeful idealism about the future and pessimism about the capabilities of the Cuban people was at the heart of medical nationalist discourse and would continue to mark struggles over how to best address the health conditions of the Cuban people. To what degree was disease the result of popular ignorance and backwardness or the result of structural poverty and racial inequality? What was the responsibility of individuals, elites, and the state? Over the coming decades, each of these questions would come to trouble health officials, medical workers, politicians, and ever-broader swaths of the urban population, as they confronted disease and faced the limits of medical nationalist hopes against the hard realities of the postcolonial economy and U.S. empire.

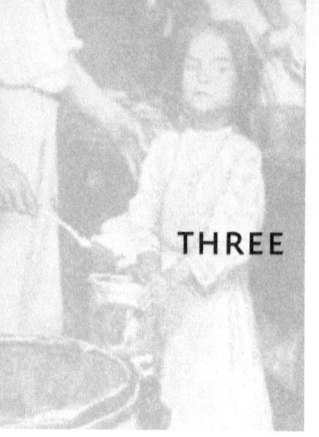

# THREE   Salus Populi Suprema Lex
## Medical Modernity, Neocolonialism, and the 1914 Bubonic Plague Outbreak

### LOVE IN THE TIME OF THE BUBONIC PLAGUE

Early Sunday evening on April 26, 1914, Gumersindo Pérez, a thirty-eight-year-old Spanish immigrant, met his girlfriend Asunción Flores and their teenage son, Emilio, in central Havana. While Emilio stayed behind at a shop on Reina Avenue, Gumersindo took Asunción on a quiet sunset stroll. From the old Campo de Marte park near the city center, the couple walked to the Malecón, Havana's great oceanfront promenade, and then along the tree-lined Paseo del Prado. They had been together for fifteen years, and Asunción always thought they would marry. But Gumersindo was a low-level worker at a food warehouse, and she worked as a maid for a physician on nearby Neptuno Street. And whether from exhaustion or inertia, they never got around to it.

The couple made their way back to the shop and their waiting son, and then the trio took a streetcar ride back to Asunción's home in the western neighborhood of Vedado. Gumersindo stayed a while, visiting with his son and girlfriend. At some point during their conversations, Gumersindo complained of pain in his legs and a lack of feeling in his hands. A member of the Centro Asturiano, the mutual aid organization for immigrants of the Asturias region of northern Spain, Gumersindo had free access to the Covadonga Hospital. But he hated going to hospitals, often saying they were where one got worse, not better. Around 11:00 P.M., Gumersindo headed back to his "home," the warehouse where he worked and slept on the corner of Obispo and Baratillo streets, near the docks of Old Havana. Asunción and Emilio would never see him again.[1]

While many details of the following two days would be under dispute, what is clear is that Gumersindo Pérez worked on Monday, at the warehouse owned by three Spanish immigrant merchants. That day he did his usual work, running deliveries from various warehouses and docks throughout the cobblestoned streets of the commercial district. He delivered ten sacks of dried garbanzo beans to one client, brought sacks of rice back to his workplace, and transported crates of dried codfish to the train station. His friends found him to be his typical jovial self, horsing around with coworkers during their group lunch break that afternoon. But that evening Pérez came down with a high fever, violent chills, a headache, and vomiting.[2] He was unable to work the following day, and when his condition dramatically worsened on Wednesday morning, his coworkers brought him to the Covadonga Hospital. By the time they arrived, Pérez was unable to walk; his friends carried him into the clinic by his shoulders. During his medical examination, the physician on call, Dr. Luis Barroso, noted a painful swelling the size of a hazelnut in the right gland in Pérez's groin. Pérez was in a stupor, running a fever of 101 degrees, and vomited repeatedly during the examination. Recognizing the symptoms of the bubonic plague, Dr. Barroso immediately transferred the patient to an observation ward and contacted the Health Department.

Within three hours, Dr. Juan Guiteras, the national health director for the Secretaría de Sanidad y Beneficencia, and Dr. Mario G. Lebredo, the noted bacteriologist and head of the National Laboratory for Scientific Investigation, arrived to examine Pérez and extract lymph cells from his swollen gland. An hour later, word arrived from the national laboratory that microscopic analysis had confirmed the plague diagnosis. Pérez was immediately transferred to an isolation unit and given 100 ccs of the Yersin antiplague serum, but his condition quickly worsened. By 4:30 P.M., Pérez was running a fever of 106.8, and his heart rate was so fast that the doctor was unable to gauge his pulse. Doctors attempted to stabilize him with injections of camphorated oil and caffeine, but these treatments had no effect. Gumersindo Pérez was pronounced dead at 5:30 in the afternoon. In order to prevent the possibility of further infection, his body was immediately wrapped in blankets soaked in formaldehyde and then enclosed in a zinc box that was then filled with formaldehyde. This box was enclosed within a wooden box, also treated with formaldehyde. In this manner, his body was transferred to the cemetery and buried that very evening.[3]

The death of Gumersindo Pérez, while widely reported in the city's press, was just one case in the months-long bubonic plague outbreak that gripped Havana in the spring and early summer of 1914. At first the outbreak was believed to have been limited to a single case in early March, rapidly identified by an activist public health service that quickly instituted a series of measures meant to eliminate the disease at its source. By late March and early April, however, a steady stream of new cases appeared across the commercial district of Old Havana, sparking widespread fear and international concern. By mid-April, as the situation seemed to be getting out of hand, Cuban public health authorities ordered a broad quarantine of seventeen blocks in the mixed commercial and residential district in the heart of Old Havana. Under widespread protest, 7,000 people were forced to leave their homes while sanitary brigades worked around the clock cleaning streets and disinfecting and fumigating homes and businesses. The Cuban army was brought out into the streets of the capital to enforce the quarantine and keep the peace in the "infected district" in the commercial core of Old Havana.

On its most basic level, the 1914 bubonic plague outbreak was a biological event predicated on the interactions between humans, rats, fleas, and the microscopic bacterium *Yersinia pestis* in an urban environment that facilitated infection. As medical researchers were just coming to learn in the early years of the twentieth century, the plague is primarily propagated by the common rat flea, *Xenopsylla cheopis*. When a flea feeds on a rodent infected with *Yersinia pestis*, the flea becomes infected and able to introduce the plague bacteria into a human host. Once in the infected human's bloodstream, *Y. pestis* multiplies rapidly, its numbers doubling every two hours, overrunning the body's lymphatic system and inflaming tissue in the liver, spleen, and lymph nodes. This latter effect gives rise to the disease's name, as many victims develop painful and massively swollen lymph nodes, known as a buboes, usually in the groin or legs. Left untreated, about half of the people infected will die as the infection overpowers their immune system, causing major organ failure and precipitating death, usually within a week of the appearance of the bubo.[4]

Outbreaks are never just biological events, however. People ascribe meaning to disease within specific historical contexts, shaped by biology but rooted in time, culture, and place. Although by any measure a relatively minor medical event resulting in only a handful of deaths over the course of several months, the 1914 bubonic plague outbreak took on outsized importance for Havana's public health officials, city press, and Spanish immigrants, sparking fierce conflicts over the authority of the new health ministry, the transnational politics of disease control, and the postcolonial legacies of Spanish power. For medical nationalist health officials, the outbreak was the first major occasion to prove the ability of the new Ministry of Health to protect Cuban lives, commerce, and even sovereignty from a dangerous infectious disease. The city press, however, interpreted the outbreak through the lens of local ethnic or party politics, and their editorials and daily reports became a forum for debating the scientific capacity and political authority of Cuban health officials.

Unlike previous outbreaks of infectious disease in Cuba, the plague seemed to implicate Spanish immigrants: the initial outbreak remained limited to the Spanish commercial district in the heart of Old Havana and primarily infected Spanish immigrant workers. The line between victim and perpetrator grew blurry, however, as health officials and city newspapers increasingly blamed the outbreak on Spanish immigrant merchants and the retrograde public health practices of Spain. Fifteen years after the end of colonial rule, the outbreak enflamed nationalist sentiment and revived the image of a Spanish threat to Cuban health and independence. More than any other event, the bubonic plague outbreak highlighted the ambiguous position of Spanish immigrants in postcolonial Cuba: at once favored white immigrants who some believed would help Cuba achieve its economic potential, they were also decried as a backward, unhygienic, and insular population whose continued economic power reflected a hated colonial past.

While Spanish-Cuban conflicts were shaping the politics of disease control on the streets of Havana, the United States was never far from the minds of the politicians and public health officials who pushed for aggressive action against the spread of the disease. Having for years bristled against U.S. sanitary supervision, health authorities were highly conscious of American eyes on the island as the sanitary campaign progressed. As the city's popular and medical press reminded their readers, the fifth article of the Platt Amendment "put in the hands of *La Sanidad cubana* the stability of the nation," for an uncontrolled outbreak "could provoke the intervention of foreign powers . . . engendering for the Cuban state a shameful wardship" only five years after the end of the second U.S. occupation of the island.[5] In organizing an aggressive response to the outbreak, health officials were simultaneously trying to stave off the possibility of further U.S. intervention, looking to highlight a modern and efficient health apparatus, and seeking to minimize the inevitable economic damage the presence of the disease would cause the island. The plague therefore put to a test both Cuban scientific progress and the capability of health authorities to meet international treaty obligations and the needs of the Cuban population. Health Department officials organized an aggressive response to the disease threat, following their motto *Salus populi suprema lex* (the health of the people is the highest law) to the protests of those whose economic interests were harmed and whose homes were intruded upon. In response, urban residents tested the limits of state authority and asserted their own understandings of personal rights. With the help of a powerful merchant class and its allies in the press, they undermined the public health campaign. The resulting conflicts give us insight into popular understandings of disease and the role of neocolonial politics and lingering anticolonial resentments in the shaping of disease control efforts on the ground.

## IMMIGRATION, RACE, AND THE THIRD PANDEMIC OF THE BUBONIC PLAGUE

In the early years of the republic, questions of disease, race, and immigration intersected as medical nationalists inserted themselves into national debates on immigration policy, and as the success of yellow fever interventions seemed to open new possibilities for "useful immigration."[6] Central to these debates was the idea that after the reconcentration, the Cuban countryside was depopulated and only with a rapid and extensive infusion of new immigrants could the country take advantage of its fertile soils and fulfill its economic potential.[7] But race was also at the heart of these debates, as politicians passed bills promoting European immigration and as newspaper editors, reformers, and physicians alike disparaged nonwhite immigrants as social, cultural, economic, and health threats to the fledgling republic.[8] European families, most analysts agreed, would most easily assimilate into Cuban society, settle in rural Cuba, and help lead it to a modern and prosperous future. But Spanish immigrants defied these expectations, settling disproportionately in urban areas, exacerbating urban labor shortages, and dominating key aspects of the urban economy. In a final irony, with the emergence of the bubonic plague in the heart of Havana's Spanish enclave, health officials were forced to confront what they increasingly saw as an intransigent immigrant population that seemed to represent not the sanitary and economic salvation of the country but a threat to its health and sovereignty.

By the turn of the twentieth century, scientists and other observers had long debated whether European bodies were compatible with the tropical environment. A predominant intellectual tradition, reinforced by countless colonial mortality reports, held the tropics to be the graveyard of Europeans, a space of death, disease, and degeneration.[9] But the stunning success of the Cuban yellow fever campaign seemed to prove that the tropics were actually tamable, that science and hygiene could defang the dangerous tropical environment. For William Crawford Gorgas, who helped lead yellow fever efforts in Cuba and Panama, the implications for white immigration were clear.

Four centuries after European colonization of the New World, American mastery over tropical nature represented a new "conquest of the tropics for the white race," proving definitively that "the white man could flourish in the tropics."[10] These sentiments were shared by many Cubans, who saw in the island's public health successes the key to "opening our depopulated countryside to the fertile life of progress" by removing the central obstacle to European immigration.[11] And Europeans did arrive in great number: in the twenty years after Spanish rule ended, the island's Spanish population increased almost fourfold, until it made up 14 percent of the national population.[12] And Havana became home to almost 100,000 Spanish citizens, a stunning 27 percent of the urban population. The bacteriologist Juan Santos Fernández hailed "the indisputable power of science" for making possible this "invasion" of "armies of immigrants" from Spain, noting with satisfaction that "not a single one had died from yellow fever" in recent years.[13]

One of the central ironies of postcolonial Cuba is that rather than signaling the end of foreign power on the island, independence merely changed its form. By 1902, the state was in Cuban hands, but after thirty years of war and a devastating reconcentration, Cuban wealth was largely destroyed. Cuba had little domestic capital, and Americans and Spaniards filled the void. But while the island's lucrative sugar industry would increasingly fall under U.S. control, the Spanish consolidated and expanded their control over the urban economy. Havana's large and increasingly powerful Spanish enclave dominated the commercial, retail, and industrial sectors of the urban economy. As the 1919 Cuban census shows, foreign whites—overwhelmingly Spaniards—were vastly overrepresented in key sectors of the urban economy, comprising two-thirds of Havana's merchants, 62 percent of those employed in manufacturing, and 69 percent of the city's clerks and sales force.[14]

The social world of these peninsular migrants was largely male and almost exclusively Spanish. Despite the best efforts of government officials to lure Spanish families to the island to settle in rural areas and become farmers, three of every four Spanish immigrants were young males, often in their late teens, without families. And rather than become farmers, they flocked to the cities, especially Havana, where they exacerbated rather than alleviated the tight urban labor market even as they left rural labor shortages largely unimproved.[15] Spanish commercial warehouse owners, shopkeepers, and factory owners almost exclusively hired other Spaniards, leading to growing resentment among native workers, especially black Cubans, who bore the brunt of unemployment and underemployment.[16] Spanish workers created a tight-knit male community, largely composed of fellow clerks and firm employees called *dependientes*, or "dependents," who usually slept in the buildings where they worked, whether behind the counters, in the back of the establishment, or in the hot, low spaces between floors of the building.[17] They lived together, ate together, and socialized together in one of the many Spanish immigrant mutual aid associations that flourished in the city in the late nineteenth and early twentieth centuries, most with their own social clubs, hospitals, and low-cost health insurance plans.[18]

But while Spaniards were largely welcomed—officially for their thrift, hard work, and capacity to assimilate and unofficially for their whiteness—other immigrant groups faced significant opposition. One of the final acts of the U.S. occupation government in 1902 was Order No. 155, which barred Chinese immigration outright, essentially extending U.S. Chinese exclusion laws to the republic.[19] Immigration and public health officials—including some prominent medical nationalists—were quite vocal in their opposition to Chinese immigration, which they opposed on economic, cultural, and public health grounds. Among the arguments made were that the Chinese were insular, unassimilable due to language and cultural differences, lazy—yet somehow they also took jobs away from Cubans—and had high rates of criminality and drug addiction. Their children were described as "rachitic, weak, and disposed to tuberculosis."[20]

Particularly striking, however, was the place of the bubonic plague among this litany of supposed ills ascribed to Chinese immigrants. In the fall of 1913, just a few months before the bubonic plague appeared in the Cuban capital, National Director of Public Health Juan Guiteras presented a paper before the Cuban Academy of Science on Chinese immigration to Cuba. While he did not try to hide his antipathy to Chinese immigration, he framed the Chinese danger in terms of "the pathological problem that Asian immigration represents." Southern China, he argued, was "the ancestral source of the bubonic plague," and Chinese port cities continued to be "intense foci" of the disease.[21] In a similar vein, in a 1909 report, Cuban immigration commissioner F. E. Menocal argued in favor of continuing restrictions on Chinese immigration. "China can be called the *mother of the plagues*," he wrote, adding that "cholera, smallpox, and the bubonic plague exist constantly in that country."[22]

While Cuban health officials would continue to stigmatize black Antillean and Chinese migrants as disease carriers, this association of the Chinese with the bubonic plague reflected new fears emerging out of what became known as the Third Pandemic of the bubonic plague. First appearing in southern China in 1894, the disease spread quickly to British-occupied Hong Kong, where with the help of steamships and infected rat stowaways, the disease followed global trade routes to major ports around the world.[23] Millions died of the disease in India and China. Postindependence health officials anxiously followed the spread of the disease, which had never appeared in the Western Hemisphere before January 1900, when it made its simultaneous appearance in Rio de Janeiro and Buenos Aires. They watched as the disease then jumped to California and then to the Pacific Mexican port of Mazatlán.

Given the important trade relations between Cuba and Mexico, health officials feared it was only a matter of time before the disease appeared in Cuban ports. Already in 1903, Enrique Barnet warned that the disease was a "grave threat to our Republic."[24] Since no Cuban physician had ever seen a case of the disease in person, Barnet argued that its nearby presence demanded that Cuban physicians and health authorities study the disease, develop adequate prophylactic measures, and outline effective methods of combating a potential outbreak. Cuban medical and public health workers would get some experience with the plague during a brief outbreak in 1912. But the 1914 outbreak, which came not from reviled China but from Spain, tested the limits of public health officials' ability to curb the spread of the disease and forced health officials to consider the cost of unrestricted trade and immigration from Spain.

## THE INITIAL OUTBREAK AND THE "INFECTED ZONE"

On Tuesday, March 6, 1914, newspapers across Havana announced a new outbreak of the dreaded bubonic plague. The initial victim was Francisco Fernández Núñez, a forty-eight-year-old Spanish immigrant who worked at a food warehouse on Oficios Street near the city's wharves. The previous Saturday, Fernández Núñez had woken up feeling "weak," so instead of going to work, he went to La Purísima Concepción, the hospital run by the mutual aid organization La Asociación de Dependientes, of which he was a member.[25] His symptoms led doctors to suspect the bubonic plague, so they isolated the patient and contacted the Infectious Diseases Commission. By Monday, microscopic medical analysis at the national laboratory confirmed the diagnosis, sparking a massive response from health officials. That afternoon, the National Board of Health held an emergency meeting authorizing that contingency funds be made available to national and local health authorities to deal with the outbreak. Health officials identified a wide "infected district," the area of the city east of Egido and Monserrate streets, or the entirety of the old intramural section of the city, as the focus of initial sanitary efforts. Dr. José Antonio Lopez del Valle, chief of the local health department for Havana, issued a bulletin informing city residents of the outbreak and the measures being taken by local and national health services, adding that while there was "no cause for alarm whatsoever in regards to this case . . . we should all contribute to our effort to cooperate with the measures adopted by the health authorities for the mastery of this infection."[26]

As with earlier outbreaks of yellow fever, health authorities combined an aggressive state response with a call for the active participation of the public in the sanitary campaign. But every infectious disease, each with its own particular manner of propagation, requires a different set of strategies to contain it. The campaign against yellow fever necessarily targeted the *Aedes aegypti* mosquito and the areas of fresh, still water where it bred. The antibubonic plague campaign, however, targeted the disease-carrying fleas that fed primarily on rats, which meant, in practice, targeting the city's rat population. While the public was required to cover or treat any areas of standing water in their homes during previous yellow fever outbreaks, the antiplague campaign demanded a much higher level of participation, especially from residents in the "infected district," who were urged to maintain the strictest level of personal and domestic hygiene. As the Health Department's initial bulletin noted,

> The bubonic plague is a disease that is combated, above all, through the careful cleaning of the home and the diligent washing of the body. . . . Each citizen can, therefore, greatly contribute to freeing himself from the illness and also contribute to the general sanitation, with a little effort. It is enough just to keep the home free of rats and fleas and garbage: to daily rinse out the floors with water and some smelling substance or disinfectant and to bathe daily, changing one's underclothes. Water and soap are the declared enemies of the plague.

Residents and business owners in the zone were given special instructions to follow strict measures of cleanliness and to daily wash and disinfect their floors, with the local Health Department offering disinfectants to any "working families without the resources to acquire them." Any business or home found with floors in bad condition would be closed down by the Health Department. All walls were to be grouted and painted, on pain of sanitary fines, and residents were required to use the new lidded garbage cans that were made available throughout the district.[27]

Meanwhile, Havana's local health department began an aggressive sanitation campaign in the "infected district." A 100-worker Disinfection Brigade began the task of fumigating every home and business in the block where Fernández Núñez worked. District health inspectors were tasked with closely monitoring kitchens, eating establishments, and dormitories and ensuring that all public establishments (including churches, theaters, and movie houses) were cleaned and disinfected twice a day. City garbage collection was to be expanded as well, with collection shifted to early evening to prevent rats from having access to garbage during the night. The streets were then to be swept and washed down immediately. The Health Department's extermination services were expanded, with a new Office of Rat Extermination established in the first floor of the customs building. Its job was to collect caught rats and send them to the national laboratory for testing as well as to receive complaints or notices from area residents on the presence of rats in their homes or nearby buildings. City sanitation workers placed hundreds of rat traps in businesses throughout the district, giving residents orders that only sanitation workers were to touch them. Finally, in an effort to destroy all potentially disease-carrying fleas in the area, sanitation workers were instructed to give chemical baths to all dogs residing in buildings close to the victim's home and work.

Local responses to the appearance of the plague varied widely. The press reported a general calm among the residents of the "infected zone," with *La Discusión* highlighting the success of the March 8 Carnaval parade as evidence of a "widespread and deep-rooted . . . public confidence" in the health authorities. Amidst the public revelry that evening, the paper asserted, "our Havana certainly looked nothing like that of a city showing signs of the frightful hobgoblin of the plague!"[28] But if local residents seem to have remained calm, the Liberal *El Triunfo* found "among the bureaucratic element, a more than normal panic."[29] Dozens of post office workers, whose offices were in the infected zone, stayed home in the aftermath of the plague declaration. Meanwhile, pharmacies wasted no time in using the plague outbreak to sell their wares: on March 6, the day newspapers reported the initial diagnosis, local papers were already running ads for disinfectants and pesticides that promised to cleanse readers' homes of the plague germ. Capitalizing on public anxieties, ads for products such as Chloro Naptholeum and Liquid "Vermingo" Worell allowed residents to take a more active role in protecting their families from the dreaded disease. Residents did, in fact take an active role in the sanitary campaign. In the days following the declaration of the disease, the chief of the Office of Rat Extermination reported receiving "an infinite number of denunciations from families in the city regarding the presence of rats in their homes."[30] But as we will see below, the declaration of the plague's appearance in the city and the subsequent sanitary control measures taken by the Health Department precipitated the protests and concerted opposition of the city's Spanish merchant class and sectors of the Liberal Party establishment.

## THE INTERNATIONAL POLITICS OF DISEASE DECLARATION

Five years after the end of the second U.S. occupation, public health remained deeply entwined with Cuban sovereignty and nationalism, and health officials took every opportunity to highlight the administrative and scientific capabilities of the new health ministry. When laboratory results confirmed the presence of the plague in Havana, national health director Juan Guiteras immediately broadcast news of the outbreak to every country where Cuba had a diplomatic presence. Guiteras knew this action would cause immediate harm to Cuban commerce; indeed, the United States immediately put quarantine measures in place against any ships coming from Havana. But with Cuba's medical reputation on the line, health officials had no choice but to adhere to international sanitary regulations and declare the presence of the disease.[31] What health authorities did not expect, however, was the level of opposition from the city's powerful Spanish merchant class, which accused the ministry of recklessly announcing the presence of the plague "to the four winds."[32] In this early dispute between health officials and Spanish immigrants, we can see how each side was unable to understand the perspective of the other, setting the stage for an increasingly acrimonious conflict.

For medical nationalist health officials like Juan Guiteras, the decision to announce the presence of the plague was an obvious one, given the importance they placed on international recognition of Cuban sanitary expertise. They were also aware of the very real consequences the island could face if Americans lost faith in the ability of Cuban officials to control infectious diseases that could threaten American lives. In fact, in the years after the end of the second U.S. occupation, Cuban health officials had faced a series of accusations of sanitary malfeasance and racist depictions of Cuban incapacity. In 1909, the New York *Medical Record* accused Cuban officials of covering up new yellow fever cases in order to avoid U.S. sanitary oversight, warning that unless the United States resumed control of the island, it would soon "sink to the level of Haity."[33] The *Army and Navy Journal* concurred, seeing this supposed sanitary cover-up as an example of "the ease with which a tropical community slips back into sloth and dirtiness" without the supervision of the United States.[34] Juan Guiteras, the ministry's National Director of Health, was furious that the U.S. medical press would publish these "unsubstantiated assertions," complaining that "everything that happens in Cuba is seen from abroad under the influence of suspicions."[35]

Guiteras was proven right in 1912 when Illinois representative George E. Foss brought before the U.S. Congress a resolution to investigate sanitary conditions in Cuba. Exasperated by these constant allegations of "menacing conditions that are supposed to exist" in Cuba, Guiteras responded with an open letter defending Cuban sanitary capabilities and criticizing the hypocrisy of American rebukes.[36] Rather than Cuba being a menace to the health of the United States, he countered, the reverse was actually true: the United States had smallpox, epidemic cerebrospinal meningitis, and infantile palsy, none of which Cuba had. The spread of smallpox in the United States, Guiteras noted, was a "constant source of anxiety" to Cuban sanitary authorities. Actually, he noted, the death rate for typhoid in Cuba was lower than in the United States, malaria rates were falling, and the general mortality rate in Cuba was lower than in the United States and significantly lower than in U.S.-controlled Puerto Rico. Frustrated with Americans taking credit for Cuban sanitary advances, Guiteras added that Cubans had sufficiently acknowledged the role played by the United States in "planting the seed" of public health: "We have repeated this many times, we have expressed our gratitude for all this in many ways; perhaps we are not as enthusiastic about it as we used to be; but it is certainly not to your credit that you constantly force us to bring these matters up, in defense of ourselves against the most unjustified and unfounded attacks."[37] In the face of these repeated attacks, it is clear why Cuban health officials doubled down on their commitment to the "frank reporting and declaration" of infectious diseases. By 1914, the open declaration of transmissible disease was established policy. It was a seemingly proven method of disease control, tied to Cuban public health authorities' international prestige, and a prerequisite for continued Cuban sovereignty.

Domestically, however, the plague declaration set off ripple effects that directly affected the tourism, trade, and commercial sectors of the urban economy. Shortly after the declaration, the conservative Havana daily La Discusión asserted that maritime traffic had been "broken" by the news.[38] The outbreak coincided with the high season for U.S. tourism, and the effects were immediate: on March 7, the steamship cruiser Laurentic, proceeding from New York with 500 tourists, upon discovering that the city was under quarantine, left Havana without even lowering its boarding ramp. La Política Cómica, the satirical Havana journal, printed a cartoon with the caption "Frightened tourists: Run or the rat will catch you!" showing an image of terrified Americans swimming away from the island toward the safety of Key West.[39] The editors of La Discusión were confident, however, that tourism would return, as potential travelers discovered the thoroughness of the sanitary authorities' public health measures. "For a country that has reached this level of health and hygiene, it is justified to declare it safe shelter for its foreign guests. The flow of 'tourism' momentarily receding from our beaches upon the first news given to the public, will, without concealments and without palliatives, return in its manner and in its usual season, because Cuba offers its visitors all the guarantees which the most scrupulous person demands in respect to sanitation and hygienic practices."[40] Beyond the loss of tourist dollars, however, the outbreak precipitated new restrictions and sanitary measures that affected Cuban trade, as American inspectors began requiring that Cuban pineapple exports be protected from rats by being shipped in protective boxes lined with metal cloth. But these measures were prohibitively costly: as La Discusión warned, if the "sanitary situation does not improve, we can give up on the shipment of pineapples for the next harvest."[41]

## GROWING CONFLICT WITH SPANISH MERCHANTS AND THE LIBERAL PRESS

As the antiplague campaign swung into full gear in the streets of Old Havana, the city's Spanish merchant class and their unlikely allies in the Liberal press became the center of opposition to the state's sanitary efforts. At first, criticism focused on the decision to publicly declare an outbreak. However, as more cases emerged over the coming weeks, these initial grumblings became an outright campaign against the sanitary authorities. On one hand, the conflicts emerged from the inevitable harm the Health Department's actions caused to local commerce, combined with a growing ethnic tension, as Spanish merchants felt unduly targeted by sanitary authorities. On the other hand, Liberal attacks represented the wages of an increasingly politicized public health apparatus, with state jobs becoming part of an ever-broader political spoils system during the Cuban Republic. Yet these conflicts also brought up the relationship between medicine and politics in the context of imperialism and disease, as doubts were cast on laboratory science and popular understandings of the spread of disease fed and shaped doubts about the intentions and actions of the Health Department.

The Liberal Party stalwart *El Triunfo* wasted no time in condemning the Conservative government of Mario Menocal for allowing the disease to gain a foothold in the country, blaming Conservative politicking for the removal of trained sanitary personnel and their replacement with Conservative supporters. Rather than keep the most proficient officials at what were supposed to be technical posts, the Menocal administration, "guided exclusively by partisan antipathies [and] not caring about scientific capacity," fired most of the officials at the ministry, "removing the most competent sanitation officers from their posts." According to the newspaper, vitally important rat extermination work was discontinued in order to save money, even while frivolous "so-called 'technical'" positions were created to be bestowed upon political supporters.[42] Of course, the Liberal paper did not mention that the previous administration had also often been accused of handing out public health and sanitation jobs to its political followers. Nevertheless, the paper continued to express support for the head of the national Health Department, Dr. Juan Guiteras, who, the paper repeatedly mentioned, was put into his position by the Liberal administration, regardless of Guiteras's ostensibly Conservative leanings—proof, the paper claimed, of Liberal high-mindedness in sanitary matters.[43]

The conservative daily El Diario Español, the voice of the city's Spanish commercial class, was also an early and vociferous opponent of the sanitary authorities' anti–bubonic plague campaign. Editors blasted both the health ministry and the city's press for even announcing the existence of the plague in the city, asserting that this publicity, not the disease itself, had "created in Cuba a most grave situation" and would inevitably "cause severe damage to the commerce of the country."[44] Rather than "cast to the four winds the announcement that in Havana this terrible epidemic disease exists," editors called for a more "prudent" approach, which they argued "is common in other nations"—neither covering up the outbreak nor confessing to its existence. Over the coming weeks, the paper would continue to claim that sanitary authorities were grossly overreacting and that their actions were far more harmful than any minor disease outbreak.

Questions over the provenance of the plague outbreak would shape the growing conflict between Spanish merchants and the Health Department. While it is impossible to prove the origins of the outbreak, Cuban health officials immediately blamed Spain for exporting the disease, which they claimed was endemic on the Canary Islands.[45] According to Juan Guiteras, Spain had been harboring cases of the plague without fulfilling its responsibilities under international sanitary regulations to make public the presence of the disease on Spanish soil. Fifteen years after the end of colonial rule, Guiteras argued, Spain was putting its "commercial interests" over the interests of "humanity," in effect "infecting her former colonies with the disease by hiding the existence of the Plague epidemic in the Canary Islands."[46] *La Discusión*, whose correspondent in Spain corroborated allegations of Spanish sanitary deception in the Canaries, called for the immediate quarantine of ships coming from the Spanish archipelago.[47] Cuban health officials quickly obliged, imposing moderate quarantine measures requiring strict sanitary inspection of any ship coming from the Canaries. Not surprisingly, *El Diario Español* took exception to the idea that Spain was responsible for the outbreak and therefore found these measures oppressive. Tensions increased on March 19, when Aristides Agramonte, the president of the Infectious Diseases Commission, bluntly expressed his frustration with Spanish sanitary deception: "I have always maintained that the bubonic plague has been imported to Cuba from Spain (from the Canary Islands), because we know that it exists there and that that Government has lied repeatedly and in a barefaced manner in regards to the issue."[48] In response to Agramonte's plain language, *El Diario Español* redoubled its complaints, calling the accusations "simply impertinent."[49]

In this growing conflict with Cuban health authorities, questions arose about how to gauge the threat the bubonic plague held for the island and whether to even trust the diagnoses. These questions, in addition to reflecting a fundamental Liberal and Spanish immigrant distrust of the current Cuban sanitary authorities, reflected popular understandings around laboratory evidence and the etiology of the disease. In the two weeks following the declaration of the disease, both *El Triunfo* and *El Diario Español* cast doubt on the scientific evidence supporting the plague diagnosis. On March 10, without any new bubonic plague cases having appeared, *El Triunfo* asserted that "very respectable persons have begun to doubt the accuracy of the diagnosis" of the plague in Francisco Fernández Núñez, and that the government, in its rush to proclaim a public health crisis, "has caused irreparable harm to the nation" without benefit to anyone but the corrupt elements in the Menocal administration. Weeks later, *El Diario Español* argued that the "capricious" search for the cause of the outbreak in other countries was a cover for the rash decision to declare the plague's presence after a single, allegedly dubious case.[50]

*El Triunfo* also cast doubt on the efficacy of the Health Department's sanitary measures, such as the insistence that residents in the infected zone use sealed metal garbage cans, while garbage trucks collecting refuse were left "open, scattering miasmas and microbes throughout the streets."[51] The implication that "miasmas" could be responsible for disease or that "microbes" from a passing truck could infect residents with the bubonic plague represented still-common pre-bacteriological understandings of disease causation. The rapid pace of new scientific discoveries meant that older conceptions of disease causation often coincided with newer ones, regardless of compatibility. Even the Health Department's measures sometimes reflected understandings of disease causation that contradicted official pronouncements. Given that the almost exclusive mode of infection with the bubonic plague is the bite of an infected flea, the insistence that area businesses and residences wash their floors twice a day with soapy water was implicitly based on the assumption that filth could facilitate the spread of the disease, but these measures served no real prophylactic purpose.

Frustrated at the continued attacks in the press, Guiteras wrote a strongly worded letter to El Diario Español responding to accusations that health authorities had invented the plague outbreak.[52] Guiteras pushed back against those in the press, including El Triunfo, that continued to sow doubt at a time when public health authorities were "endeavoring . . . to save the country from the wretched consequences that the propagation of this disease could bring us." To explain the process of modern medical diagnostics, Guiteras gave El Diario Español a short lesson in laboratory bacteriology, explaining that the "autograph" of the bacillus was "written in the cultures in the test tubes" in the department's laboratory. He wrote, "You say that we should concretely prove the existence of the Plague, [but the] necessary experiments were completed when we announced the first case. The [results] are in the Laboratory as permanent documents for those who wish to see. What more do you want for us to do? Shall we infect with the microbe some of those who still doubt?" As a veteran of the successful anti–yellow fever campaigns, which also were met with opposition, Guiteras was incredulous that sectors of the urban population continued to oppose the antiplague campaign: "Given the history of the Department of Health, it did not seem possible that today those aggressive campaigns against the initiatives that finished with the Yellow Fever would come back to life." Guiteras pled for cooperation from the press and the public and reminded them that those most at risk from the current outbreak were Spanish immigrants themselves: "Help us in the ways that you can. Do not allow that these deeds be distorted in order to sow mistrust in the public. . . . I ask in the names of those brave workers who come from Spain and have been, until now, the most threatened."[53]

## "¡DURO CON ELLOS!": PLAGUE AND THE
## HYGIENIC ORDERING OF CIVILIZATION

As new plague cases—all targeting Spanish immigrant commercial warehouse workers—began appearing in the heart of the Spanish commercial district, discussions about the outbreak began to change. Some publications expressed growing frustration with Spanish immigrant merchants, who were increasingly depicted as avaricious, backward, dirty, and putting their economic self-interests above the lives of native Cubans or even Cuban sovereignty. Together with a growing discourse of the disease itself as a foreign invader propagated by ignorance and filth, the stage was increasingly set for a confrontation with the city's Spanish immigrants.

La Lucha invoked the trope of the miserly Spanish immigrant when it took aim at merchants who "cunningly seek to save four miserable pesetas" by claiming "that the danger of the epidemic is and has been exaggerated." For such merchants, the paper added, "nothing comes before the pecuniary interests represented by a few hundred sacks or boxes of merchandise."[54] El Mundo excoriated those, like El Diario Español, that complained of the ministry's decision to publicly declare the presence of the disease. Invoking the threat of the Platt Amendment, the paper reminded its readers that concealing the presence of the plague would "authorize the United States to intervene in Cuba." For anyone who complained about the "vigor" of Cuban health measures, they added, "perhaps they would find even more intolerable or harsh those that the United States could impose upon us."[55]

This image of an intransigent group of Spanish immigrants could also be seen in the political cartoons of the time. "Be Hard on Them!," published in La Lucha, expresses what seems to have been a popular sense of frustration with the resistance of this wealthy immigrant sector to Health Department mandates.[56] The cartoon shows a caricatured mustachioed Spaniard in his warehouse, surrounded by sacks and barrels of merchandise. He is tied down on a chair, in his long underwear, next to a dead rat with another rat's tail poking up from behind a sack. The Spaniard is surrounded by smoking skillets—representing the burning of sulfur as an unpleasant pesticidal fumigant meant to kill rat fleas—including one in the hands of a sanitary brigade worker who is holding it up to the face of the Spaniard. The caption reads, "To those that don't want disinfection . . . three skillets!" If images like these signaled that anti-Spanish sentiment was heating up, Spanish merchants would come to feel increasingly targeted as the outbreak expanded through the city in the coming weeks, and as health authorities took increasingly harsh measures to prevent the spread of a disease that remained largely contained within the Spanish enclave.

Throughout the outbreak, public health officials and other physicians took every opportunity to remind the public of the importance of protective measures for all Cubans. As they did during the U.S. occupation, they reinforced the medical nationalist message that explicitly linked hygiene to modernity, civilization, and care for their fellow citizens. In mid-March, the popular weekly magazine El Fígaro published the first in a series of articles on the bubonic plague, as part of a regular column by Dr. Enrique Barnet called "Chats with the Doctor."[57] Meant to educate readers about the etiology of the disease and effective prophylactic measures, the series explained laboratory science, emphasized the dangers of rats and fleas, and urged readers to follow the instructions of local and national health departments. The series made effective use of illustrations to help explain medical or public health concepts, reproducing, for example, enlarged images of the microscopic Y. pestis bacteria and images of autopsied rats showing the telltale physical signs of a bubonic plague infection. The series also reproduced ideas about hygiene, culture, and the propagation of disease that organized societies along a scale of civilization according to adherence to elite visions of sanitary practice. One column posited that "the scale of civilization of a people is actually measured by the amount of soap and water its inhabitants use to bathe themselves. . . . Filth and epidemics go hand in hand. Clean people are rarely attacked by the plague."[58] Of course, the dubious claim that "the clean" were safer from the plague reinforced the idea that the diseased were guilty, whether because of ignorance or vice, but these beliefs reflected long-standing discourses equating cleanliness with modernity and dirt with disease and backwardness.

Public health officials also sometimes echoed the scientifically dubious claim that hygienic habits would prevent the plague from becoming endemic to the island. In an interview with La Lucha, Juan Guiteras and José Antonio López del Valle asserted that the "bubonic plague should not develop in civilized populations, clean, [and] loving of hygiene. 'Dramatic' epidemics of this infection cannot take hold except among people who lack sanitary conditions, in those who do not follow sanitary precepts. Havana is a clean, healthy city. Its population is distinguished precisely by its culture, its devotion to hygiene."[59] In contrast to places where the disease had become endemic, such as India, China, and allegedly the Canary Islands, the sanitary consciousness of the Cuban people would safeguard them from a similar fate. But while Cuban officials expressed confidence in the culture of hygiene

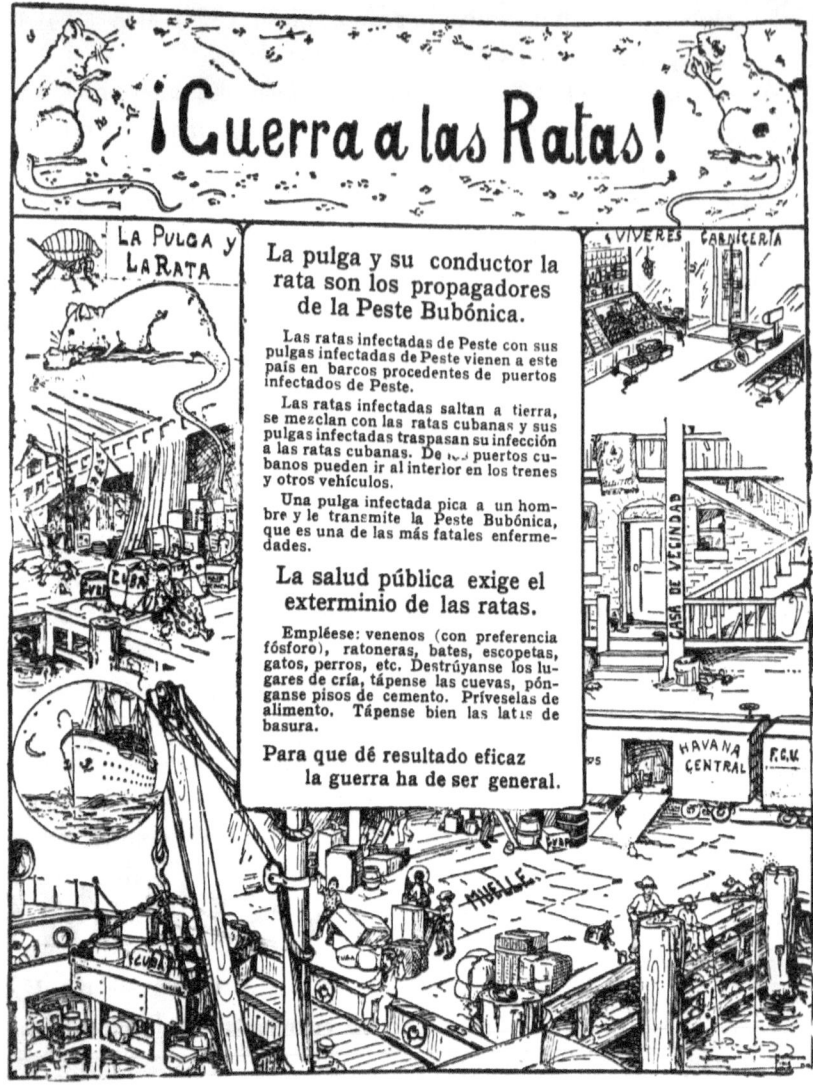

*Figure 3.1* "War on the Rats!" (from Enrique Barnet's *Conversaciones del doctor*, reproduced from El Fígaro, March 15, 1914)

among the urban residents, the state would continue to enforce its sanitary surveillance of the disproportionately Spanish immigrant residents of the infected zone: "We carefully monitor the people's homes, that they remain clean. We make them wash the floor of their homes, twice a day, with water and petroleum, and we avoid fleas and garbage. The washing of the floor has to be done scrupulously, moving objects and furniture, so that no corner remains dry and dirty."[60]

This set of associations linking the disease to filth, foreigners, and especially the Spanish is evident in the March 15 edition of "Chats with the Doctor," which featured the illustration captioned "¡Guerra a las Ratas!" (War on the Rats!) (see figure 3.1). The image presents an imagined visual history of the plague's movement through space. Moving counterclockwise, rats run rampant along a Chinese wharf with boxes of merchandise marked for Cuba; among the boxes are passed-out men with hair in queues: presumably Chinese opium addicts. The disease arrives on Cuban shores, as those boxes are unloaded at the city's docks, from where they might travel by train to any part of the island. The presumably infected rats are then seen at a *casa de vecindad*, the racially coded tenement buildings notorious as spaces of disease, and finally appear among boxes of fruits and merchandise at a bodega. The illustration reproduces common early-twentieth-century Cuban discourses of Chinese immigrants and the poor as vectors of disease, but the discourse of the hygienic threat of the Spanish *bodeguero* seems to have arisen specifically during the bubonic plague outbreak. Together with Barnet's "Conversaciones del Doctor" series, newspaper editorials, and public pronouncements from national health officials, this amounted to a surprisingly coherent discourse of a modern and hygienic Cuban population whose lives and national sovereignty were now threatened by Spanish immigrant merchants. In creating this vision of hygienic order, Cubans could claim a modern, civilized status that their former colonial masters, whose actions betrayed a dangerous sanitary carelessness, could not hope to claim.

## CRISIS AND QUARANTINE

In April, the Health Department's work continued apace: fumigation brigades made their way through the "infected district" and street sweepers and garbage collectors worked night and day to keep the streets free of garbage. But despite the around-the-clock sanitation work of the Health Department, the next few weeks saw the appearance of a dozen new cases in the capital; soon, additional cases would appear in the outlying towns and in the eastern city of Santiago de Cuba. With new infections rapidly appearing, city and national health departments felt the situation slipping out of control. Between April 12 and 14, three more cases appeared in the capital; the victims were all Spanish immigrant workers employed in a warehouse in the infected zone, on Inquisidor Street. Under pressure, health officials felt they needed to take extreme action in order to keep the outbreak from getting further out of control. At first, three city blocks around where these Spanish workers lived and worked were ordered quarantined, but the following day, fearing that this would be insufficient to contain the disease, health officials put a full seventeen city blocks, the heart of the capital's commercial warehouse district, under quarantine. Residents were ordered to evacuate, while businesses were shuttered. The entire quarantine zone was to be systematically disinfected and fumigated, with the goal of killing all rats and fleas within the zone, eliminating future sources of infection. In order to enforce the quarantine, the army was ordered onto the streets of the "infected district."

Over 7,000 residents were forced to leave their homes.[61] Those who could not afford to rent a room elsewhere were sent to the quarantine station at Triscornia, east of the city. All residents of the quarantine zone were required to keep the Health Department informed as to their current whereabouts. Residents were given one day to evacuate their homes. All traffic through the zone was to be prohibited: carts, wagons, and horse-drawn carts were barred from entering or exiting the zone. The only vehicles allowed transit through the quarantine zone were electric streetcars, their windows firmly shut as they sped through the district, with conductors prohibited from picking up or dropping off any passengers in the zone.

As Juan Guiteras explained to the press, the quarantine was necessary to prevent the spread of the disease. Previous sanitary measures had proved insufficient, he argued, because residents of warehouses in the zone kept getting infected "due to [their] lack of care, [as the residents], upon noting the presence of rats, did not notify the Health Department."[62] Worse, Guiteras alleged, warehouse owners were trying to conceal the cases of illness among their workers. The intransigence, foot dragging, and deception of the Spanish merchants in the face of a growing health crisis was too much for Cuban health authorities. Every case of the plague so far had occurred among Spanish-owned wholesale food warehouses, and every victim so far had been a Spanish immigrant worker. But health authorities were getting little cooperation from warehouse workers and active opposition from their Spanish merchant employers. With the quarantine of the commercial district and the expulsion of its residents, health authorities argued, sanitary brigades would be able to work unimpeded. Guiteras acknowledged to the press that the quarantine would cause damage to local commerce, but he saw no other way to resolve the crisis.[63]

On the morning of April 14, residents of Old Havana woke up to the sound of two artillery companies of the Cuban army taking possession of the streets of the quarantine zone. Overnight, Marcelino Trueba, one of the recently infected Spanish workers, had died after two days of fever and delirium at the

Covadonga Hospital. And yet another case of the plague had been confirmed. Throughout that day, workers and residents began to evacuate the quarantine zone, and the streets were busy with a flurry of movement and confusion. Disinfection brigades began their work in the first three evacuated blocks, as the streets were thronged with curious onlookers "not driven back by the fear of contagion so long as they could be close to and see the cleaning and disinfection operations."[64] The crowd grew so large that the police had to clear the streets. But while the flurry of activity of the sanitary campaign fascinated passersby, for residents of the quarantine zone, the situation was getting out of hand.

The forced evacuations affected residents according to their economic means. While many families from the quarantined blocks were able to find other places to stay within the infected zone of Old Havana, others, the poorest and most desperate, were sent to the Triscornia immigration camp, where they were to be given food and shelter by the government. According to La Discusión, "The greatest number of these were men, and almost all of them Spaniards, who, from the look of them seemed recent arrivals to this country."[65] Anyone who went to Triscornia was barred from leaving the camp for the duration of the quarantine period, so people with jobs outside the quarantined zone often refused to go, and several let their children go without them so they could more easily find a place to stay and be able to keep their jobs. A reporter from La Discusión described a "pathetic scene" where "a group of women, four or five, a paralyzed man and a battalion of kids" without a place to stay were thrown out of their home on Calle Sol. One of the women, who worked at a nearby bookstore, feared the eviction would cause her to lose her job. For single women with children, the situation was particularly precarious, as accepting passage to Triscornia could mean losing the means to support their families.

But for those who did not go to Triscornia, housing was difficult to find. While Health Department officials proclaimed that the residents posed no threat, landlords feared that potential lodgers from the quarantine zone could bring with them the plague germ. According to reporters, residents made "many inquiries in different tenements and inns, but that these proved unfruitful, since in all of those places where they went they were told they would not be admitted, out of fear that a case of the plague could present itself among one of them, leading the Health Department to close down the building and quarantine the block where they were located."[66] Some families sought shelter in the neighboring towns of Regla and Guanabacoa, but there too they were met with fear. According to La Discusión, residents in Guanabacoa, alarmed that they were being inundated with residents from the infected zone, "saw in the clothes of each of these individuals the microbe of the horrible disease."[67] The local health officer of Guanabacoa, together with the mayor and police department, set up surveillance at the train station. Anyone disembarking at the station who was not a resident of Guanabacoa was stopped and questioned, and those arriving from the infected zone of Havana were forced to have their clothes and possessions fumigated. The same measures were soon put in place in Regla.

### "LA RECONCENTRACIÓN" IN REVERSE

While residents of the zone eventually evacuated, many did not leave quietly. Protests, especially from Spanish merchants in the district, began as soon as the quarantine plans were announced, as business owners feared the financial harm the closures would inevitably engender. Merchants found the closure orders extreme and unreasonable, the costs to commerce far outweighing the damage caused by the outbreak. A correspondent from El Triunfo reportedly spoke with several business owners in the infected zone who "uniformly agreed that the La Sanidad is crazy."[68] According to La Discusión, Health Department chief Juan Guiteras was "completely besieged by different commissions of property owners, residents and merchants" from the zone seeking exemptions from the quarantine orders.[69] One group was led by Cuban senator and former vice president Domingo Méndez Capote, who with a representative of Álvarez, Valdés & Co. sought to have the quarantine order reversed entirely. Finding Guiteras "inflexible," the delegation sought guarantees as to the duration of the quarantine and even offered additional workers and money toward the sanitation campaign. But Guiteras was unyielding, noting that "although it was unfortunate, they would have to accept it for the good of all."[70] Nevertheless, he promised that the quarantine would be as short as possible.

One group of Spanish merchants, still convinced that the plague outbreak was a hoax, devised a plan to bring a commission of doctors from British-controlled India (where the plague was endemic) to examine the patients in Havana; these businessmen were "hopeful that the medical opinion [of the British] would be contrary to that of our Health Department."[71] La Discusión found the plan to signify an "irritating lack of confidence in our serious, competent, and zealous Health Department and in the scientific capacity of the eminent doctors that lead it."[72] Asserting confidence in Cuban health officials and upholding the significance of laboratory proof, the paper noted that the department's orders were based not on "abstract opinion" but on concrete "bacteriological analysis of the blood extracted from the buboes of the afflicted." In order to understand this, the paper asserted, one "does not need the knowledge of a professional, but just the possession of a little common sense."

But doubts about the plague diagnosis continued to be widespread among the Spanish merchant class. As *La Discusión* noted, "It is precisely in a certain part of the Spanish business class where the greatest resistance to the Health Department is to be found and where doubts about the truth of the diagnoses are the greatest." *La Discusión*, in order to allay these doubts, interviewed the Spanish minister, who expressed his full confidence in the diagnosis of the bubonic plague by the Cuban sanitary authorities. The Spanish minister counseled the merchants in the zone to follow the orders of the Cuban health officials "first, because they are the authority of the country in which they reside, and should be complied with loyally; and second, because these measures are necessary." The minister did, however, deny that the current Cuban outbreak was imported from the Canary Islands.

The quarantine orders created scenes of confusion and anger among residents and merchants. Some residents saw the orders to leave as an "outrage and an abuse of authority without precedent," and they refused to leave their homes until forced to by the police.[73] Others, such as the owner of a café on Inquisidor who refused to close down his shop, were fined.[74] Eventually, all the residents of the seventeen quarantined blocks evacuated the zone. By the afternoon of April 14, soldiers were stationed at each corner within the quarantine zone, weapons in arms, under orders to inspect all passersby and make sure they were authorized to enter and exit the zone. Sometimes conflicts arose out of confusion with the sanitary orders, such as when, on the morning of April 15, an ice cream peddler entered the quarantine zone for "a few brief and fateful minutes" to sell ice cream to evacuating residents. Unfortunately, the soldiers guarding the edge of the zone then barred the "sad and regretful" peddler from leaving the quarantine zone with his cart.[75] A correspondent from *La Lucha* described the district as "a devastating scene" with whole "families sobbing as they left their homes, accompanied by their children. . . . It was appalling."[76] These images of scared families fleeing their homes under orders from the state brought to mind the infamous policies of the Spanish during the War of Independence. For the correspondent from *El Triunfo*, the evacuations reproduced "scenes from the reconcentration," but in reverse, with Cuban authorities forcing the evacuation of Spanish women and children. A reporter from *La Lucha* echoed this imagery: "Families with their children, carrying large bundles of clothing, gave us an idea of that famous reconcentration ordered by the general Weyler."[77]

By the night of April 15, the streets of the quarantine zone were eerily quiet. A reporter from La Discusión described the scene: "The disorder and confusion of the coming and going of the carts from the warehouses, that gave so much life to that part of the city, had disappeared. The animation and the life had ended and only the patrols of workers sheathed in their protective boots were to be seen on these streets. Every now and again a group of persons emerged from a private residence. These were neighbors complying with the Health Department's orders and silently abandoning their homes in search of others where their health would not be endangered."[78]

## THE LIMITS OF SALUS POPULI SUPREMA LEX

The quarantine of the core of the city's commercial district did not prevent the bubonic plague from spreading. In the days and weeks to come, another seventeen cases appeared in the city and its outskirts. While most of the new infections occurred among Spanish workers within the infected zone of Old Havana, five Cubans also contracted the disease. But even as the plague continued to spread, sanitary authorities did not extend the quarantine beyond the original seventeen blocks. Faced with the redoubled protests of the Spanish merchant class, the growing belief that the Health Department had gone "too far" in its aggressive quarantine measures, and the noticeable effects of the quarantine measures on state customs receipts, the Health Department attenuated its response to the new waves of infections. In the coming weeks, sanitary authorities would come to target specific buildings, rather than entire neighborhoods, for disinfection and fumigation. The resulting shift shows the limits of the Health Department's power to impose its hygienic vision on an increasingly unwilling population. While still claiming Salus populi suprema lex, the republic's health authorities would in practice come to take a more pragmatic approach that would limit damage to commerce, undercutting the main source of popular disaffection with the sanitary campaign.

With the new plague infections, El Diario Español stopped publishing articles casting doubt on the existence of the disease, but in the face of the quarantine, the paper redoubled its criticisms of the course of the sanitary campaign. While recognizing that the worsening plague situation could require "radical" measures to end the outbreak, in the coming weeks the paper published over a dozen articles and editorials demanding compensation for the damages and for loss of business resulting from the sanitary measures and quarantine. "If by chance," the paper asked, a merchant "should have the misfortune that their warehouse shelters the plague, [should] they have to suffer the material damages which originate in the prophylactic measures? Logically, of course not."[79] But as no compensation had been offered to the merchants of the quarantine zone, the editors defended the right of merchants to "defend themselves." In response to the criticism that some residents of the infected zone were actively "putting obstacles in the way of [sanitary] measures and disobeying its orders," the paper asked what could be expected, "if nothing is ever talked about but sacrifices?" Rather than being a sign of a "lack of culture," as proponents of the sanitary campaign argued, resistance to the Health Department's measures was a "defense" that, if "there existed indemnifications . . . would not manifest."[80]

As the editors of El Diario Español understood, the question of indemnification was complicated by the fact that most of the businesses in the quarantine zone were Spanish-owned, and many Cubans blamed Spaniards for the outbreak. "The way in which these issues became mixed with nationality," the editors noted, "engendered a loss of all reason. . . . Because the Spanish were those most directly harmed because of the bubonic plague, no one spoke about the measures by La Sanidad in themselves, in an independent manner, but in relation to the elements against which they were adopted or would be adopted." And since the Cuban government insisted that the plague was imported from the Canaries, the editors argued, "all of the measures employed [by the sanitary authorities] were excessively applauded."[81] Nevertheless, in the context of constant protests and a series of delegations of Spanish businessmen, Cuban politicians, and neighborhood business associations, the Health Department did announce, on April 16, that businesses subjected to fumigation and disinfection by the sanitary brigades would be compensated for damages caused to merchandise from the procedures. The government would not, however, to the consternation of merchants and El Diario Español, compensate businesses for loss of revenue resulting from the forced closures.

The animosity and distrust between the Health Department and the Spanish merchant class, which El Diario Español had done so much to foster, wound up harming the interests of both the merchant class and the sanitary campaign. As Juan Guiteras would later assert in his assessment of the 1914 outbreak, the resistance of the merchant class to the sanitary campaign was responsible for helping spread the bubonic plague beyond the confines of the quarantine zone. Merchants, fearful of the losses that would result from closure and fumigation, would attempt to get rid of as much merchandise as they could before the arrival of the sanitary authorities. In at least three incidents, police were called to investigate the illegal transfer of merchandise from food warehouses that were under closure orders or where new cases of the disease had been found.[82] According to the Health Department, illegal transfers of food merchandise led to the appearance of the disease in Artemisa, a small town outside Havana, where a Spanish grocer became ill with the plague after having received a shipment from the quarantine zone. Similar incidents occurred at a bakery on Calle Sanidad and at a horseshoe-making shop on Calle Concha.[83] From the perspective of Cuban health officials, Spanish merchants actively impeded the antiplague campaign with their constant protests, purposefully broke the quarantine, and even hid cases of disease—all of which exacerbated the outbreak and endangered Cuban lives and sovereignty. In this context, the Health Department refused to even entertain the idea that merchants would be recompensed for the loss of business the closures and quarantine inevitably caused. In turn, of course, Spanish merchants continued to undermine the sanitary campaign that harmed their business interests.

In the coming days and weeks, however, even as new cases of infection appeared across the city, health authorities did not extend the quarantine beyond the initial seventeen blocks. For many residents of Havana, the state's sanitary campaign seemed an extreme response to an uncertain danger. The forced evacuation of seventeen city blocks in the heart of the commercial district, the relocation of 7,000 residents, and the military occupation of the streets of the capital—all in response to what was then only a handful of infections and two deaths—seemed out of proportion to the threat posed by the outbreak. As El Diario Español succinctly put it, "If for two deaths they quarantine seventeen blocks, the day that the cases increase . . . they will have to quarantine entire cities."[84] With the calling of the quarantine, the Liberal El Triunfo renewed with vigor its campaign against what it again called "La Sanidad Conservadora." Even worse than the bubonic plague, the newspaper argued, the Health Department itself had become a "scourge" for the "poor souls" who were expelled from their homes in the commercial district."[85] While such opposition from Spanish merchants and political opponents of the Menocal government were expected, soon even the most ardent supporters of the Ministry began expressing doubts about the quarantine. The magazine Vida Nueva, published to educate the Cuban people on questions of hygiene and science and usually a vocal advocate for the Health Department, found the quarantine measures to be "extreme."[86] Finally, *La Lucha*, which was also always a vocal supporter of the sanitary campaign, began to criticize what it saw as a double standard on the part of the health authorities: while private individuals and businesses were forced to keep their properties in the highest levels of hygiene, government buildings were left teeming with rats.[87]

In the end, the state could not long endure the loss of revenue from an expanded quarantine. By the middle of April, the sanitary campaign was already having an impact on customs receipts, as merchants suspended orders in order to protect themselves from further loss.[88] Importantly, given the warped taxation system prevailing in Cuba, import duties on merchandise brought into Cuba accounted for 85 percent of the national budget.[89] An extended quarantine of the commercial heart of the capital was unsustainable.

With each new infection, the Health Department's sanitary work became more targeted. Rather than a neighborhood or even a block, single buildings would be evacuated, disinfected, fumigated, and then returned to their occupants as quickly as possible. As *El Diario Español* correctly put it on April 21, since the quarantine and the subsequent protests, the Health Department "has attempted to proceed more prudently, softening the measures which had been rigorous. For two cases [of the plague] seventeen blocks were quarantined. Soon after, for one more case (that on Tenerife Street), three blocks were quarantined and no more. Tomorrow, if another case appears, the house of the plague victim will be quarantined and thank you."[90] The quarantine measures were surely effective in giving the Health Department the space for a thorough fumigation and sanitation campaign in what was always "ground zero" of the 1914 bubonic plague outbreak. But the political, social, and economic realities around which the anti–bubonic plague campaign had to maneuver proved decisive in forcing the Health Department to moderate its tactics. In the end, the Health Department realized that it could not simply impose its will on the public.

Any public health campaign needs the active support of the public in order to be effective, but in its zeal to crush the bubonic plague, the department's tactics wound up alienating key segments of the urban population. The image of *La Sanidad*, propagated by newspapers supportive of strong sanitary action, as a decisive singular force battling against a foreign and deadly disease was a myth. The anti–bubonic plague campaign, like any public health campaign, was socially situated, requiring the participation, or at least acquiescence, of broad sectors of the population. When its support, even among previous backers, eroded over the month of April, it could no longer pretend to impose its hygienic vision on Havana.

As Louis A. Pérez Jr. has argued, late-nineteenth- and early-twentieth-century Cuban conceptions of modernity, in large part drawn from U.S. cultural influences, were always defined in contrast to the perceived backwardness of Spain and the Spanish.[91] Central to Cuban anticolonial discourse, conceptions of Spanish backwardness shaped the medical nationalism of the reformers who, by 1914, were in charge of the Cuban public health apparatus.[92] When the bubonic plague, a disease rife with associations of medieval filth and ignorance, appeared in the heart of the Spanish commercial district and threatened Cuban independence under the provisions of the Platt Amendment, the stage was set for an acrimonious conflict between sanitary authorities and the Spanish merchants.

As historians of medicine often point out, epidemics are events that can serve to highlight the social fissures that until then have stayed relatively below the surface. In the case of the 1914 bubonic plague outbreak, long-standing resentments between the Spanish merchant class and Cubans came to the fore, with each distrustful of the other. Cuban public health authorities waged an aggressive campaign not just against the plague but also against what they deemed the ignorance and dangerous sanitary obstruction of the city's Spanish merchant class. That the disease took root in the Spanish-dominated commercial sector made it easier for the Health Department to be unrelenting at first—a foreign population made an easier target for thorough and aggressive sanitary measures—but with the centrality of Spanish-dominated commerce to the broader economy, the Health Department's aggressive policies were unsustainable. The neocolonial development of the Cuban economy, along with the constant protests of those affected by the measures, limited the freedom of the Health Department to act. But while these conflicts illuminate the often ambivalent relationship Cubans had with Spanish immigrants, just as illuminating are the actions officials chose not to take: although Spanish immigrants were at the center of a conflict that seemed to threaten the lives of native-born Cubans and even the very sovereignty of the nation, Cuban officials made no efforts to curb the rapid flow of Spanish immigration. And despite the conviction of health authorities that Spain continued to flout international sanitary law by hiding cases of infectious disease, trade with Spain continued much as it did before.

Less than two years after the bubonic plague outbreak, however, Cuban health officials mandated a fifteen-day quarantine for all black West Indians coming into the country, citing concerns about the role that Haitian and Jamaican migrant workers played in the country's growing malaria problem.[93] Despite the fact that malaria was endemic to Spain and despite the prevalence of the disease among Spanish immigrants on the island, they were never targeted as vectors of the disease or subject to onerous quarantine measures. But in the coming years, Chinese, Jamaican, and Haitian migrants and immigrants would consistently be singled out as particular dangers, as "grave sanitary and social threats to the Republic," who "infected Spaniards and native Cubans" with everything from beriberi and malaria to smallpox and the plague.[94] Cuban health officials, scientists, and politicians continued to cite public health reasons for continuing to bar Chinese immigrants and proposed similar measures to bar the immigration of Afro-Antilleans. Not surprisingly, these attacks were rooted more in racial fears than health concerns. Haitians were decried for "contaminating black Cubans" with their traditions of "witchcraft" and "Voodu," while the Chinese continued to be labeled as vice-driven opium addicts who "inculcated [Cuban] youth" with their drug habits.[95] And the *Diario de la Marina*, which consistently lauded the contributions of Spanish immigrants, described the scourge of disease, violent crime, and a host of other problems that Cuba "must confront due to the invasion of Chinese, Jamaicans, and Haitians."[96]

This contrast between the treatment of Spanish immigrants and their West Indian and Chinese counterparts clearly illuminates the intertwined medical, racial, and class politics that shaped immigration debates in early-twentieth-century Cuba. As Alan Kraut has argued, one of the major themes in the history of disease and immigration has been the "medicalization of pre-existing prejudice," the ways in which outbreaks serve to reinforce existing power relations as persons on the margins of society bear the brunt of blame and stigma.[97] The Third Pandemic of the bubonic plague is itself a global case study for how outbreaks magnify existing power relations. As the disease traveled across the world after 1894, health officials targeted Chinese immigrants in Hawaii and San Francisco, and Afro–Puerto Ricans were subject to the harshest disease measures in San Juan, as were black South Africans in Capetown.[98] But in Cuba, despite the unhygienic habits sometimes attributed to Spanish immigrants, their higher rates of malaria, and their association with the 1914 plague outbreak, in the end they seemed to benefit from a kind of class and racial immunity to the stigmas that so easily attached themselves to black and Chinese immigrants. Despite their sometimes ambiguous position in the postcolonial order, Spaniards were, it seemed, always the "right kind" of immigrant. They were culturally assimilable and racially preferable. And, of course, they were vital nodes in the transnational economy that funded government health work.

Fifteen years after the plague outbreak, in his *Compilación sanitaria de Cuba*, Dr. Edualdo Gómez described the 1914 bubonic plague campaign as representing the "most resonant success of our health authorities."[99] And indeed, despite the protests of Spanish immigrant merchants, the Ministry of Health's aggressive actions to limit the spread of the disease were a success. In many ways, however, the 1914 campaign represented the last gasp of a broadly interventionist public health apparatus. There would be no more expansive urban quarantines, no more major efforts akin to the plague or yellow fever campaigns to eradicate a specific microbe from the urban environment. Public health authorities' ability to impose sanitary authority over the Cuban capital seemed to be exhausted. In the aftermath of the 1914 campaign, health officials largely avoided sanitary reforms that could harm the material interests of the powerful, focusing instead on disease prevention through public health education. By the 1920s, however, it became increasingly clear to the nurses and physicians who worked most closely with the poor that beyond the habits of the poor, it was the Cuban economy itself that was responsible for so much disease and death in the capital.

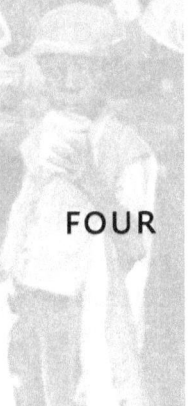

FOUR   The Dangers That Surround the Child
Gendered Poverty and the Fight against
Infant Mortality

ON A WARM SATURDAY morning in 1912, Havana's residents woke up to the usual sounds and smells of the busy city. Street sweepers, their once-white uniforms caked in dust from a long night's work, noisily rolled barrels filled with refuse down cobbled roads, while dockworkers unloaded heavy crates of salted codfish and potatoes destined for Spanish-owned bodegas and Cuban dinner tables. In the dense neighborhoods of central Havana, children teased dogs and shouted for their friends to come down to play while itinerant fruit sellers sang their distinctive songs to entice hungry customers. Horse-drawn delivery carts clip-clopped down alleylike streets while trolley cars clanged their bells to alert absentminded pedestrians. It was a Saturday like any other.

Residents who picked up a copy of the Havana daily El Mundo on their morning rounds might have learned, tucked away in the Civil Register notice at the bottom of page 4, that Nicolás Fernández Coronado had recently wed María Bordes Torres. But just below this welcome news, readers also learned of the eighteen fellow habaneros who had died in the previous twenty-four hours. Like Ricardo Soler, a newborn just one month old, who died of gastroenteritis in his family's Centro Habana home. Or Juan Clemente Sánchez, a seven-month-old from the neighborhood of El Cerro, who died of "congenital weakness." Or Little Nila Garrido, at eleven months, who succumbed to enteritis, or nine-month-old Leando Plá, whose severely malnourished body also failed him that day. All together, half of the city residents who died in the previous twenty-four hours were babies under two years of age, and almost all of these deaths were attributed to gastrointestinal ailments or severe malnutrition.[1]

We know little about these nine young lives prematurely cut short or the families they left behind. The brief notice in the daily paper omits the web of relationships in which these young lives were embedded and tells us nothing about the meaning their early deaths held for loved ones. To most readers of El Mundo that morning, the notice would likely have caused little stir, for this day was like so many others, and child death was an everyday occurrence in early-twentieth-century Havana. In a kind of somber alchemy, however, the little details included in the Civil Register—age, address, and cause of death—were shed of pain and personal meaning and transmuted into the city's annual infant mortality statistics. These sterile grids of lines and numbers told their own stories and took on increasingly urgent meaning for a growing cohort of health officials, nurses, feminist reformers, and journalists, who saw in them not personal loss but national shame. As the numbers indicated, the problem was of tremendous proportions: between 1904 and 1913, over 12,000 children under the age of one died in the Cuban capital, an average of over 100 infants dying per month in a city of less than 300,000 inhabitants.[2]

Of these, the majority of the deaths were the result of infantile enteritis. Enteritis and gastroenteritis are gastrointestinal ailments often caused by bacteria-laden water, milk, and food and can be particularly deadly for young children with still-developing immune and digestive systems.[3] Afflicted children can develop acute diarrhea, and without the antibiotics and intravenous fluids that today are the common therapeutic response, many died quickly of dehydration. In a grimly regular cycle, the city's death rate for young children would spike every summer, as the hot weather facilitated the growth of foodborne bacteria, leading to a sharp increase in dangerous gastrointestinal disorders.[4] In the years after independence, reformers, physicians, and health officials routinely decried this situation, which seemed an increasingly intolerable embarrassment for a country that had eliminated yellow fever, transformed its sanitary reputation, and created the first Ministry of Health in the world. But despite overall improvement in urban health statistics, infant death rates remained gallingly high. As physician Domingo F. Ramos wrote, "There is no reason why Cuba, which is at present such a healthy country for inhabitants over five years of age, both native and foreign, should prove so unfavorable to children under this age."[5]

There were, in fact, many reasons why young children died so regularly in early-twentieth-century Havana. Infant mortality, unlike yellow fever and the bubonic plague, cannot be stopped by something as straightforward as eliminating mosquito breeding areas or exterminating rats. In early-twentieth-century Havana, infant mortality emerged out of a complex set of largely structural problems rooted in the postcolonial economy. While child deaths affected families of all classes, they were overwhelmingly clustered among the poorest households, often those without the support of a male breadwinner. Infant mortality was, as much as any metric, a reflection of gendered poverty in republican Havana. The capital's notoriously high cost of living forced poor women into the labor market, but in early-twentieth-century Cuba, women's labor was so poorly valued that many single women were unable to properly feed themselves or provide decent housing for their families. This was especially true for women of color, who were relegated to the lowest rungs of the urban economy. This gendered and racialized geography of labor left its imprint on the city's mortality statistics, as work requirements prevented many women from breastfeeding their infants, leaving them susceptible to dangerous gastrointestinal disorders. Low wages, poor housing conditions, adulterated milk supplies, lack of childcare options, and high cost of living all worked together to increase the likelihood that the infants of the city's poorest women would not reach their first birthday.

Over the first two decades of the twentieth century, the fight against infant mortality took on transcendental importance in Havana, drawing the participation of new women's groups, the city press, medical workers, public health officials, politicians, and the working women whose children were most at risk. But while all seemed united in the medical nationalist project to save Cuban babies, there were deep divisions over the appropriate public responses to the public health crisis. These differences reflected a still-developing epidemiological picture of infantile enteritis, but they also highlight long-standing divides among medical nationalists over how to best lead Cuba to health and modernity. We can identify three main positions that various advocates adopted. The first group, including the inveterate reformer Manuel Delfín and a growing cohort of women's organizations, most stridently called attention to the economic roots of the problem in women's poverty, poor housing conditions, hunger, and the early weaning of young children. For this group, the answer lay in antipoverty work and the provision of direct services such as free childcare, food aid, and economic assistance to offset the high cost of living in Havana. While this group initially focused on private organizational efforts, perennial funding shortfalls limited the reach of their work, and over time they increasingly advocated for far-reaching state interventions into the gendered economy as the answer to infant mortality.

Most public health officials, however, saw such economic issues as out of the purview of the Ministry of Health. Rather than tackle national-level economic realities or directly intervene in the gendered urban economy, then, state efforts focused instead on regulating the mothering practices of the poor. Economic explanations for child death were subordinated to cultural interpretations, based on the assumption that poor women rejected expert hygienic counsel and endangered the lives of their children by improperly feeding them and that early weaning was a choice rooted not in economic necessity but in maternal ignorance. New health education campaigns therefore targeted poor urban women in order to extirpate "colonial habits" and inculcate the new techniques of modern scientific mothering. The campaign against infant mortality that developed in the 1910s represented the state's profound intrusion into the home and made the most intimate relationship between mother and child an object of elite surveillance and scrutiny. But it did little to improve the material conditions of poor families. By the 1920s, a third group entered these debates. For a growing cohort of eugenicists like Domingo F. Ramos, the root cause of infant mortality was neither economic nor cultural but fundamentally "racial" or biological. The answer, therefore, lay not in support for working mothers or hygienic education but in preventing those deemed "unfit" from reproducing.

These debates over the causes of and solutions to the infant mortality crisis were not just about appropriate public health practice or the limits of state responsibility; they also were, at their heart, about the meanings of motherhood, children's lives, and women's poverty in postindependence Cuba. As with the battle against yellow fever or the plague, the campaign against infant mortality resonated in multiple national and transnational registers. Emerging as the most extensive long-term health campaign after the creation of the new ministry, infant health work was deeply embedded in the nationalist politics of Cuban medicine. With the tens of thousands of Cuban children killed during the reconcentration still in living memory, this work came to represent the fulfillment of the medical nationalist promise of a state and society that cared for rather than ignored its youngest. But it also represented the battle to cement Cuba's place among "civilized" nations, as the infant mortality rate was already becoming a signifier of what would eventually be termed "underdevelopment."[6] Finally, the reduction of infant mortality would increase population growth, thereby reducing the need for immigrant workers. As Health Minister Enrique Nuñez argued, "Saving Cuban children from poverty, sickness, and death is patriotic work preferable to that of promoting the immigration of unknown individuals, degenerated by social and physical maladies, completely lacking the ties that unite one to the land in which they are born."[7] At the center of this campaign—as the objects of both scorn and intermittent support—were the working women of the city. They fed and cared for their children as best they could and sought medical services when they fell ill. But with officials vacillating between blaming poor women and recognizing the economic roots of the crisis, the campaign against infant mortality was never able to commit to a set of policies that could have significantly reduced infant death.

## GENDERED POVERTY AND THE LIMITS OF PRIVATE PHILANTHROPY

In the hot summer months of 1904, little flyers began appearing in small shops and open-air markets, public medical clinics, and Spanish-run bodegas across the city. They announced the opening of a new organization: La Casa del Pobre, or House of the Poor. Founded by the inveterate reformer and physician Manuel Delfín, its mission was to give aid to the city's poorest women and children. Whether by coming across one of these notices or increasingly, through word of mouth, poor women across the city learned that La Casa del Pobre might help them secure some basic resources—food, bedsheets, maybe even funds to cover a few months' rent during especially hard times—as well as basic medical services and useful tips for keeping their families healthy. They might enroll their children in the free breakfast program run by Delfín's Dispensario La Caridad, get help finding a decent job, or even borrow work implements like a sewing machine, an iron, or a small oven, which would allow them to earn money from sewing or taking in laundry or making small confections—anything that would help them support their families.[8] As is evident from this list of services, La Casa del Pobre was primarily an antipoverty organization, but one whose real goal was to reduce the city's exorbitant infant mortality and tuberculosis rates.

In many ways, Manuel Delfín was an early proponent of what today are called the "social determinants of health," a model for understanding disease that eschews a narrow biomedical focus on microscopic disease vectors and focuses less on individual behaviors than on the social and economic contexts that facilitate ill health. Delfín had written often and eloquently in the pages of La Higiene of the plight of the poor and ill of Havana, creating portraits of the destitute children and women who turned to his Dispensario La Caridad that he hoped would spur his readers to actively support this work. Daily contact with these families seems to have shaped his thinking, as Delfín's writing increasingly reflected an understanding of the relationship between disease and gendered poverty. Many early articles in La Higiene painted a picture of willful maternal ignorance as the cause of the city's high infant mortality rates, but Delfín's later writings focused much more on the structural causes of women's poverty and disease.[9] As Delfín came to understand, disease control efforts were of little use if they did not also address the role of poverty in spreading illness. But gendered poverty itself was the product of a society that devalued women's labor and made it profoundly difficult for single women to support themselves and their families.

There were, in early-twentieth-century Havana, few economic opportunities for women. For those without the support of male breadwinners—single women with children, widows, and women abandoned by their husbands—life was often quite precarious. Census data from 1907 show a gendered urban labor market that relegated women, especially women of color, to the lowest-paying work. More than three-quarters of working women were employed as *costureras*, *lavanderas*, and *criadas*, but the wages that sewing, laundry, and domestic labor garnered barely covered the basics for a single woman, let alone a family. Almost 10 percent of working women were lucky enough to find work in a tobacco factory, but here, too, women were stuck in the lowest-paying jobs.[10] Reflecting the racialized urban labor market, the worst-paying jobs were disproportionately relegated to women of color: although making up only 30 percent of the city's female population, women of color comprised 57 percent of all female domestic workers, 88 percent of laundresses, and 74 percent of seamstresses.[11] And, as Anasa Hicks has shown, employers regularly paid black domestic workers less than native white Cubans or Spaniards for the same work.[12] Low wages did not go far in notoriously expensive Havana, whose tight housing market allowed landlords to charge exorbitant rents. Exacerbating matters, much of the city's food supply was imported and therefore subject to high duties that were disproportionately felt by the city's poorest families.[13] The result, in Delfín's words, was that a single mother could "not earn, even making miracles, enough for the sustenance of her children."[14]

The gendered and racialized urban economy left its mark on the bodies of poor women, as hunger, exhaustion, and stress weakened their immune systems and poor housing conditions facilitated the spread of infection. As Delfín noted,

> [For] a woman stuck to the sewing machine or to the washing trough from dawn to midnight, who eats poorly, who lives in a cave-like room where within its circumference can be heard the moans of her hungry children; her work efforts, far from contributing to her subsistence, drain her body and prepare her for gynecological afflictions or for the terrible tuberculosis. And this ensues because what she is paid for her labor barely suffices to pay for the horrible little room in which she lives, without leaving anything to nourish herself and her children.[15]

Literary flourishes aside, Delfín's analysis is largely correct. Depressed wages and few social safety measures meant that life expectancy for the city's poorest families was grim. We can see this most clearly in the racialized breakdown of infant mortality. According to the 350-page study of infant mortality that Rafael Fosalba presented to the Cuban Academy of Science in 1914, babies of color were extraordinarily more likely to die within their first year than white babies.[16] While the overall death rate for infants of color was double that for white children, within the first two weeks after birth, newborns of color were 3.8 times as likely to die than white newborns. Further, women of color had 66 percent more stillbirths than white women. As Fosalba explained, these numbers reflected the precarious living conditions—lack of healthy housing, insufficient nutrition, overwork, and greater stress—that women of color faced in the early republic.[17] But for Fosalba, it was women's work outside the home that most directly contributed to infant death, for "any form of work or other reason that separates the mother from the newborn increases the likelihood that it will lose its life."[18] It was precisely this nexus of gender, poverty, and disease that Delfín hoped to address in creating La Casa del Pobre. Delfín believed that by providing basic resources and improving the living conditions of the poor, disease rates across the city could decrease. Tuberculosis, for example, could "be reduced to the most minimum expression" if "we could abundantly feed poor families and avoid their being cast out every month from the extremely modest shelters that they occupy."[19]

While Manuel Delfín primarily sought private donations for La Casa del Pobre, he knew that government funding would ensure its long-term success. And it seemed obvious that the government would support the mission of the organization, whose stated goal was to help the poor "avoid the [public] Hospital and make the asylum unnecessary" by providing preventative health services and basic economic resources.[20] But securing state support proved extremely difficult. During the second U.S. occupation, Delfín wrote to the provisional governor of Cuba, Charles Magoon, asking for state funding for La Casa del Pobre, as the needs of urban residents had rapidly outpaced the organization's resources.[21] In less than three years, over 1,000 families, representing 3,159 women and 4,213 children, had turned to La Casa del Pobre for assistance. For Delfín, the "miserable situation of such a rapidly growing number of destitute merit[ed] the attention of the public powers." But no financial support from the provisional government would be forthcoming. In a terse statement to Governor Magoon, government advisor E. St. Greble wrote that La Casa del Pobre "does no work which could legitimately be asked to be done by the Government." Reflecting perennial American concerns about the dangers of state support for private charities, Greble recommended "that no aid be extended to this society. It is strictly a private one and if the income is not sufficient to cover the expenses, it should do as every other private society does—retrench in its expenses."[22]

In the coming years, even as the numbers of poor families seeking La Casa del Pobre's aid swelled, elite support for the organization plunged.[23] With philanthropic spending fluctuating with the broader economy, small organizations like Delfín's struggled. By 1913, donations were less than a fourth of what they had been just three years prior. The following year the organization's board dissolved for lack of participation, leaving the entire work of the organization in the hands of its aging president, Manuel Delfín, and its secretary, Ramón Ramírez.[24] Despite years of petitions and pleas to state officials, the organization received no government support aside from the small, if steady, monthly subvention from the Havana City Council. The organization's work, as a result, suffered considerably. Amid growing financial struggles, support given to each family dwindled. Food rations were cut significantly, so that the Casa's meager funds could aid more families, even at a lower rate.[25] As Delfín wrote in 1913, "We have not been able to fulfill our program due to lack of public patronage and due to the scant cooperation that the State, Province, and Municipality have lent us." Reflecting his deep disappointment with the lack of government support for a potentially lifesaving antipoverty measure, he added, "Here the State has always been little concerned with these things that look toward the future."[26]

But even as Delfín was writing these lines, an expansive new public campaign to address infant mortality was being organized in the capital. The health ministry's new Servicio de Higiene Infantil, or Children's Health Service, represented, in the words of an American observer, "nothing less than a complete state department of child welfare."[27] Based largely on the work of Cuban physicians Eusebio Hernández and Domingo F. Ramos, the Children's Health Service was meant to improve maternal and children's health through hygienic education and new health care institutions, but unlike Delfín's innovative work, it did not directly address the role of poverty in creating the conditions for disease and infant death.

## A MOST POWERFUL AID TO THE HEALTH AUTHORITIES

In many ways, obstetrician and military general Eusebio Hernández Pérez represents the ideal figure of Cuba's early-twentieth-century medical nationalism. Of impeccable *independentista* credentials, Hernández was famous for his revolutionary activities during Cuba's long struggle against Spain. He fought in all three anticolonial wars, beginning at the age of sixteen, when he took up arms during the Ten Years War. When that war ended with both slavery and the island's colonial ties intact, he refused to recognize the peace agreement and helped organize the short-lived Guerra Chiquita. Over the following years in exile, he balanced medical duties and revolutionary work, serving as medical director of a hospital in Tegucigalpa, Honduras, while helping build the exiled revolutionary movement. He finally returned to the island in 1896 to fight in the final War of Independence, where he gained acclaim as a military surgeon and was eventually promoted to the rank of general in the Liberation Army.[28]

In the interim, Hernández traveled to Europe to further his medical education, studying obstetrics in Paris under the famous French obstetrician and social reformer Adolphe Pinard. In Paris, the revolutionary Cuban physician was able to participate in the obstetrical revolution initiated by Pinard, including the development of manual version to aid in the delivery of a breached fetus and new medical treatments for placenta previa.[29] But for Hernández, Pinard's influence extended far beyond his obstetrical work. As a prominent medical reformer whose work addressed infant and maternal mortality and morbidity, and as an influential figure in the development of puericulture, Pinard's work helped shape Hernández's efforts to use the benefits of medical science to transform Cuban society. Derived from the Latin for "the cultivation of the child," "puericulture" was defined by Pinard as "the science that has for its object the investigation of the facts relative to the reproduction, conservation, and betterment of the human species." In practice, puericulturists focused on maternal and child care, sexual and hygienic education of parents, and aid to poor families. As a scientific agenda that centered around reproductive and child health, and as a model for organizing public support for new health care institutions, puericulture would have an enormous influence on Hernández and, later, on Cuban health work.

During the first decade after independence, Eusebio Hernández was able to direct his nationalist politics and medical expertise to some of the major health problems facing the young republic. As professor of obstetrics at the University of Havana, he began what would be three decades of preparing new generations of Cuban obstetricians. For Hernández, being a physician and a scientist did not mean separating oneself from the problems of society. According to one of his medical students, he would often pause in the middle of his scientific lectures and express his indignation with the terrible living conditions of the poor, the country's high infant mortality rates, illiteracy, and malnutrition, "as if to make clear that a physician, even a specialist, must contemporaneously develop their social conscience, which would culminate in an urgent sense of duty" to the nation.[30]

While he would continue to participate in Cuban politics, teach, and publish scientific articles, perhaps his most important socio-medical contribution was the creation of homiculture. Derived from Latin meaning "the cultivation of the individual," homiculture elaborated on the work of Pinard, incorporating puericulture but extending its reach to all aspects of human health and development. Together with his student and protégé Domingo F. Ramos, Hernández developed homiculture as a comprehensive science of human heredity and reproduction, linking maternal and infant health to the study of environmental factors in pregnancy and early childhood that affected child development, as well as exploring genetic influences on health and reproduction.

In their 1911 book *Homicultura*, Ramos and Hernández outlined an expansive national project organized around the new science to address maternal and child health in Cuba.[31] They argued that infant mortality could only be brought under control through the kind of specialized government campaign that helped rid the island of yellow fever, linking scientific research and public health action, hygienic education and direct medical care. They proposed the vast expansion of maternal health services in Havana, including a comprehensive maternity hospital and new home health services. The plan also included a virtual sampler of policies based on innovative foreign models, including home births assisted by licensed midwives under the supervision of a clinic obstetrician, as was then the practice in New York City; *Kinderschutzen*, or asylums for women who had just given birth; *gouttes de lait*, or distribution centers where free pasteurized milk would be given out to poor mothers; and crèches, or day nurseries where women could leave their children when they went to work. The plan also advocated the passing of laws similar to the Roussel Law of France, which regulated wet nurses and "defended the children's rights to their mother's milk."[32]

That Hernández and Ramos's work was steeped in transnational debates over how to organize maternal and infant health services is obvious. As the above list of proposals makes clear, the Cuban homiculturists had a catholic interest in foreign health laws and institutions. As they were well aware, the United States was making strides in consumer protection laws that helped reduce its infant mortality rates. German *Kinderschutzen* and U.S. day nurseries were valuable institutions that, Hernández and Ramos believed, could be fruitfully replicated in Cuba. But the strongest influence on their plan was certainly the tradition of French maternal and child protection laws, crèches, *gouttes de lait*, and obstetrical and pediatric innovations that both doctors had seen firsthand in their studies in France.[33] But their goal was never to simply reproduce European and North American institutions and medical projects. As their elaboration of puericulture into the science of *homicultura* makes clear, Hernández and Ramos did not see themselves as imitators or junior partners in transnational medical debates. Instead, they sought to expand the work of their European and U.S. counterparts, do innovative scientific research, and create health institutions that responded to specific Cuban conditions.

As Nancy Stepan, Alejandra Bronfman, and others have shown, homiculture was an important influence on Cuban and Latin American eugenics and played an important role in national and transnational scientific debates in the 1910s and 1920s.[34] But it emerged first as a response to the capital's troubling infant mortality rates and shaped new on-the-ground institutions that affected the lives of tens of thousands of urban residents. Indeed, the goal of this new science was always to provide a framework for organizing state and private efforts to reduce infant mortality. For years, Hernández had been frustrated by the lack of government support for his work. After returning to Havana at the end of the final War of Independence, Hernández hoped to found Havana's first, and much needed, modern obstetrics clinic, but he received no support from the first U.S. occupation government. Although the Havana City Council approved funds to support it, the "American authorities did not find themselves willing to cede me one of the many unoccupied buildings the State possessed."[35] When he was finally given space for an obstetrics clinic at Mercedes Hospital, it was much smaller than he had hoped and met neither the needs of an obstetrics research and teaching hospital nor the needs of the city's residents: "What should have begun as a lying-in hospital in the capital of our young republic, was reduced to a simple ward in a general Hospital where my students receive a deficient instruction, which is all that can be furnished with such few elements."[36]

With the creation of Cuba's new Ministry of Health, Hernández's work finally began to receive the attention of public officials. From the earliest days of the ministry, children's health work was articulated as a priority, but it was divided among various projects, like tuberculosis education and the health inspection of children in schools. But in homiculture, health officials saw a viable research agenda and institutional framework for improving children's and maternal health throughout the island. Declaring his support for Hernández's "patriotic and humanitarian plans," Secretary of Health

Manuel Varona Suárez requested targeted funding from the president and appointed Hernández and Ramos to a special committee to oversee the best means of putting their proposals on infant and maternal health into practice.[37] The minister proposed that the first step would be to construct a new hospital that would serve as the national center for the organization of homiculture, with obstetrics, children's health, and gynecological services as well as dispensaries and clinics. It would be not just a hospital for children and women but "a school for mothers" that would teach women how to care hygienically for their infants and preserve their health. In honor of the founder of homiculture and as a sign of the influence of French thought on Cuban obstetrics and pediatrics, Varona Suárez proposed calling this new hospital the Pinard-Hernández Palace of Homiculture.[38] As Hernández wrote in 1911, "The indifference which I have encountered on the part of the public authorities of the country has now been followed by a period of attention, first, and afterwards of enthusiasm. I believe that my ideal is on the way to its realization."[39]

Eusebio Hernández and Domingo Ramos had reason to be optimistic. By 1910, Ramos was in charge of the health ministry's new puericulture office, where he was busy conducting research and analyzing health statistics. Hernández and Ramos headed a special commission to advise the ministry on how to put their maternal and child health program into practice. But under the presidency of José Miguel Gómez (1909–13), funding for the expansion of health services would be difficult to come by. In 1911, Health Secretary Miguel Varona Suárez sent a terse letter to President Gómez complaining of his shrinking budget, even as new laws called for the expansion of health and sanitary services.[40] While other, non-health-related government projects were moving forward, budget cuts forced public health reforms to be put on hold. "It is lamentable," he wrote, "that the demands of other Government Departments do not permit me to expand my budget in order to address the [country's public health] deficiencies, as Hygiene and modern Science demand, for the benefit of the public's health." It would take another two years and the election of a new president before any substantial work on maternal and infant health would begin.

ON JULY 18, 1913, at the height of the dangerous summer season and less than two months after taking office, President Mario Menocal signed a decree establishing the Children's Health Service within the Ministry of Health. According to its preamble, the goal of Decree No. 441 was to "diminish as far as possible the present high percentage of infant mortality which prevails . . .

in the capital of the Republic."[41] To that end, it incorporated many of the proposals put forth by Hernández and Ramos, including the registration and inspection of wet nurses, the expansion of milk inspections, and the creation of a special sanatorium for tubercular children. It established the Consultorio de Higiene Infantil, or Children's Health Clinic, which provided free medical care as well food donations to poor children and their mothers.[42] With the decree encouraging physical education and outdoor activities for maintaining children's health, the government funded the creation of the Colony for Children's Sanitary Defense at the Triscornia Immigration Center and the new Granja de Verano, a summer health camp for poor children organized by Manuel Delfín. Medical inspectors attached to the service were responsible for much of the ministry's infant and maternal health work, from overseeing the children's vaccinations to promoting physical education and providing basic health care to pregnant women and children.

While the new Children's Health Service provided some important new health care services, the program was much more limited than the expansive state health action that Hernández and Ramos had envisioned. Like many other ostensibly "national" public health campaigns of the period, the reach of the campaign was limited to the capital, with the Children's Health Service placed under the authority of Havana's local Department of Public Health. Rather than substantially expand state health services or create a modern maternity or children's hospital, as Hernández and Ramos advocated, the main thrust of the law was a vigorous surveillance regime. Medical inspectors, almost always nurses working with the Children's Health Service, would inspect schools, crèches, and asylums at regular intervals and submit reports on the condition of each. But while these institutions were subject to government inspection and oversight, the core of the new surveillance regime focused on women whom public health authorities believed to be most directly responsible for the city's infant mortality crisis: unlicensed midwives and wet nurses and "ignorant" popular-class mothers. As the decree announced, "poor women during their pregnancy and rearing of their offspring" during their first two years of life would now be subject to "inspection and sanitary instruction."[43] Inspectors were to "give special attention to the dwelling places of poor people, exacting perfect cleanliness of their rooms, halls, corridors, stairs and yards." They were also to investigate midwives in their area and report any unlicensed midwifery to the courts. And they were to make sure all area wet nurses remained in strict compliance with sanitary regulations and undergo regular health examinations, including submitting samples of their breast milk for bacteriological examination.[44] Any wet nurse found "not in the proper condition to suckle a child" would be denounced to the courts, "charged with fraud, deception, and as a danger to public health."[45]

Some programs were later added to address the deeper causes of child death, including a new school breakfast program meant to help protect poor children from "diseases brought about by organic weakness."[46] And mothers bringing their babies to the ministry's Children's Health Clinic could receive free cans of condensed milk, which provided a sanitary alternative to breast milk for times when they would be away from their children. Indeed, each month the clinic would give out thousands of cans of condensed milk, as well as conduct routine maternal and infant medical exams and perform the occasional circumcision.[47] But these consultations were also an opportunity for the nurses and physicians at the clinic to give "conferences and advice to mothers" about the hygienic rearing of their children.[48] Pregnant women were taught "the hygienic principles of pregnancy," and mothers with children under two years old were urged to breastfeed their children. As we will see below, convincing Cuban women to nurse their babies was "the fundamental point of the entire children's hygiene campaign."[49]

## "DO NOT KILL YOUR LITTLE CHILD": MILK, MODERNITY, AND SCIENTIFIC MOTHERING

As Cuba's medical researchers repeatedly showed, infantile enteritis was the greatest cause of infant death on the island. Yet its solution seemed clear. Researchers pointed to the improper nourishment of young children as the primary cause of the often fatal gastrointestinal ailments of Cuban babies.[50] The problem, they all agreed, was that Cuban mothers were weaning their children too early, substituting cow's milk of uncertain quality for the breast milk that medical reformers saw as the "right" of Cuban children. In order to tackle the problem, reformers and health officials worked on two fronts: on one hand, they would strengthen the oversight and regulation of milk production and distribution to ensure that urban residents were not exposed to adulterated, spoiled, or tainted milk; on the other hand, reformers organized a multipronged health education offensive, aimed at the city's women, to transform popular childrearing habits. A broad array of *higienistas*, public health officials, home inspection nurses, and crèche workers urged mothers to exclusively breastfeed their infants, to consult medical experts before attempting to wean their children, and to take extreme care with introducing cow's milk to their babies. Together, these two initiatives sought to ensure that the city's children would be given healthy and safe nourishment "appropriate to their age."

The argument for breastfeeding infants was simple: the still-developing digestive systems of young babies were too delicate for any other forms of nutrition, and cow's milk was a potentially deadly substitute. With much of Havana's milk traveling long distances from farm to city, with dairy and milk delivery workers of dubious hygiene, and with home refrigeration still extremely rare in the homes of the poor, there were just too many potential sources of bacteriological infection to assure parents that cow's milk would be safe for their young children. As a 1914 study presented at the Cuban Academy of Science argued, the milk supply in Havana, while nutritionally sound, was "bacteriologically tainted by improper manipulation."[51] There were many points of bacteriological infection, from filthy conditions in dairies to sick workers handling the milk to the reuse of bottles without disinfection. But even in the best conditions, as Cuban *higienistas* strove to make clear to their readers, cow's milk was "one of the best mediums for the cultivation of microbes."[52]

The first order of business for the sanitary campaign, then, was the regulation and oversight of the city's milk supply. Medical inspectors were responsible for visiting the city's cow stables, dairies, and ice cream establishments, making sure they were in "rigid compliance" with the health codes and ensuring that all establishments were "maintained in proper hygienic condition."[53] Inspectors would regularly examine milk from any establishment that sold it and send the samples to the ministry's Bromotological Service for microscopic analysis if the milk was suspected of being adulterated or of bad quality.[54] Cows would be inspected to ensure their health, and even milk delivery, café, and dairy workers were subject to hygienic inspection: those "attacked by any transmissible disease . . . [or] suffer[ing] from an ailment of the skin of any kind" would be "retire[d] from such work."[55] Printed cards outlining the new sanitary ordinances were distributed to all sectors of the city's dairy industry.

Workers in these industries resented this expanded sanitary surveillance. Like the Spanish commercial sector that complained of the economic damage caused by the anti–bubonic plague campaign, dairy industry workers saw the sanitary campaign as a threat to their economic interests and an unnecessary intrusion of the state. According to Enrique Barnet, *lecheros* "grumbled a great deal" about the new oversight "and cursed the health department," saying the new regulations were "bad for business."[56] Barnet wrote scathing articles about milkmen, accusing them of being, in the majority, "poisoners of the public" who regularly adulterated the milk they sold, watering it down with unsafe water in order to increase their profits and caring nothing about contaminating the public.[57] For milkmen, Barnet wrote, "what is important is the business. If half of humanity gets sick and dies, what does it matter?"[58] Regardless of the actual prevalence of adulterated milk or unscrupulous milkmen, it is clear that medical inspectors sometimes provoked the ire of those whose products they inspected. According to court documents, in 1922, a medical inspector visited El Malecón café "in order to recover some samples of milk for analysis." The café owner, however, "tried to prevent him from doing so . . . insulted him, threatened him, and taking a revolver out of a drawer attempted to assault him." Luckily for the medical inspector, an "unknown person" grabbed the café owner's hand, preventing him from shooting.[59] While attempted murder of medical inspectors was thankfully rare, increased state oversight surely angered many in the dairy industry.

But if the regulation of milk supplies was fairly straightforward (if sometimes dangerous), changing the childrearing practices of the Cuban people would prove more complicated. To help spread the gospel of breastfeeding and supplement the "hygienic advice" that visiting nurses gave popular-class women during home inspections, the health ministry sought the aid of the city's newspapers and popular magazines. One new source of popular health education was Enrique Barnet's column "Conversations with the Doctor," published in the Havana weekly *El Figaro* and distributed for free by the Health Department. With an evangelist's zeal, Barnet pushed the importance of breastfeeding and warned mothers of the myriad everyday dangers that surrounded their children. His column was filled with vivid illustrations: a mother weeps over an empty crib; a grotesquely oversized fly sits atop a child's plate; a sitting infant is encircled by a ghastly group of dancing diseases; an improperly fed "sickly, sad" baby sits beside a "healthy, happy" infant raised exclusively on breast milk, with the caption imploring mothers, "Do not kill your little child!" In one column, Barnet outlined the many potential points of contamination between farm and home that made cow's milk so dangerous for young children.[60] The adjoining illustration shows a long tube stretching from a cow's udder and passing through train station, train, wholesaler, dairy, and milkman and finally reaching "the victim," a sickly child nursing from a bottle of tainted milk. This dangerous trek from cow to child, full of unseen points of possible infection, is counterposed to an image of a mother serenely nursing her child, reinforcing the safety and naturalness of breastfeeding. The caption reads, "God's Law: A Mother's Milk is for her Baby, A Cow's Milk is for her Calf," and the text at the bottom of the image warns, "Do not flout God's Law! For the good of your baby, give it the breast!" Nevertheless, he warned, while "all the doctors incessantly preached" this message, "few mothers listened."[61]

Indeed, Cuban women's inattentiveness to the hygienic counseling of Cuban doctors was a regular refrain during this period. Barnet and others regularly complained that although "few mothers really [knew] how to take care of their children," they listened to the advice of "ignorant" neighbors over their medical counsel.[62] Since the end of Spanish rule, Cubans had made great sanitary strides, actively participating in urban health campaigns against yellow fever and the bubonic plague. But Cuban mothering, reformers groused, remained embedded in colonial habits and superstitions. Havana-based physician Juan Valdés complained that young mothers often "imprudently listen to the advice of those around them, almost always old women. In this way old errors and backwardness reproduce themselves generation after generation."[63] On a similar note, Barnet complained that "many mothers let themselves be completely guided by the counsel and superstitions of the neighborhood grandmothers, of nosy midwives, and their wet nurse friends. This is a great error, sustained by ignorance."[64] For *higienistas* like Barnet and Valdés, who sought to assert physicians' professional authority over questions of child health and maternal practice, the answer lay in the "difficult struggle against customs, prejudices and superstitions" of women, replacing the trusted counsel of grandmothers and neighbors with the medical authority of the physician.[65]

In asserting their professional expertise over mothering practices and pushing women to nurse their infants, Cuban health workers were part of a growing transnational movement to modernize motherhood, replacing ostensibly backward habits with the medical benefits of scientific motherhood. From Porfirian Mexico to Progressive Era United States, across Europe and throughout the British empire, physicians, nurses, and health officials extolled the benefits of breastfeeding and sought to educate women in the hygienic care of their offspring.[66] In each historical context, however, these efforts took on different associations and meanings, and in Cuba the mothering practices of the poor became the central front in the medical nationalist project of saving children. Whether through magazine columns like Barnet's and journals like *La Higiene* or through home visits by nurses and doctors or trips to the city's dispensaries and clinics, women in Havana were increasingly exposed to the new hygienic commandments. Posters in clinics, articles in newspapers, and workers in crèches all spoke in one voice, exhorting women to exclusively breastfeed their babies until they were old enough for solid foods. One particularly blunt image from Enrique Barnet's "Conversations with the Doctor" series commanded mothers not to "kill their little children" by denying them breast milk.

The campaign against infant mortality therefore balanced new programs with punitive supervision, support with blame. For women who ignored hygienic counsel, the physician Juan Valdés proposed punitive measures. While he advocated for the expansion of public services to support mothers with food aid and expanded health services, Valdés believed that women should be compelled to nurse their young. He proposed that the state mandate that mothers be required to breastfeed their children, arguing that mothers who do not are guilty of murder: "One of the most powerful resources on which we could rely to greatly reduce infant mortality is legislation that would obligate mothers to nurse their children, as is their duty, with the milk that nature provides them, which it the best nourishment of the child . . . The mother that is able to nurse her child but does not give him the milk that belongs to him has committed infanticide."[67] While such legislation was not forthcoming, official discourse constantly reminded new mothers that it was their moral and medical responsibility to nurse their infants.

These discourses were meant to denaturalize child death and show mothers that their actions mattered, that they had the power to defend their children from disease and early death, if they only took the correct action. But they also placed blame on women who could not nurse their children due to work requirements or medical issues, as well as women who chose not to nurse. Unfortunately, sources are largely silent on how poor women felt about these efforts to transform their childrearing habits, although Domingo F. Ramos admits that "at the beginning, they were poorly received by the public."[68] Of course, women fed their children as best they could according to methods they learned from trusted sources. Better to listen to trusted neighbors than the intrusive medical inspectors who entered their homes with the purpose of changing their habits, telling them that the ways they cared for their babies could make them sick or kill them. And, of course, what most of these conversations ignored were the reasons why many poor women weaned their infants early: they often had no choice but to immediately return to whatever paid work they could find, often leaving their newborns in the care of relatives. In public, however, health officials asserted that poverty was no barrier to breastfeeding, that women simply needed to embrace their fundamental social role as mothers and commit themselves to their essential maternal task. This confounding disconnect between economic reality and public health policy was perhaps most clearly revealed in the ministry's newest effort to curb infant mortality, the Concurso Nacional de Maternidad, or National Motherhood Competition.

ON JANUARY 1, 1918, the Ministry of Health held its third annual Concurso Nacional de Maternidad. That morning an enormous crowd gathered at the ministry's headquarters, which despite the building's size soon became virtually impassable. In the building's central courtyard, large wooden bleachers adorned with flowers and palms filled with close to 600 mothers holding hundreds of young infants in their arms.[69] Their babies had been weighed, measured, and examined by a team of official judges from the ministry who carefully wrote down their measurements and pored over the reports that the visiting nurses of the Children's Health Service had compiled over months of periodic observation of these infants and their mothers in their homes across the city. On the morning of the competition, President Menocal personally presented the top honors to the three poor mothers who had been judged to best exemplify the fundamental goals of the event. These were women who had exclusively breastfed their children, who had closely followed the counsel of the ministry's visiting nurses, and whose infants evinced the chubby healthfulness the judges deemed indicative of exemplary maternal care. In all, dozens of prizes were awarded, from new Prizes for Fecundity for women with large, healthy families to prizes for poor women whose homes were judged by visiting nurses to be kept in as pristine hygienic condition as their often cramped spaces allowed.

Inspired by the growing trend of Better Baby Contests in the United States and England, the National Motherhood Competitions rapidly gained the interest of Cubans from across the island.[70] Wealthy families, city councils, local businesses, and elite clubs donated prize money, and by 1918, most municipalities were holding their own regular local *concursos*.[71] And local industry took advantage of their popularity by using pictures of corpulent prizewinning infants to sell malted beer to nursing mothers (see figure 4.1). While established by the Ministry of Health as a kind of "school for mothers" whose primary goal was to promote breastfeeding among the country's poorest women, it is easy to see why the contests captured the public imagination and drew the participation and support of Cubans of all classes.[72] Observers describe the throng of babies, "all cheerful, happy, and strong" as inspiring collective joy and pride, cementing community and national bonds.[73] And surely the pride of having their infants presented to a supportive public and their often thankless daily maternal labor recognized and lauded attracted the hundreds of poor women who participated each year, as did the potential

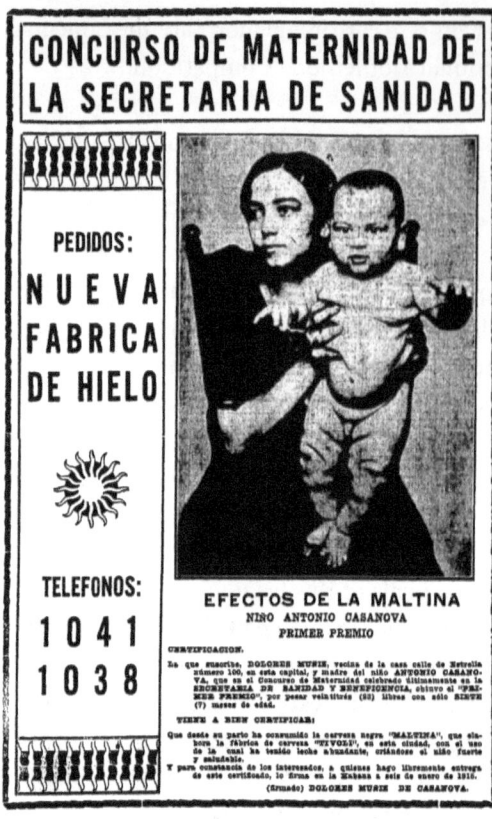

*Figure 4.1* Advertisement for Maltina malted beer, which promised lactating mothers "abundant milk" and "strong and healthy babies." (El Mundo, January 4, 1915)

to earn much-needed prize money. Beginning in 1918, wealthy families were also included, and well-to-do mothers brought their infants to be weighed and measured for honorary prizes. In a postcolonial society increasingly divided along class and race lines, then, the concursos brought together rich and poor, black and white, in a shared nationalist celebration of Cuban mother and child.

The National Motherhood Competitions reinforced the idea that mothers had a natural, moral, and even patriotic duty to nurse their young: indeed, as the mothers in attendance were told during the 1918 competition, "The future of the Nation depends, in large part, on the results of your endeavors."[74] But in elevating poor mothers who were nevertheless able to nurse their young and presenting them as "models of maternity" for all Cuban women, the health officials downplayed economic barriers to breastfeeding.[75] Sometimes they were explicit that there were no economic barriers at all. For José Antonio López del Valle, the director of Havana's local Department of Health, "the concursos present[ed] the spectacular example of mothers who, despite the difficult economic situations in which they find themselves, of the privations and heartbreaking struggles they experience due to their lack of resources, have nevertheless nursed their children at their own breast and complied with the health regulations, proving in this way that poverty does not prevent these practices." For López del Valle, proper health education and a nationalist embrace of "their most sacred duties" as mothers were all that was required to ensure the health of Cuban children. But poverty was most certainly a barrier to breastfeeding, as reports published by the Ministry of Health made clear. Indeed, in his 1917 study on infant mortality, Mario Lebredo admitted that poor urban women, forced by economic necessity to work in factories or in domestic labor, "cannot nurse their children with their own milk."[76] What was needed more than anything, he argued, was "the creation of crèches and shelters to care for young children" while their mothers "worked to earn a living."[77] By 1917, several crèches, or free daycare centers, did exist in the capital, providing an important source of free childcare for working women. But, as we will see, a lack of government support stymied this institution, leaving it out of reach for all but those mothers lucky enough to secure one of the limited spots.

## ORGANIZING FOR CHILDREN'S HEALTH: CRÈCHES, INFANT MORTALITY, AND THE LIMITS OF STATE SUPPORT

While the new Children's Health Service represented a narrow vision of state action to combat infant mortality, health officials hoped that private organizations would emerge to complement the state's limited role. In Havana, groups of middle- and upper-class women took up the call for action and formed a collection of new organizations that had as their central task protecting the health of poor children. Through these new organizations—including separate Women's Committees for the Protection of Children for the neighborhoods of Vedado and Habana Nueva, the National Congress of Cuban Mothers, and a Women's Committee made up of women employed by the Ministry of Health—elite *habaneras* formed an institutional framework for their participation in a health campaign of national importance and helped shape an emerging women's movement. Combining traditional maternal charity with modern medical nationalism, these new institutions gave these women an important platform for participating in national politics.[78] But they also created on-the-ground institutions that provided food, health care, and security for the city's children and gave Havana's working mothers safe places to leave their children while they worked in the city's factories, workshops, and upper-class homes. Once again, however, a lack of elite support and limited state funding hampered the ability of these new organizations to curb the city's infant death rate.

The National Congress of Cuban Mothers and the Habana Nueva Women's Committee for the Protection of Children provide two contrasting trajectories for elite women's involvement in child health and welfare issues in the 1910s and 1920s. Organized in response to the problem of infant mortality in the capital, the National Women's Congress had its roots in the work of the National Congress of Mothers, the U.S.-based child welfare organization. The National Congress of Cuban Mothers was Cuba's most elite women's philanthropical organization, bringing together the highest echelons of the Havana oligarchy.[79] Being very well connected, the National Congress of Cuban Mothers was able to secure the donation of the Hospital de Higiene —the recently shuttered state hospital for prostitutes—for use as an asylum and crèche.[80] That the Menocal government turned the state hospital for prostitutes into an organization for child health and welfare highlights the shifting priorities of the Cuban public health system, which had recently ended the state regulation of prostitution, often criticized as an immoral vestige of the colonial public health system. The new Asilo Menocal, with a staff of paid employees and Sisters of Charity, supported eighty children in its crèche and over fifty children in its asylum. In addition to the use of the building, the Asilo Menocal continued to receive regular financial support from the government.

Not all organizations, however, were as well connected. The Habana Nueva Women's Committee for the Protection of Children had a similarly auspicious beginning. In February 1914, a group of women from the Centro Habana neighborhood—including Angeles Mesa de Hernández, the wife of the revolutionary obstetrician and homiculturist Eusebio Hernández—set out to organize a crèche as part of the new movement to curb the city's high infant mortality rate.[81] In addition to caring for poor children while their mothers worked, the crèche offered nutritious food, free medical consults for children and pregnant women, and "health counseling for children of all ages." In line with the Children's Health Service campaign, the crèche's staff took extra care to counsel mothers "about the best manner to nurture and nurse their children," urging breastfeeding as the best method to ensure the health of their infants and "trying through all possible means to propagate maternal lactation." Mothers "who could not nurse their children, either due to a total lack of milk or an insufficient milk supply," would be given "excellent quality pasteurized milk" for their children.[82]

While the documentary record for the Crèche Habana Nueva is slight, reports from the Children's Health Service show that the crèche usually cared for thirty to forty children every day, filling the small space that was donated by the Health Ministry. The créche was clearly a key local institution, relied upon by the dozens of neighborhood women who every morning dropped their children off at the little childcare facility, knowing that their children would be fed and cared for while they worked in nearby factories, workshops, and elite households. But unlike the well-resourced Asilo Menocal, with its Sisters of Charity and regular government subventions, the Crèche Habana Nueva relied almost exclusively on the work of its volunteer board and the physicians who provided free medical consults for the crèche's children and their mothers. By the early 1920s, with funds stretched to their limit and the board exhausted, the Women's Committee began looking for a way out. As records from an emergency meeting held in 1924 attest, the crèche was barely surviving for lack of funds: "For a long time now, all the members have known that the Crèche was having a very insecure life, sustaining itself providentially, since members' dues only reached the insignificant sum of 30 pesos per month, more or less."[83] The issue was serious, especially for the forty children who attended the crèche every day, "who would be left abandoned were the crèche to close its doors, which would be lamentable given that these children are the sons and daughters of poor mothers, and receive there appropriate food, care, and instruction." But unable to maintain the crèche due to a lack of funding, and exhausted from the work of maintaining a volunteer organization in the face of government indifference, the governing board voted to join with and turn over the crèche to the Bando de Piedad, the organization run by the Sociedad Humanitaria de Cuba, which had been "very desirous of having its own crèche."[84]

The plan worked to save the crèche, which continued its work for decades, but the organization's financial crisis highlights both the importance that elite reformers attached to child health and welfare work, as they labored intensively to keep their financially strapped institution running, and the limits of the government's efforts to tackle infant mortality. As all observers agreed, the crèches were an important front in the fight against infant and child mortality, providing much-needed daycare, nutritious food, and medical care for poor children and medical consults for pregnant women and mothers. As Children's Health Service reports made clear, given the extreme poverty of many families, even the simple provision of healthy meals had important health effects: as one health inspector noted in 1917, "One can see the difference in favor of the children who have been attending [the crèche] for some time. There are some that when they were admitted could barely hold themselves up for lack of nourishment."[85]

But even though it provided essential health services, and even with its elite membership and strong connections to Eusebio Hernández and other health officials, the Crèche Habana Nueva was denied government financial support. In a 1924 letter to the city's director of *beneficencia*, the crèche's director noted that the organization "did not receive subventions or monetary assistance of any kind from the government. . . . On several occasions and under distinct Public Administrations, this aid had been requested, but always without success."[86] This lack of government support for all but the most politically connected organizations is emblematic of a child and maternal health program that focused more on surveillance, health education, and gathering statistics than on the provision of needed services to the urban (let alone rural) poor. As a 1915 report from the health ministry attested, two years after the much-heralded inauguration of the Children's Health Service, "very little has been done by the State to support . . . destitute children."[87] In discussing the work of the crèches, the report recommended the creation of more crèches to meet the needs of the urban poor and urged the minister of health to "urge the municipal governments of the island to allocate in their budgets annual subventions to these kinds of organizations."[88] But little changed in the coming years, as Rafaela Mederos de Fernández of the Congreso Nacional de Madres noted during the first National Women's Conference in 1923.[89] Although Havana's private crèches, asylums, and dispensaries did "aid many children, they were insufficient and incomplete. The army of destitute little ones that cannot obtain a spot [in these institutions] is numerous."[90] In the end, the crèches supported a very small percentage of the children of working mothers, underscoring, rather than meeting, the needs of the urban poor.

## EUGENICS, RACE, AND INFANT HEALTH

In 1924, while on an official visit to Paris, Cuban health official José Antonio López del Valle gave a lecture on "The Sanitary Advances of Cuba," in which he noted the great debt Cuban maternal and infant health policy owed to French medicine, especially to famous French obstetrician and puericulturist Adolphe Pinard.[91] Surely Cuba's Children's Health Service owed much to Pinard's influence on Cuban homiculture, especially through his student Eusebio Hernández. But by the early 1920s, French influence—which emphasized proper nutrition, health education, and access to medical care—was being eclipsed by the growing sway of North American eugenics. Efforts to promote proper childcare continued unabated, and new hospitals were opened for children and pregnant women. But for a growing segment of Cuban health officials and medical reformers, led by Domingo F. Ramos, improving the health conditions of Cuban children was not enough; what was needed was to prevent the "unfit" from reproducing to begin with. While infant health work would continue, Ramos would spearhead new plans to "improve the Cuban race" by imposing a series of eugenic laws limiting marriage to the healthy, restricting immigration, and forcibly sterilizing those deemed "unfit."

The growing influence of hard-line North American eugenics on Cuban science reflected and reinforced long-standing tensions within Cuban medical nationalism, which contained within it a range of perspectives about the best ways to use medical science to improve Cuban health and advance the Cuban nation. Eusebio Hernández had long emphasized the effects of poverty on maternal and infant health and advocated for legislation to protect workers' rights, reduce the cost of expensive primary goods, and address the exorbitant cost of living in the nation's capital. He loathed the country's growing economic inequality, the class and caste privileges of the urban elite, and the neocolonial influence of the United States. He believed that the health of the Cuban people could be improved through intelligent state interventions, the provision of social services, and a more equitable economic system.[92] In this, Hernández echoed the concerns of Cuban doctors and nurses throughout the republic. But by the late 1910s and early 1920s his protégé Domingo Ramos increasingly looked to North American racial science for answers to Cuba's long-standing health problems.

In 1921, Domingo F. Ramos was sent by the Ministry of Health to the Second International Congress of Eugenics in New York City, where he lectured on homiculture and its relation to eugenics. After the conference, Ramos began a long correspondence with the prominent American eugenicist Charles Davenport, and he would increasingly come to share Davenport's views on the importance of racial purity for the health and progress of the nation. If homiculture emphasized the positive influences hygienic reforms could have on the population, Ramos grew increasingly convinced that without limiting what he saw as "dysgenic" reproduction, progressive health reforms were actually counterproductive.[93] As he would later argue, it was not enough to protect the child; what was needed was to protect the child from a dysgenic birth.[94] For Ramos, improving health conditions, the terrain of homiculture, was of little use if an individual's "germ plasm" was faulty, since it would allow the unfit to reproduce, thereby spreading genetic "ills" throughout the population. But limiting reproduction to the genetically fit was also not enough, since "nothing comes from a good seed that has not been well cultivated." Public health reforms therefore needed to work in tandem with eugenic legislation to improve the "health of the race."[95]

Throughout the decade, Domingo Ramos and his allies in the Ministry of Health would try to popularize eugenic concepts in Cuba. They organized national and international conferences on eugenics, wrote articles in the local Havana press, sponsored public-private organizations such as the Social Hygiene League, and pushed for the passage of eugenics-inspired legislation, including the sterilization of criminals and the insane. During the First Pan-American Conference on Eugenics and Homiculture, held in Havana in 1927, Ramos urged delegates from across Latin America to press for laws restricting the reproduction of persons deemed genetically "harmful" and rejected the idea of national progress through *mestizaje*.[96] In 1927, the Ministry of Health began a campaign to restrict marriage to the genetically "fit," through the passage of a eugenic marriage certificate law.[97] But despite the explicitly white supremacist agenda of the North American eugenics that so influenced Ramos, on the ground, infant health programs continued to serve urban residents regardless of race and seem to have been especially utilized by Cubans of color.

Cuban scientists had noted since the early 1910s that infant mortality rates were consistently higher among Cubans of color, but public debates rarely addressed the racial dynamics of the problem.[98] This dynamic began to shift in the late 1920s, especially after a 1926 speech by Ángel Arturo Aballí at the National University brought new public attention to the rate at which black babies were dying in the Cuban capital.[99] Aballí was well positioned to propel the topic into public consciousness. As the island's preeminent pediatrician, Aballí had founded Cuba's first pediatrics clinic at Mercedes Hospital, was professor of pediatrics at the National University, and would go on to found the Cuban Society of Pediatrics. Aballí had spent decades studying the main causes of infant mortality, publishing works on infant gastrointestinal illness, malnutrition, and pediatric tuberculosis. In his 1926 speech, Aballí rejected racist explanations for black infant mortality as rooted in biology or the poor mothering habits of Cubans of color. Instead, he saw differential mortality as emerging out of economic conditions on the ground: an economy that relegated black women to the lowest-paying jobs, the highest levels of unemployment, and the worst housing conditions. The disproportionate death of black babies highlighted what was, at best, the

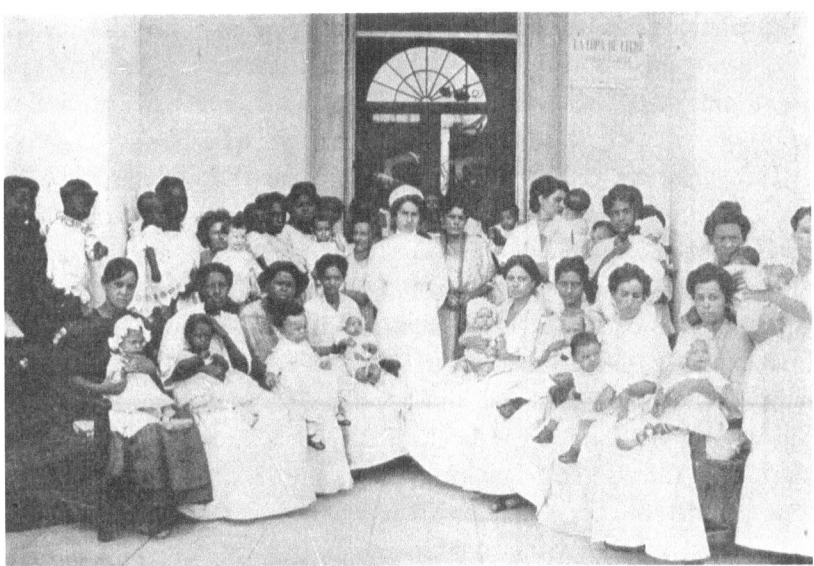

Figure 4.2 Mothers and their babies attending the Consultorio de Higiene Infantil, 1914. (Boletín Oficial de la Secretaría de Sanidad y Beneficencia de la Isla de Cuba, November 1914, 627)

partial reach of government health programs and the utter insufficiency of the city's private crèche system to meet the needs of poor women, among whom women of color predominated. But it was precisely the economic conditions that structured black mortality that made the city's few public medical institutions so important for black families.

While the records of the Health Ministry are largely silent about the demographics of those who utilized children's health services, evidence suggests that women of color sought these institutions out at rates higher than their percentage of the urban population. This surely reflects their higher rates of poverty compared with white women, who could more often pay for private medical care. But this also hints at the meaning these institutions held for the women who relied on them to safeguard their children's health, who increasingly looked to them for guidance on feeding and caring for their infants, or who relied on donations of canned food to supplement what they could purchase with their slim wages. Through their engagement with new children's health services, however, black women turned on its head the idea that poor women made poor mothers. Published photographs show the Children's Health Clinic filled with women and children of color, and black mothers won special prizes for highest regular attendance at the clinic and actively participated in National Motherhood Competitions, presenting their children as models of vibrant infant health and themselves as models of Cuban motherhood.[100] In short, they asserted their own definitions of respectable motherhood, based on their engagement with new state health institutions that would help them care for their children.

Throughout the early years of the republic, there was broad agreement that aggressive action was necessary to confront the crisis of infant mortality. But there were considerable differences of opinion over both the causes of the problem and the appropriate action to be taken. Was the problem primarily the ignorance of poor women, who did not know how to feed or care for their young children, or structural issues of poverty, which condemned impoverished women and their children to malnutrition and disease? And what kind of public resources should be expended to address the problem? The new Children's Health Service created by the Ministry of Health in 1914 was an impressive start. But the program was hobbled from the beginning by a perception that poor women themselves were primarily responsible for the diseases that decimated Cuban children. If officials hoped Cuban mothers would breastfeed their infants for the first nine months of their lives, they provided little access to services like childcare or support to stay at home, which could have aided mothers in doing so. Havana's working mothers faced a difficult bind in the early decades of the twentieth century. Forced to work to support their families in an expensive city, many had to wean their babies early. But where to leave them and whom to trust for advice on what to feed them? In the days before powdered infant formula and pasteurized powdered milk, these were choices with terrible implications.

If we trace the institutions and discourses that shaped early-twentieth-century Cuban maternal and infant health work, we gain a sense of the broader shifts that Cuban public health underwent during the first decades after independence. For medical reformers like Manuel Delfín and Eusebio Hernández, the immediate postindependence period was a time of great expectation and hope; the successful campaign against yellow fever was a sign of the wondrous benefits concerted public health and medical reforms could achieve in an independent Cuba. Infant mortality represented a special case study, however, for the ability of Cuban health institutions to achieve the kind of medical modernity envisioned by early medical nationalists. With infant mortality an important internationally recognized index, medical nationalists were eager to highlight the effectiveness of innovative Cuban health institutions, and the lives of poor urban children took on greater national significance. But health officials could not reproduce the success of the yellow fever or bubonic plague campaigns, for the causes of infant death were much more complex and required much more substantive economic interventions. The middle-class women who organized and struggled to keep open that first generation of crèches understood that infant mortality was fundamentally caused by women's poverty, and that only by supporting women—by providing food aid and no-cost childcare—could they hope to make an impact. But need always far outstripped availability, and the city's monthly mortality statistics served as a constant reminder of the utter insufficiency of these efforts. Nevertheless, as Cubans confronted the obstinate reality of disease in postcolonial Cuba, the connections between economic relations and health became increasingly clear, shaping medical discourse and opening new possibilities for public health action.

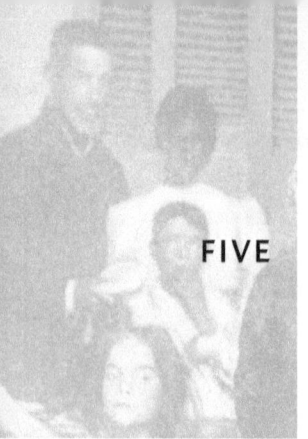

## FIVE   With All, and for the Good of All
### Race, Poverty, and Tuberculosis

ON AUGUST 18, 1929, the *Diario de la Marina* published "La tuberculosis en la raza negra."[1] Written by the prominent black journalist and politician Primitivo Ramírez Ros in "Ideales de una Raza," the weekly page dedicated to issues of concern to Cubans of color, the article was a powerful call to arms for Cuban society to tackle the problem of tuberculosis among Havana's black population. In the years since independence, a series of new public institutions and private organizations had emerged to reduce tuberculosis mortality in the Cuban capital, from the expansive national sanatorium and smaller institutions targeting "pretubercular" children to private organizations like the Cuban Anti-Tuberculosis League and the elite Damas Isabelinas. But while tuberculosis mortality had dropped from its turn-of-the-century heights, it remained frustratingly high, continuing to rank as the greatest cause of death in the Cuban capital. Moreover, the risk of death by consumption was not equal, with Cubans of color dying of the disease at much higher rates than white Cubans. As Ramírez Ros argued, "The odious white plague, in relation to the colored population of Cuba, could well be called the *black plague*."[2]

The article set off months of debate in the columns of "Ideales de una Raza" as Cuban journalists, physicians, and philanthropists debated the meaning and implications of the country's disproportionately black tuberculosis mortality. Were these deaths due to black ignorance or disregard for hygiene, as some elite observers alleged, or was the root cause an economic system that relegated Cubans of color to the lowest-paid jobs? What role should the state or private organizations take in curbing the city's high rates of infection and grim yearly death toll? These debates brought into the open long-standing issues at the heart of the city's public health landscape, highlighting both the complex social and biological causes of disease and the often fraught politics of health care in postindependence Cuba. More than any other disease in the early twentieth century, tuberculosis provides a lens onto the broader social and economic dynamics that shaped the health conditions of the Cuban people. Havana's disease landscape mirrored—even emerged out of—the city's racial economy, with Cubans of color relegated to lower wages, higher levels of unemployment, and substandard housing. As health experts regularly expounded, the key determinants of tuberculosis mortality were proper nutrition, sufficient rest, and adequate living conditions. As Ramírez Ros reminded his readers, however, for "the black race of Cuba . . . subjected against its will to a situation of poverty, habitual economic crisis, [and] a low standard of living," these basics conditions were often out of reach.

This was particularly true in the case of housing. Ramírez Ros, like many other reformers of the era, singled out the *solar*—the quintessential Cuban tenement. Housing in the Cuban capital was exorbitantly expensive, forcing poorer Cubans to live in cramped, overcrowded *solares* whose close quarters and terrible conditions, observers all agreed, facilitated the spread of tuberculosis. Reflecting the mix of overt moralizing and social concern of most elite observers, Ramírez Ros decried "the infected, nauseating *solar*, where a very great part of the Cuban population lives piled up, lacking air, lacking hygiene, in terrifying physical and moral promiscuity. The greater part of which IS BLACK."[3] For some public health officials and elite white observers, the *solar*—read as a black space of disease and poverty—was proof of black backwardness, immorality, and imperviousness to hygienic precepts. But for the journalists and politicians of color who increasingly pushed the government to put extra effort into tackling the disease among the city's black residents, disproportionate tuberculosis mortality rates represented more than just another troubling health statistic. Rather, the disease stood as an indictment of an economic and political system that kept Cubans of color in conditions of poverty and disease.

Tuberculosis is a disease of poverty. Despite its nineteenth-century reputation as a romantic disease of the wealthy, globally by the beginning of the twentieth century people who got sick (as opposed to just infected) with tuberculosis were overwhelmingly poor.[4] In most cases, tuberculosis is spread when people with active cases of the disease cough or sneeze or otherwise expel into the air droplets full of *Mycobacterium tuberculosis*. Transmission occurs when these droplets, which can remain airborne for several hours, are inhaled and make their way to the alveoli of the lungs. Factors that influence the probability of transmission include proximity, frequency, and duration of exposure, as well as environmental factors such as space and ventilation. Most often, initial infection results in the latent (asymptomatic and nontransmissible) form of the disease, but in some people—especially those with immune systems compromised by the stress, poor nutrition, overwork, and insufficient rest that marked the lives of the urban poor—the tubercle bacilli overcome the immune system, resulting in an active case of the disease. Active cases of tuberculosis can occur years, even decades, after initial exposure. Symptoms include terrible bouts of coughing, chest pain and difficulty breathing, fever and chills, numbing fatigue, and loss of appetite. It was and is a terrible wasting disease. Sick individuals become gaunt, weak, and wracked with a debilitating cough. As these symptoms worsen, work becomes impossible, and the subsequent loss of income plunges the family into subsequent cycles of poverty, hunger, disease, and death. In Cuba as everywhere, the highest rates of mortality were for those in the prime of their lives, between the ages of twenty and thirty-nine, making the progression from relative strength to wasting death all the more stark.[5]

All statistics tell stories. Perhaps the most revealing ones for early-twentieth-century Cuba are Havana's monthly mortality statistics published haphazardly in the Ministry of Health's official *Boletín*. These reports give us a glimpse into the living conditions of the urban poor, allowing us to see the effects of the city's gendered and racial economy, with low wages and high unemployment a determining factor in the ability of poor Cubans to feed, clothe, and shelter their families. The results, clearly shown in the mortality reports, were thousands cut down by a dreaded disease in the prime of their lives, often leaving behind sick children with dwindling prospects. They show us that while Cubans of color died of tuberculosis at alarmingly disproportionate rates, the problem was even worse for women of color. According to the 1929 mortality statistics for Havana, Cubans of color as a whole were 1.87 times as likely to die of tuberculosis than white Cubans. But women of color were a staggering 2.77 times as likely to die of tuberculosis than white women.[6] When we look into the national census data and see what kinds of jobs men and women of color in Havana held, especially in comparison with white Cubans, these numbers begin to tell a story of the devastating health effects of racial inequality in a country ostensibly committed to racial egalitarianism, as women of color, relegated to the lowest-paying jobs, bore the greatest burden of disease and death.

Yet there is much that these statistics do not tell us, and for that we must turn to other sources. It is well known that the poor often leave few traces with which historians can reconstruct their experiences, their ideas, their daily struggles with illness, and their difficulties making monthly rent payments. Generally, elites in Cuba did not much concern themselves with the lives of the poor. As public health official José López del Valle noted in 1924, the problem of urban housing was largely ignored by Cuban society. "It appears," he lamented, "that no one notices the bitter tears of the victims of these economic struggles."[7] But throughout the 1910s and 1920s, a small but steady trickle of newspaper and magazine articles and public health reports, and one book-length study, addressed the relationship between poverty, living conditions, and disease in the Cuban capital. These pieces were most often written by individuals with experience entering the homes of the poor—especially visiting nurses and doctors—who then became the most vocal proponents of aggressive social action, spurring further research and slowly making the issue one of greater public concern.

As historian Samuel K. Roberts writes, "Poor housing [is] what public health scholars would call a 'fundamental cause' of tuberculosis."[8] With fully a third of Havana's population living in unhealthy, overcrowded tenements, there was perhaps no greater issue affecting the day-to-day lives of urban residents.[9] Exposure to the disease in tight, enclosed spaces with poor ventilation increases the likelihood of transmission: with families crowded into small, dark, one-room apartments in early-twentieth-century Havana, a single member sick with the disease could quickly infect the rest of the household.[10] The roots of the housing crisis were many, but the general dynamic was well known: the combination of low wages and exorbitant rents—the latter exacerbated by real estate speculation, local corruption, and rural-to-urban migration—led to cycles of eviction, overcrowding, and disease for the city's poorest residents.

The discourse of medical nationalism came up against precisely these underlying structural issues and was unable to overcome them. As observers increasingly noted, if the root cause of the city's disturbingly high tuberculosis rate was economic, then what was needed was more than new hospital beds or dispensaries. Over the 1910s and 1920s, there began to emerge a growing sense of the need for deep structural reforms: new public medical institutions to address the immediate health care needs of the poor combined with broad economic reforms to increase wages and bring down rents and the cost of basic necessities. These reforms would, advocates hoped, help ameliorate the health effects of Cuban poverty. But as the debate in "Ideales de una Raza" made clear, neither poverty nor disease were colorblind. Unlike earlier medical nationalist debates, then, the fight against tuberculosis forced Cubans to confront the economic and racial dimensions of disease, rooted in a postcolonial order that condemned Cubans of color to greater suffering and death.

This reality of systemic racialized poverty and disease was at odds with the egalitarian raceless nationalism forged during Cuba's long anticolonial struggle, which had promised, in the words of José Martí, a nation "with all, and for the good of all." These debates therefore refracted a series of questions at the heart of republican politics, touching on the terms of black citizenship in a republic formally committed to racial egalitarianism: the degree to which the state should intervene in the market to guarantee a living wage, affordable housing, and low-cost food; and fundamentally whether health was a right of citizenship to be protected by the state or a privilege, with access to care determined by the market and supplemented by private charities. As we have seen, Cuban medical nationalists had for decades held a variety of positions on the appropriate scope of state or private responsibility for achieving their shared goal of a healthy republic. Whether shaped by racial and class biases born of their elite backgrounds or unwilling to confront the economic and political clout of local private interests, few public health officials pushed for the kinds of structural reforms that would have alleviated the disproportionate mortality of the city's poorest families. Health officials focused instead on the same policies that seemed so successful at the turn of the century: vector control, the isolation of individuals sick with infectious disease, and especially hygienic education campaigns to "modernize" the habits of the poor. By the late 1910 and 1920s, however, a growing chorus of nurses, health officials, journalists, and activists of color rejected the idea that tuberculosis could be "solved" through these traditional means, and they increasingly demanded economic interventions to reduce the cost of living and improve living standards. These kinds of reforms were outside the scope of private charities, however; they required firm state action. As we can see in the decades-long struggle against tuberculosis, Cubans of all classes increasingly took up the language of medical nationalism, latched onto the discourse of a healthy republic, and demanded health as a right rather than a privilege.

### EL SOLAR HABANERO:
### RACE, HOUSING, AND POVERTY IN HAVANA

In the decades after independence, the housing of the poor took on multiple, conflicting meanings. For the tens of thousands of Cubans who made their homes in Havana's *casas de vecindad, solares,* or *ciudadelas* (different terms used to describe tenement houses), these were where they raised their children, found religious community, took care of one another, sometimes fought, and often—disproportionately—got sick. But for most Cuban elites, these complex social spaces were reduced to a flat symbol of backwardness, vice, criminality, and disease. In newspaper and magazine articles, papers presented at the National Academy of Science, and book-length studies, Cuban physicians, elite feminist reformers, and public officials all decried the pernicious influence of these tenements on the island's health and morals. *Casas de vecindad* came in several forms. Some were old mansions subdivided over time to house many families, while others were constructed for that purpose—usually as a one-or two-story building with a central long patio lined with single-room apartments on either side (see figure 5.1). What they all held in common, as the esteemed medical figure Diego Tamayo noted in 1907, was their "general principle: store in the least space the maximum number of individuals."[11] They were also increasingly associated with the city's black population. Indeed, over time the term *solar* became closely tied to blackness, along with a host of social and health problems, from prostitution to gambling, ñañiguismo to illegitimacy, and gonorrhea to tuberculosis. For some, the *solar* became a potent symbol of the failure of the republic to reshape the morals of the Cuban people and achieve the kind of hygienic modernity envisaged by the first generation of medical nationalists. But for others, especially radical reformers and intellectuals of color, *solares* were an indictment of a corrupt racist system that relegated poor Cubans of color to substandard housing and disease.

Among the most important figures in republican debates over Havana's housing crisis was the black lawyer and writer Juan Manuel Chailloux Cardona, who in 1945 published his *Síntesis histórica de la vivienda popular: Los horrores del solar habanero.* Born in the rural outskirts of the far eastern town of Guantánamo, Chailloux was the son of a veteran of the wars of independence who fought under the famous black general Quintín Bandera. The elder Chailloux later rose up in the failed insurrection of the Partido Independiente de Color, which fought to address entrenched racial inequality in the republic. Chailloux's formal education was interrupted by poverty and political turmoil. Despite this, after years working as a shoemaker, clerk, and salesman, he moved to the capital, where he finished his high school education at night and eventually gained entrance to the University of Havana. During his early years in Havana, and throughout his time at the university, Chailloux struggled financially and lived in a *solar* in Habana Vieja. With his university schedule preventing him from continuing his work in shoe factories, Chailloux made ends meet selling knickknacks in the city's *solares*. And he was an excellent student, winning prizes for his work that allowed him to purchase the jacket, tie, and collared shirt that made up the required uniform at the university. *Síntesis histórica de la vivienda popular* was his final thesis, and it reflects both his years of study and personal experiences in the city's *solares*.

By the 1920s and 1930s, when Chailloux was working and living in the capital, the vast majority of the city's *solares* were in the central neighborhoods of Habana Vieja and Centro Habana. As wealthy families moved out to the tony western suburbs in the early decades of the twentieth century, their old mansions in the city center were increasingly turned into tenements.[12] But given the city's tight housing market, *solares* increasingly appeared wherever enterprising landlords could subdivide old mansions and generate a quick profit, even the more upscale neighborhoods of Vedado and Jesus del Monte.[13] And subdivide they did. Observers described how shrewd landlords took advantage of the city's housing shortage to rent any available space, including hallways or closets, and subdividing rooms in order to maximize their profits.[14] Chailloux describes old colonial mansions, "once occupied by a single family [and] now, deteriorated over time and divided and subdivided, home to more than one hundred persons." Those who could afford a little more were given the largest spaces and rooms with windows, while "those who can afford the least are given corners and nooks" with spaces divided "with cardboard or discolored cloth."[15] Sometimes landlords would take advantage of the high ceilings of old colonial structures—meant to facilitate the circulation of air during the hot summer months—to build mid-level lofts called *barbacoas*, effectively doubling the space available to rent while subjecting residents to stiflingly hot, low-ceilinged dwellings.[16] As the architect Pelayo Pérez put it, the attitude of the "modern urban landlord" was to pack tenants into smaller and smaller spaces, like "sardines in a barrel."[17]

Chailloux's work is unique for its sustained analysis of the racial contours of housing in Havana. Cubans of color made up a majority of *solar* residents and the "extraordinary majority" in the *solares* with the worst conditions: indeed, Chailloux found that an overwhelming 95.7 percent of those residing in the worst *solares* were black and mestizo.[18] Even in racially mixed tenements, the larger, better-kept rooms (for example, those with windows or direct access to the street) housed families—usually white—who could pay a little more for the better amenities. Moreover, some tenements—especially those in better condition—refused to rent rooms "out to blacks, by virtue of a tacit agreement which the renters of those apartments observe, regardless of the constitutional precepts that prohibit discrimination on the basis of race or color." The result was that even families of color with the economic resources to rent a "dignified apartment" often had difficulty finding decent housing.[19] That Cubans of color were forced to live in these conditions was, for Chailloux, an affront to the nationalist goals of racial equality that his father had fought for during the Wars of Independence and then later during the 1912 Partido Independiente de Color uprising.[20]

By the 1910s, journalists of color were increasingly calling attention to the city's exorbitant rents, writing articles about black families facing eviction whose possessions were thrown into the streets, and decrying perpetual governmental indifference to the living conditions of the city's disproportionately black poor.[21] But given the city's racialized labor market, there were few options for many families other than the *solar*. As Alejandro de la Fuente has shown, in the decades after independence, Cubans of color faced fierce competition for jobs in Havana, especially with Spanish immigrants controlling the transportation and commercial sectors and almost exclusively hiring other Spaniards for positions in these key sectors of the urban economy.[22] Labor data from the 1919 census highlight the racial disparities by profession in the capital, with Cubans of color disproportionately working as servants, dressmakers, and laundry workers and virtually locked out of the higher-paying professions. While men of color were well-represented among tobacco factory workers and trades like carpentry and masonry, women of color faced significant hurdles in a labor market that relegated them to the lowest-paying jobs.[23] As black feminist journalist Catalina Pozo Gato wrote, even for university-educated women like herself, who were "equally prepared and qualified, it is difficult for the black woman to find the opportunity to demonstrate her aptitude . . . because the reality is that racial prejudice—which is eating away at Cuban nationhood—annuls her efforts, makes sterile her actions, and embitters her life."[24] As Pozo Gato makes clear, even well-educated women of color were forced to take jobs "with such meager pay that they only provide enough to live in . . . *solares*." For the majority of women of color in Havana—without the privilege of a university education or professional training—poverty and the *solar* seemed all but certain.

But for elite white Cubans, removed from the daily struggles of women and men of color, the *solar* became more cultural symbol than physical structure, its imputed social effects more important than its health consequences. Elites linked the *solar* to a host of social problems, from a low marriage rate to illegitimate births, prostitution, gambling, and overall criminality, and all of this represented a "ferment of immorality," a "school of vice," a dangerous "way of being and way of life."[25] Of course, it is impossible to divorce these social concerns from elites' racial anxieties and the identification of *solares* with Cubans of color. While the *solares* were almost always racially mixed spaces, they became a stand-in for blackness, criminality, and vice. As Alejandro de la Fuente has written, "The identification of solares as black spaces was a construct aimed at excluding the poorest from the city's geography and society, a cultural validation of social hierarchies. In the mainstream press, the slums were linked to marginality, crime, and promiscuity—attributes frequently used to characterize blackness."[26] Indeed, as the feminist writer Mariblanca Sabas Alomá wrote in 1929, Cuban elites believed *solar* residents to be the "detritus of society." "The favored insult of the bourgeoisie," she continued, was to say that someone "looked like people from *solares*."[27] As Sabas Alomá made clear, the term was a euphemism for Cubans of color, a way of linking marginality, poverty, and blackness without explicitly articulating racial terminology.[28]

Sometimes, however, elites were explicit in linking the "danger" of *solares* to their racial heterogeneity. As Ada Ferrer has shown, the discourse of raceless Cuban nationalism emerged and gained wide purchase in the late nineteenth century as Cuban intellectuals celebrated the mutual sacrifice of black and white soldiers who fought side by side in the independence struggle.[29] But while nationalist writers like José Martí and Juan Gualberto Gómez celebrated the union of black and white Cubans on the battlefields of the independence struggle, for postindependence elites the commingling of black and white in the tenements of the Cuban capital was a source of profound anxiety. According to Dr. Alberto García Mendoza, the "terrible moral conditions" of the *solar* represented "the fecund germ of degradation" for Cuban society as a whole.[30]

Indeed, for many elite professionals in the postindependence period, commitment to universal suffrage came up against an entrenched belief in white racial superiority that was increasingly buttressed by the transnational currents of racial science.[31] Many Cuban elites had been ambivalent at best about universal suffrage being instituted less than two decades after emancipation. For an important sector of Cuban medical nationalists, including such luminaries as Diego Tamayo and Fernando Méndez Capote, Cuba's constitutional liberties were ill suited for a population whose morals and culture were not sufficiently advanced. In a 1915 speech before the Cuban National Academy of Science that was later reprinted in Tamayo's *Vida Nueva*, the future secretary of health Fernando Méndez Capote argued that the social effects of race-mixing in the city's *solares* represented a threat to the viability of Cuban democracy itself. For Capote, universal suffrage was a "weapon imprudently handed over to that multitudinous element that emerges from the *ciudadela*."[32] For figures like Capote, Tamayo, and García Mendoza, then, the *solar* was a central point of moral and cultural infection in early republican Havana, where Cubans of color exerted a pernicious influence on the body politic.

Inextricable from white racial fears of cultural and moral contagion was the fear that the very bodies of *solar* residents represented a threat to the rest of the population. Health experts and reformers regularly singled out *solares* as "seedbeds of tuberculosis," as perhaps the central nodes of infection for the entire city, "wreaking havoc in their neighborhoods."[33] But rather than spreading infection far and wide, those most at risk from the disease were family members, people who nursed and shared living quarters with the sick. Havana's *solares* were therefore natural incubators of the disease, forming, in the words of Juan M. Chailloux, "a formidable bastion of tuberculosis" in the Cuban capital.[34] With whole families sleeping in small, poorly ventilated rooms and often sharing utensils, infection was almost impossible to ward off. Once an individual was infected, proper rest and nutrition were essential for recovery. But with inconsistent access to clean water and nutritious food, and without the economic or material means to ensure sufficient rest for those who became ill, persons sick with tuberculosis would often continue to get worse, their wracking coughs spreading the bacillus to everyone around them. Indeed, tuberculosis was rampant in the city's tenements. According to the 1905 *Manual de Practica Sanitaria*, more than 62 percent of patients in the city's tuberculosis dispensary lived in *casas de vecindad*, while a later study found that three-quarters of tubercular patients at the J. L. Jacobsen Dispensary lived in "poor hygienic conditions," such as those found in *solares*.[35]

In a speech before the Sixth National Conference on Charities and Corrections, Diego Tamayo made clear the danger the city's tubercular tenement residents posed to the greater population. Painting a grim picture of this disease threat, he described gaunt, pale figures with burning skin, "who cough frequently and spit upon the floor and wall that yellowish sputum, which flattens and drips across the wall where it appears to write, with its elastic fibers and its albuminous veins, coagulated with Koch's bacillus, the curse that a misery poisoned with all the unhappiness be launched against those who boast of enjoying the pleasures of a comfortable life." His meaning was clear: wealth and privilege offered limited protection from this infectious

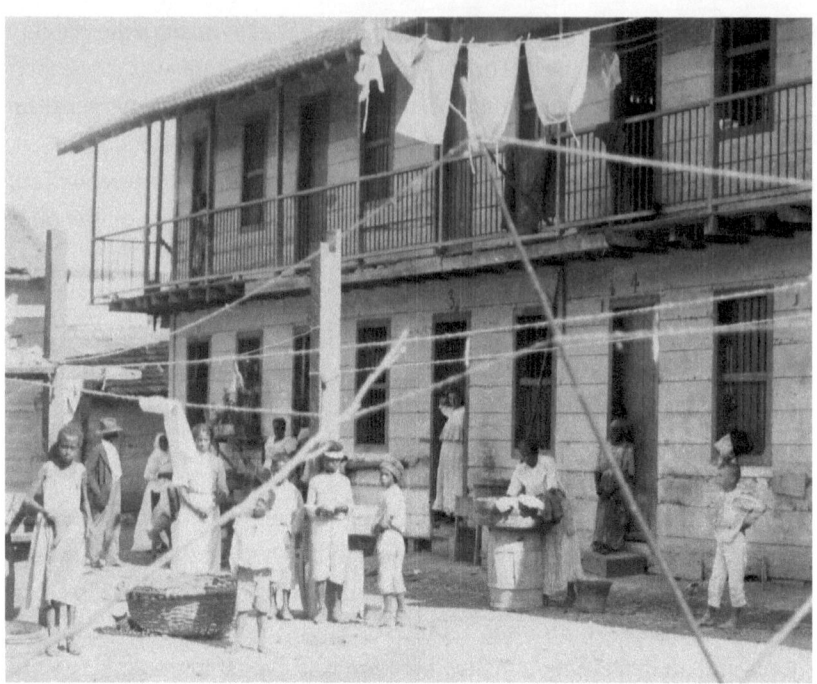

*Figure 5.1* Residents of the Solar Poloni in Centro Habana. Detail from "Tenement building 'Poloni,' San Rafael Street, Corner Oquedo, Cuba—an exterior view of the building on laundry day, with the inhabitants outside. Photograph, 1902." (Wellcome Collection)

disease. Aggressive public health action to address the tuberculosis crisis was therefore not charity, but in the self-interest of the Cuban elite. "Think clearly about this," he told his audience, either the housing conditions of the poor are improved or they die, "but [they] die spreading around them their germs of death which respect neither the rich nor the powerful."[36]

Of course, *solares* were more than the symbolic terrain upon which other Cubans made arguments about universal suffrage or the need for public health action. Again, photographs from the period are revealing. While often taken and published as evidence for a city that elites wished would soon disappear, early-twentieth-century photographs provide a glimpse of the complex social lives of the city's tenement dwellers. In one photograph (figure 5.1), women wash clothes by hand and hang white linens along clotheslines far above the dusty ground of the patio. A group of children stare at the camera, while a cat rests in the shade of a laundry basket. A woman catches a cool breeze in her doorway, beside the houseplants carefully displayed by her apartment window. In another photo (figure 5.2), neighbors line up along the

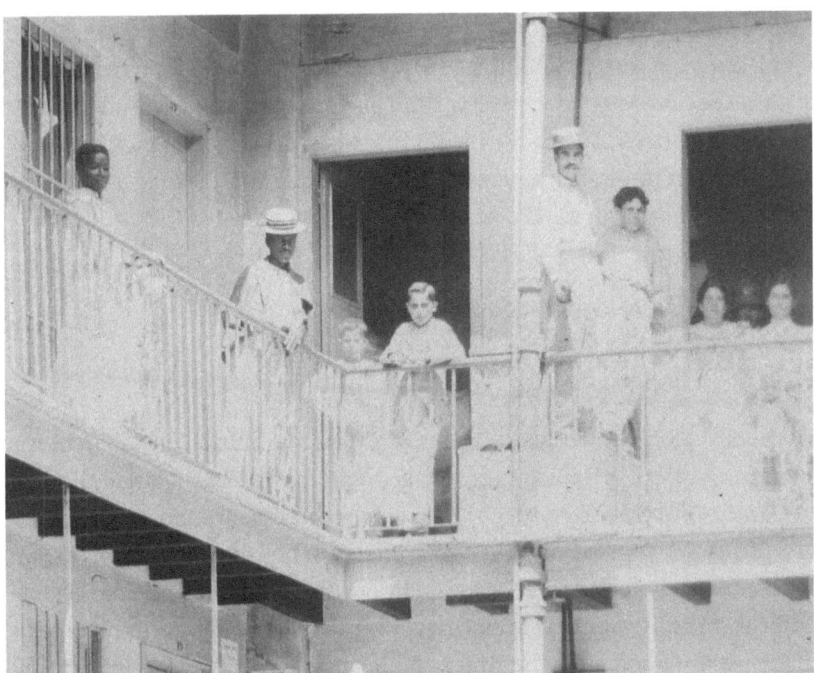

*Figure 5.2* Residents of a tenement in Centro Habana look over the courtyard. Detail from "Tenement building, Aquila [sic] Street, 116, Cuba—a view of the courtyard, with inhabitants standing on balconies at each floor. Photograph, 1902." (Wellcome Collection)

railings of the third floor, dressed in their Sunday finest for what was surely the rare occasion of being photographed. A young woman stands proudly before the Cuban flag. Black, white, and mestizo tenement residents lived side by side. Their children played together in patios and ran along balconies. They shared gossip as they hung up their laundry and shared *cocimientos* when family members got sick. They celebrated important life events with rum and sweets. They watched each other's children, got pregnant, and shared tips for caring for their infants. They fell in love and sometimes fought. They took pride in their homes and maintained them as well as material conditions allowed.

But as observers as different as Juan M. Chailloux and Diego Tamayo point out, the physical conditions in which these families lived predisposed them to sickness, worked against recovery, and caused many to have unnaturally short lives. Compared with wealthy families in El Vedado, these children playing in the patio were more likely to die before reaching adulthood, their mothers and fathers much more likely to succumb to tuberculosis. This reality, hidden in these photographs, reflected material conditions that were themselves the result of political decisions over whether and how to intervene in the economy, how much to fund public health services, and whether to address entrenched racist hiring practices. As observers increasingly recognized, if the state had a responsibility to care for its citizens, then the conditions that gave rise to disease and early death needed to be addressed.

## "WE ARE POOR AND DO NOT HAVE SERVANTS TO TAKE CARE OF US": POVERTY AND THE LIMITS OF TUBERCULOSIS CARE

By the late 1920s, Cuba had decades of experience in the antituberculosis struggle. A mix of private initiatives and public institutions—largely limited to Havana—worked to stem the spread of the disease, primarily through education campaigns, but also through a system of housing inspections meant to ensure that buildings met basic public health standards. The central node of the campaign was the Dispensario Furbush, the national antituberculosis dispensary named after the American health official Dr. Charles Lincoln Furbush, an early supporter of Cuban antituberculosis work during the first U.S. occupation. By the mid-1920s, over 400 people a day would visit the Dispensario Furbush, housed by the central train station on the outskirts of Old Havana.[37] Some sought a diagnosis for their respiratory ailments; others, knowing or suspecting they had tuberculosis, hoped to be granted admission to the national sanatorium, La Esperanza, or "Hope" (see figure 5.3). Others, the gravest cases, desperately hoped to gain admittance to the Romay Clinic for Advanced Cases of the disease. In order to extend the reach of the tuberculosis dispensary, a group of ten visiting nurses, each assigned a neighborhood district, would regularly visit the homes of residents diagnosed with the disease. During their visits, they would keep track of the development of the illness and teach families how to care for the sick and the proper hygienic practices for preventing the spread of the disease. In the years before effective antibiotic treatment, prevention through education was the primary method available for tuberculosis control. As the dispensary's director noted, the goal of the entire antituberculosis program was to give Cubans, "especially the poor, the necessary information to prevent the spread of the disease, so that they are not a danger to the rest of the collectivity."[38]

Health regulations and sanitary inspections formed an important part of the government's fight against tuberculosis. Regulations explicitly forbade

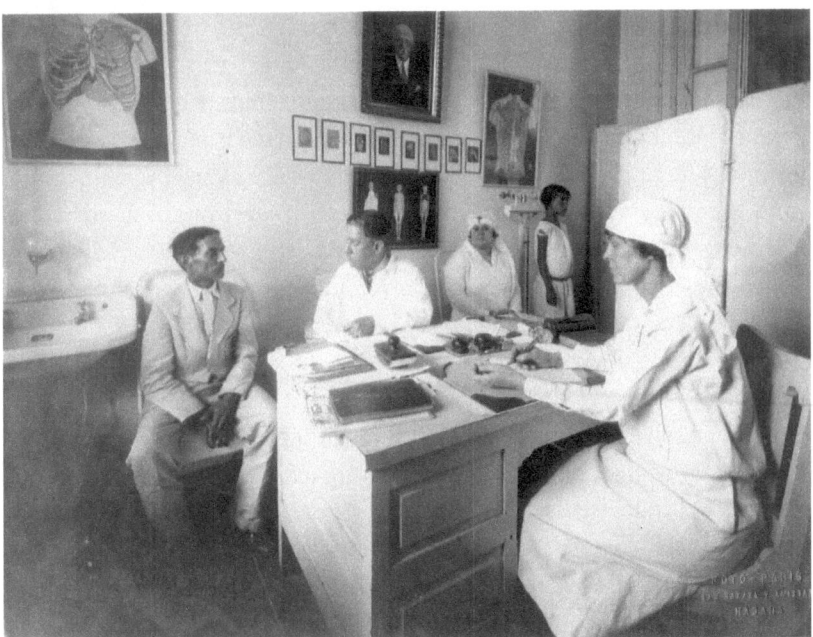

*Figure 5.3* Tuberculosis consultation at La Esperanza. (Archivo Nacional de Cuba, La Habana, Fototeca, caja 133, sobre 117, registro 4330)

public spitting—and all public establishments were required to post signs to that effect—and streetcar and train conductors were authorized to kick out any passenger who spat on the floor despite being warned. Indeed, anyone caught spitting on the floor was supposed to be given a small printed card with the text "PLEASE do not spit on the floor again. IT IS PROBABLE that you did it unawares. THIS habit is damaging to the public health and spreads tuberculosis among other diseases."[39] More importantly, tenement buildings were subject to strict sanitary oversight, with health inspectors tasked with regularly visiting the city's *solares* and *casas de vecindad* to ensure compliance with health codes. Health inspectors were to ensure that rooms were not subdivided, that spaces not built for habitation were not illegally rented out, and that tenants were not illicitly making confections in their cramped rooms to sell on the streets.[40] Each tenement had an *encargado*, a person in charge of collecting rent and maintaining proper conditions in the building. The Health Department required *encargados* to keep hallways and central patios clean and clear of obstructions, provide one regularly cleaned spittoon for every twenty residents, and ensure all shared bathrooms and urinals were clean and in working order.[41] Not surprisingly, each of these regulations was regularly flouted.

According to his 1917 report to the Ministry of Health on *casas de vecindad*, José Antonio López del Valle asserted that the ministry had "been fighting for years to improve these things and make tenements comply with the Sanitary Ordenances." Some improvements had been made: "More than one thousand rental houses have been shut down due to bad hygienic conditions," he wrote, adding that "periodic sanitary inspections of these homes have been completed." But "despite all of our efforts," they encountered "sometimes insuperable obstacles" due to the "passive resistance" of private interests.[42] Resistance, it seems, was widespread, as tenants avoided regulations preventing them from making confections, and tenement owners and supervisors conspired to rent out as much space as possible and disregard regulations regarding cleaning, painting, and providing running water.[43] The sanitary engineer José A. Cosculluela argued that the problem was not a lack of health legislation. "Everything that can be prohibited is officially prohibited." But "here in Havana there are regulations that no one follows, as their infraction is not punished."[44] Despite the best efforts of some reformers within the Ministry of Health, a combination of entrenched economic power of landlords and a weak enforcement regime hobbled efforts to use a regulatory framework to address the city's tuberculosis crisis.

Far more impactful was the work of visiting nurses, who spread across the city, entering the homes of residents diagnosed with tuberculosis and helping them find ways to manage the illness and prevent further infection. Their regular visits allowed them to check the progress of the tubercular residents in their assigned areas. As with their work to reduce infant mortality among the city's poorest families, however, their main task was to "instill in the habits and customs of the people new [scientific] theories and educate them in the laws necessary for healthy living."[45] Mary Eugénie Hibbard, the American-born chief of tuberculosis nursing for the Ministry of Health, understood that this was delicate work, requiring "good judgment and skill" in order to make those under their care adopt new habits, such as avoiding coughing or talking close to others, spitting only in spittoons treated with antiseptic solution, and covering their mouths and noses with a handkerchief when coughing or sneezing.[46] To take one example, the tuberculosis nurse Emma Deulofeu wrote that while fresh air was essential to treating tuberculosis, the custom among Cubans had always been to avoid fresh air when sick. "In this country, the majority of families were afraid of the air." Through their regular visits and compassionate nudging, she argued, visiting nurses had managed to transform the habits of their patients, until "ninety percent of them know that what is necessary to attack the disease is exactly fresh air."⁴⁷ It seems that this work of entering the homes of the poor and working closely with them to improve their chances of survival affected the nurses themselves, as they became among the most vocal proponents of legislative action to improve the lives of the poor.⁴⁸

For a small percentage of the newly diagnosed, the national tuberculosis sanatorium, La Esperanza (Hope), held the promise of recovery and cure. La Esperanza was reserved for incipient cases of the disease—individuals who had been diagnosed but who, it was hoped, had sought treatment at an early enough stage that the prescribed six-to-eight-month stay at the sanatorium would result in remission. While La Esperanza originally served only 50 patients, by the late 1920s, up to 150 people at a time were treated there free of charge. Like other sanatoriums in the decades before effective antibiotic treatment for tuberculosis, La Esperanza provided residents the ideal conditions for the body's immune system to combat the infection: rest, nutrition, and fresh air. Just as important, however, was its educational function. La Esperanza was envisioned as a kind of "antituberculosis school," teaching its residents how to improve their chances of putting the disease in remission and how to avoid infecting others. Of course, given the enormity of the tuberculosis problem in Havana alone, the national sanatorium's 150 beds were woefully inadequate. As Luis Bay y Sevilla noted in 1924, its capacity was "minuscule in relation to the number of sick that exist."⁴⁹ Making matters worse, the health sector's rampant patronage system increasingly shaped access to the sanatorium. As Kelly Urban has shown, by the late 1920s, "many of those who had gained access to treatment at the sanatorium had done so through political connections."⁵⁰

While demographic data on the sanatorium's patients are extremely spotty, they do give us some idea of who was able to gain admittance. According to admission and discharge records for July 1918, those who passed through La Esperanza skewed female, white, and young. Women made up over two-thirds of the patients, and 78 percent were in their teens or twenties. It makes sense that sanatorium patients would skew younger, since the facility was officially reserved for incipient cases, and the disease tended to take the heaviest toll on those in their peak working years. But the gender disparity is noteworthy and suggests that it was harder for young men to take the six- or eight-month break from work to recuperate in the sanatorium. Further, the fact that the overwhelming majority of women were unmarried, and therefore more likely to be childless, suggests that those with greater family responsibilities were less able to enter the sanatorium.⁵¹ Strikingly, women of color gained admittance at rates far below their need, especially in comparison with white women. Women of color were twice as likely to die of tuberculosis as white women, and yet white women entered the sanatorium at more than three times the rate of black and mestiza women.[52] There are a few possible explanations for this disparity. Perhaps women of color had additional familial responsibilities and were less likely to be able to spend the six months needed to recuperate. Or perhaps white women were more likely to visit the tuberculosis dispensary and get diagnosed at an early enough stage to gain admittance to the sanatorium. Another possibility was that white families were disproportionately able to use their political connections to secure a coveted bed at La Esperanza. Likely, it was a combination of these factors. What is clear is that the national tuberculosis sanatorium, the central government institution capable of giving tubercular Cubans a better chance at recuperation, disproportionately served white Cubans at the expense of Cubans of color, who continued to die at much higher rates.

While those lucky—or politically connected—enough to get access to a coveted spot at the sanatorium did get the opportunity to rest, eat healthy foods, and breathe fresh air, the entire educational thrust of the antituberculosis program was predicated on the idea that these conditions could be achieved within the home. However, as the health ministry's own nurses understood, for the Cuban poor, these conditions were often impossible to meet. Ample rest was a central component of any treatment plan for tuberculosis, but as María Merelles, one of the ministry's tuberculosis nurses, wrote in 1912, "We find that, when we make our regular visits, that many of the sick do not maintain the proper rest, because, as they tell us, they cannot do so, as they need to work to take care of their basic needs."[53] Merelles describes patients coughing up bloody sputum, who, when advised to maintain rest, would respond incredulously: "Who is going to take care of the children, hang the laundry and take care of the cooking? We are poor and do not have servants to take care of us."[54] As Merelles noted, "Many times we had no response," because, of course, "it is often impossible for poor patients" to maintain the necessary conditions for improvement.[55] In the face of the cramped living quarters of the poor, visiting nurses would sometimes recommend that the sick "move outside of the city" into more ample housing.[56] Of course, those who lived in the city's *solares* were often in no position to move into better housing. Against these clear economic constraints, visiting nurses could only hope their hygienic counsel would prevent, to some degree, subsequent disease transmission.

Even as new public hospitals and dispensaries opened and private organizations like the Cuban Anti-Tuberculosis League and the Damas Isabelinas spread their hygienic counsel to whoever would listen, tuberculosis mortality remained remarkably consistent, regularly topping 1,000 deaths per year in the capital alone. And Cubans of color continued to get ill and die at disproportionate rates. Certainly, more money was needed for public tuberculosis work, and figures like Joaquín Jacobsen tirelessly petitioned the national government for more public investment in the antituberculosis campaign. But if, as a growing number of observers noted, tuberculosis was at its root as much an economic issue as a medical one, then—as the editors of the popular weekly magazine *Carteles* put it—"combating tuberculosis with sanatoriums, dispensaries, and lectures on hygiene is simply to dodge the problem, ignoring its primary causes. The success of the campaign against yellow fever was due precisely to the fact that it attacked the disease at its roots, suppressing the generating cause. The unsatisfactory results of the antituberculosis struggle must be attributed to the adoption of the wrong tactics."[57] Any successful campaign would have to take on the underlying economic conditions that shaped the spread of the tubercle bacillus, like the city's skewed housing market, terrible living conditions, and the poverty wages earned by so many workers. But as Cubans of color regularly noted, these conditions were not distributed equally. Given the de facto racial segregation of Havana's worst *solares* and the lower wages and higher levels of unemployment that Cubans of color faced, then of course Cubans of color would bear the brunt of the city's most deadly scourge. The question then became, given the disproportionate black mortality and failures of state and private efforts to effectively combat it, what did "black tuberculosis" say about Cuba's formal commitment to racial equality?

## ASKING NOT FOR PRIVILEGES, BUT THE SOCIAL JUSTICE THEY ARE OWED

In the summer of 1929, the young physician Gustavo Adolfo Aldereguía gave a speech at the Sociedad de Torcedores, the anarcho-syndicalist union of the city's tobacco workers, highlighting the disproportionate rates at which Cubans of color were dying of tuberculosis. By 1929, Aldereguía was becoming increasingly well-known both for his work as a lung specialist focused on tuberculosis and for his political activities as a student radical and communist physician. His thinking on tuberculosis, social medicine, and the possibilities of reform under the Machado dictatorship were shaped by his politics. He was a student of the revolutionary obstetrician Eusebio Hernández and was a close associate of the recently assassinated Julio Antonio Mella, the founder of the Cuban Communist Party. As a founding member of the Ala Izquierda Estudiantil (Student Left Wing), Aldereguía would be imprisoned for his opposition to the dictatorship of President Machado. Aldereguía's commitment to ending tuberculosis was also shaped by his family's history, as his mother died of pulmonary tuberculosis when he was still an infant. Aldereguía was among a growing number of physicians, journalists, and politicians who had been calling attention to the problem of tuberculosis and the failures of existing public and private health campaigns to curb the spread of the disease. This was not especially controversial, nor was his focus on the disproportionate mortality rate among Cubans of color. What was controversial and set off a months-long debate in the pages of "Ideales de una Raza" was his suggestion that Cubans of color form their own organizations to tackle the health crisis.

In his 1929 speech, Aldereguía proposed the creation of a Liga Negra Contra la Tuberculosis, or Black Anti-Tuberculosis League—modeled after the Cuban Anti-Tuberculosis League—which would raise funds for this work and centralize activities, as well as educate Cubans of color in how to avoid infection and care for the sick. He hoped that this organization would create a tuberculosis dispensary, which would serve as the "first scientific center in our country exclusively dedicated to the study, understanding, and repression of tuberculosis" among Cubans of color.[58] As Aldereguía noted, there were already many *sociedades de color* in Cuba—fraternal organizations made up of Cubans of color—formed on social or cultural bases. Why not one that took on issues of health?[59]

For the black journalists and intellectuals who wrote of "Ideales de una Raza," however, the call for separate health institutions was an affront to the ideals of racial unity that underlay the Cuban independence struggle. As Alejandro de la Fuente has shown, the discourse of raceless nationalism—that the very idea of Cubanness was predicated on making no racial distinctions—held powerful sway over postindependence political life.[60] During the Cuban Republic, the language of raceless nationalism served as a powerful discursive tool for framing black demands for full inclusion, even as it served to quash attempts for autonomous black political organizing, most infamously with the brutal repression of the Partido Independiente de Color in 1912.[61] Channeling this discourse, the columnists strongly rejected the idea of separate health institutions as anti-Cuban. Gustavo E. Urrutia found the proposal to be "not concordant with Cuban ideology" and tantamount to "voluntarily sanctioning and perpetuating the existent [racial] division."[62] Primitivo Ramírez Ros added that Cuban intellectuals of color, from venerable black politician and writer Juan Gualberto Gómez to acclaimed poet Nicolás Guillén, were horrified by any move toward racial isolationism.[63] The health of black Cubans, these writers argued, was not just the responsibility of Cubans of color. As citizens of an ostensibly racially egalitarian republic that had made health a central pillar of the state's responsibility, they demanded state action to stem the rates of black tuberculosis.

That this debate unfolded in the weekly columns of "Ideales de una Raza" propelled the topic to a broad national audience. As we have seen, since the end of Spanish rule, the city press had become a central forum for discussing the health needs of the Cuban people and debating the meanings of disease and public health action. But the "Ideales de una Raza" tuberculosis debate explicitly put these medical nationalist debates into direct conversation with Cuba's long-standing raceless nationalist politics, in a forum read by white and black Cubans alike.

From 1928 to 1931—the years that "Ideales de una Raza" ran in the Sunday edition of *Diario de la Marina*—the page was without a doubt the most prominent forum for intellectuals of color in Cuba. It was spearheaded by Gustavo E. Urrutia, a former accountant, salesman, and architect who began his fourth successful career as a public intellectual and journalist at the age of forty-eight, when he approached Pepín Rivero, the owner and editor of the archconservative *Diario de la Marina*, with the idea to have a weekly column dedicated to discussing issues of importance to Cubans of African descent. Surprisingly, Rivero agreed, giving Urrutia a powerful national platform with the potential to reach the tens of thousands of readers of the country's most prominent newspaper. Urrutia used his position to bring in other important black voices, including Juan Gualberto Gómez, the venerable writer/activist/politician who had been the most well-known intellectual of color during Cuba's decades-long independence struggle; Primitivo Ramírez Ros, the newspaper editor and former Conservative Party politician; and the up-and-coming young poet Nicolás Guillén, whose career was launched in the pages of "Ideales de una Raza."[64] Week after week, Urrutia used "Ideales" to promote black culture and discuss the problems of Cuban racism from a wide variety of perspectives, but during the summer and fall of 1929, the page was dominated by the debate over what should be done to combat the scourge of tuberculosis for Cubans of color.

The debate brought out into the open the de facto racial segregation of the city's private medical system, which provided significantly more health care options for white Cubans than for those of African descent. As Primitivo Ramírez Ros noted, while all Cubans had access to public health care institutions, such as "hospitals, preventoriums, sanatoriums, clinics, and crèches, etc.," whites also had exclusive access to the city's robust Spanish immigrant private mutual aid medical system, "with their numerous medical corps and inexhaustible economic resources."[65] As discussed in the following chapter, the Spanish mutual aid clinics were the backbone of the city's private medical system, with almost 40 percent of the city's residents covered under one of the Spanish immigrant mutual aid clinics' low-cost insurance plans. Membership was limited to Spanish immigrants and those who could claim Spanish ancestry, which, in practice, meant white Cubans only. While Ramírez Ros and Urrutia were careful not to directly criticize the existence of these institutions in the pages of the conservative and pro-Spanish immigrant *Diario de la Marina*, the implication was clear: these institutions embodied precisely the kind of racial isolationism that they decried as anti-Cuban. (Indeed, in the coming years, this argument would be made in more explicit terms by the Cuban Medical Federation.)[66] In practice, then, Cubans of color were forced to rely on the inadequate and underfunded public medical system and compete with poor and working-class whites for a hospital bed or a coveted spot at the national sanatorium. But these spots were often reserved for persons with political connections, adding an additional layer of hardship for those seeking care for themselves or a family member.

Beyond the idea that having separate institutions was a repudiation of the egalitarian nationalist promise of Cuban independence, Ramírez Ros and Urrutia also rejected the idea on more practical terms. If, as all agreed, the disproportionate tuberculosis mortality was largely due to the disproportionate poverty of Cubans of color, who were forced to live in substandard housing and subsist on low-wage labor, then how would they be able to raise the funds to create their own health care institutions? As Ramírez Ros put it, the "economic powerlessness" of Cubans of color precluded it: "In what way can black Cubans create a private clinic, which even white Cubans have not been able to build for themselves?"[67]

For Ramírez Ros, the idea spoke to how out of touch even sympathetic white Cubans were to the daily realities of Cubans of color. For example, the elite Cuban antituberculosis philanthropist Consuelo Morillo de Govantes suggested that Cubans of color should "leave the *solar* and go with their offspring to live in the suburbs. There are some homes there," she added, "and they should take advantage."[68] Ramírez Ros, incredulous, responded, "Ay, señora de Govantes! But the black Cuban can barely [afford to] live in the *solar*. How is it possible for them to go with their offspring to live in the suburbs?" Regarding the idea that "there are homes" in the suburbs and

Cubans of color should "take advantage of them," he added, "allow me to very respectfully advise the most dignified lady not to announce that she knows where these may be found, because I assure her that she will have to call the police reserves at the station assigned to her elegant residence, to not see it invaded by [a throng of Cubans] requesting please some of these available houses."[69] For Ramírez Ros, elite philanthropists like Consuelo Morillo de Govantes—whose organization the Damas Isabelinas had no women of color among their ranks—would "never be able to understand the true situation of tuberculosis in the black race" without the guidance of Cubans of color.[70]

This back-and-forth highlighted the fact that crucial educational efforts like those of the Damas Isabelinas nevertheless only addressed the surface of the problem. Surely it was still important to continue to spread knowledge about how tuberculosis was contracted and how to best avoid infection. And the Damas Isabelinas certainly lauded their own work as "the most transcendental and humanitarian work in modern times" in Cuba.[71] Although their regular radio addresses and home visits allowed their gospel of hygiene to reach a broad swath of the city's poor, the organization's narrow educational focus and blindness to the structural and racial dimensions of the problem limited the impact of their work. The high rate of tuberculosis in the country's *solares* was not, as the work of the Damas Isabelinas seemed to suggest, due to the "low culture" of their residents; rather, Gustavo E. Urrutia pointed out, the root causes were "fundamentally socio-economic."[72] But the Damas Isabelinas treated tuberculosis as if it were a matter of imparting the correct information to the Cuban poor, leaving it up to them to apply that knowledge to their particular circumstances. As Ramírez Ros's frustration suggested, this was an insufficient response to a much greater problem.

As the debate in "Ideales de una Raza" highlighted, one of the main questions facing Cuban health advocates was whether tackling the tuberculosis crisis was primarily the responsibility of the government and what the proper role was of private organizations like the Damas Isabelinas. This debate over the appropriate sphere of the government in promoting or protecting the health of the Cuban people had been going on for decades, but nowhere was it as central to health debates as with tuberculosis. In fact, this issue was at the heart of Joaquín Jacobsen's address before the Sixth International Congress on Tuberculosis, held in Washington, D.C., in 1908. As the founder of the Cuban Anti-Tuberculosis League, Jacobsen was naturally a proponent of broad social action to combat the disease. Indeed, he spoke in glowing terms of the rich associational life and philanthropic culture that supported private health work in the United States during the height of the Progressive Era. Yet the United States, he argued, was "an exception to [the] rule" and could not be the model for a country still emerging from colonial rule.[73] As Jacobsen made clear, this was largely an issue of funding: "Private associations, in Cuba at least, and our own League among them, have not been able to carry on by their own efforts really profitable work of education. A social work of this scope must be backed by resources larger than those of private associations, public charity, and even municipalities; it must be supported by the State." Looking across the Atlantic for successful models, Jacobsen noted that in Great Britain and Germany "the State assumes the responsibility" for reducing tuberculosis mortality, with "brilliant" results.[74]

For private health organizations to thrive in Cuba, Jacobsen argued, they needed robust government support. But in Cuba, such support was generally weak and vulnerable to shifting political tides. As Jacobsen admitted, the Anti-Tuberculosis League had little to show for its years of work: "I do not deny that some good has been done, but it is not worth comparing with the time employed, nor with the exertions that have been made."[75] Indeed, seventeen years later, José A. Cosculluela offered an even grimmer assessment: "Has the Anti-Tuberculosis League accomplished anything practical to avoid or combat [tuberculosis] in the capital?"[76] The problem, as Joaquín Jacobsen understood, was a lack of philanthropic support from wealthy Cubans, combined with inconsistent government support. As we saw with Manuel Delfín's Casa del Pobre and with the city's private crèches, most private organizations struggled to find donors to cover basic costs, while the privileged few, with close connections to the government, had relative success and longevity.[77]

But while some state funding was available for children's welfare work, there was little public enthusiasm for supporting private medical charities. As Alberto Sánchez de Fuentes, the director of the Dispensario Furbush and the person in charge of the government's antituberculosis work, put it: "In our country, as occurs in the majority of Latin America, the very rich—those who possess great fortunes—bequeath little, very little, to the promotion and creation of institutions of a medical character and the State must undertake these complicated problems by itself, which always proves very costly."[78] With elites providing little support to private medical charities, health work oriented toward the poor fell to the Cuban government. Indeed, the fact that there were no private charitable options for poor tubercular Cubans was a source of annoyance to the reformer and architect Luis Bay y Sevilla. Bay found it to be "absolutely absurd to expect that the public Treasury bear all of the costs, when the entire country should contribute" to fight against tuberculosis. But, as he argued, Cubans "leave everything to the Government."[79]

In this discussion over private versus public tuberculosis work, we begin to see how health care was increasingly understood and articulated as a right of citizenship over the course of the postindependence decades. During the U.S. occupation, American officials worried constantly about the "medical pauperization" of the Cuban people, that they would come to see health care as a right rather than a privilege. They feared that when the government took responsibility for the hospitalization of the poor or providing direct aid to the hungry, then Cubans would come to claim these as rights. But Cuban health advocates turned this formulation on its head and regularly pointed to health and social policy during the first occupation as a model for state action to combat tuberculosis. For example, Juan B. Fuentes, the chief of the tuberculosis section of the Department of Health, proposed that the government could open shops where the cost of basic food items would be subsidized for the poor, as had been done under the first U.S. occupation, ensuring that hunger would no longer be a factor in predisposing the poor to tuberculosis.[80] And health advocates regularly pointed to the successful yellow fever campaign as a model for state action to eradicate tuberculosis. For Joaquín Jacobsen, the "only thing needful for success is an earnest pledge to fight tuberculosis, a determination to carry on the fight with as much energy as has been shown in that against yellow fever."[81]

Throughout the early republic, medical nationalists regularly expounded the idea that the government had a responsibility to safeguard the health of the Cuban people. Joaquín Jacobsen, for example, argued that "the State ought to protect the life and property of its citizens; ought to come to the defense of the poor and to the assistance of the sick." He was explicit that the healthy have "a right to the protection of their life and health," while "the consumptive, for his part, has also the right to ask the State: Can you admit me to a special establishment where I cannot be of any danger to the rest of the people and wherein I can be taken care of?"[82] Mary Eugénie Hibbard argued that just as the state was responsible for safeguarding the economic interests of the nation, it should also be responsible for protecting the health of its citizens.[83] This required more than just additional dispensaries or hospital beds, however. Juan B. Pons, the first director of La Esperanza, advocated for the building of more government health care institutions to care for the sick, but he admitted that these would not get at the root of the problem. "What is needed," he argued, "is to improve the living conditions of our working people, providing hygienic housing instead of those caverns without air and light that we call *casas de vecindad* . . . [and] make cheaper '*artículos de primera necesidad*,' especially foodstuffs."[84]

As the "Ideales de una Raza" debate made clear, these ideas had gained much wider purchase by the late 1920s. As most agreed, beyond health education, what was needed was significant state investment in public medical services and national legislation to improve the living conditions of the poor. "The problem is deeper," argued Primitivo Ramírez Ros, than the possibilities afforded by private charity. Rather, the fight against tuberculosis required the dramatic expansion of the public health system and greater state intervention in the economy: "It is a matter of social defense, of legislation of an economic character, of the expansion of social welfare [*beneficencia pública*], of the multiplication of adequate establishments to combat this disease: preventoriums, sanatoriums, hospitals, crèches—on a greater scale, if possible, than what is currently being done."[85] Gustavo Aldereguía, while advocating for private initiatives on the part of Cubans of color, was explicit in articulating the idea that Cubans had "the right to live in health" and that this emerged out of the "immanent right of all sick people in every civilized society to efficiently receive medical attention."[86] And the feminist Mariblanca Sabas Alomá argued that what was needed in the city's *solares* was to convince their residents that "we all have the right, not just to suffrage, but to health . . . and well-being." But, she warned, these rights would not "be given as gifts" but would have to be "conquered" through collective action.[87]

As Gustavo Urrutia and Primitivo Ramírez Ros made clear, the statistics on black tuberculosis death were an indictment of a republican economic, political, and health system that had failed Cubans of color. To them, racialized poverty and disease were neither natural nor inevitable but, rather, emerged out of specific historical relations. As Ramírez Ros declared, black Cubans were "not idle or lazy." Indeed, enslaved black labor had been "indispensable for the creation of the splendid colonial factory, and the sweat of their brow enriched the white Cuban patrician."[88] But despite the egalitarian promise of independence, in postindependence Cuba, whites continued to enjoy a privileged position within the economy and, therefore, an abundant diet, better living conditions, and "greater organic resistance to the disease."[89] The wealth and health of white Cubans and the poverty and disease of Cubans of color were therefore interdependent facts emerging out of the same racialized economic system dating back to the colonial plantation economy. Therefore, when Cubans of color sought government action to improve their material and health conditions, it was "not asking for privileges" but rather demanding "the social justice they are owed."[90]

In the coming years this discourse of a right to health continued to penetrate Cuban society and frame political claims making. One striking example is the 1936 program for the National Convention of Cuban Societies of the Race of Color.[91] With roots in postabolition mutual aid organizations, by the early republic black fraternal societies became central institutions shaping urban middle-class black life. They provided a range of social and educational opportunities and routes to professional advancement for black politicians, writers, lawyers, physicians, and other professionals. Their publications were forums for black intellectuals to address national political issues, but they also gave space to mark important events such as a wedding or the graduation of black doctors and pharmacists from the university. As Melina Pappademos has shown, these societies also shaped black engagement with the state, providing support for local and national politicians in exchange for promises of employment and state support for black institutions. In the 1930s, however, black fraternal societies were subject to the same social forces transforming Cuban politics more broadly. Reflecting the radicalism of the 1933 revolution that ousted President Gerardo Machado, new radical black societies like Club Adelante and the Directorio Social Revolucionario "Renacimiento" emerged to challenge what they saw as the conservatism of the most prominent black fraternal societies and push for more radical policies that would benefit the most marginalized Cubans.

Prepared by an organizing committee representing black fraternal societies from across the country, the 1936 program put forth a strident vision of state responsibility for the health and welfare of the poor and echoed Urrutia and Ramírez Ros in articulating the right to health within a structural and historical analysis of racialized Cuban poverty and disease.[92] At the heart of the document was a profound critique of the failures of the Cuban Republic, which saw not the advance of Cubans of color but their growing economic and social marginalization. For the drafters of the program, the "fundamental function of the State . . . and legitimate basis for its existence" was to promote "the general welfare of all the groups that comprise the Nation."[93] Yet in that essential task, the Cuban state had failed. This was evidenced by the island's economic indices that showed that 86 percent of the unemployed and 91 percent of Cubans so poor as to require state support were black. Rather than simply reflecting the general economic problems of the neocolonial economy, however, the program was clear that these conditions were rooted in racial discrimination and a history of economic disenfranchisement rooted in the island's slave past. It was these conditions—reflected in the racialized wealth gap, the growing shantytowns ringing the capital whose inhabitants were almost all black, and the disproportionate disease and death of Cubans of color—that the Cuban state would need to remedy.

The program was primarily comprised of a series of ambitious proposals for political reforms, which ran the gamut from political changes to make the government more accountable to its citizens, to a constitutional amendment banning discrimination on the basis of race, class, or sex, to economic and immigration reforms that would disproportionately help Cubans of color, such as land reform and requiring that at least half of all employees be native Cubans.[94] But the program ended with a twelve-point list of what it called "fundamental reforms of a sanitary-hygienic character," which would transform the practice of medicine on the island, vastly increase the role of the state in regulating medical education and practice, and work toward meeting the health needs of the poorest Cubans. This vision for state involvement in medicine was far reaching. Medical practice would essentially be nationalized: all branches of medical practice would be declared "a social necessity," and a constitutional amendment would grant the state the power to regulate medical practice in order to meet the health needs of all Cubans. After an islandwide health survey, medical workers would be sent where they were most needed. Emphasis was placed on rural health care, with a two-year plan to combat intestinal parasites among campesinos and new scholarships to medical students who promised to work in the countryside. In the cities, the plan called for greater public funding for public health. Private health clinics (like those run by Spanish mutual aid societies) would be subordinated to public need and obligated by the state to attend to all patients in cases of emergency. Further, the state would fund and organize national social security insurance for tuberculosis and cancer that would provide necessary support to families who lost income due to illness.

As the next chapter will show, many of these proposals dovetailed with those put forth by the Ala Izquierda Médica, or the Medical Left Wing of the Cuban Medical Federation, which also proposed the expansion of state medical practice in order to meet the health needs of the Cuban poor and the employment needs of Cuban doctors. But here the proposals were rooted in the specific economic conditions and disease experiences of Cubans of color. These demands were based on a clear understanding of the structural failings of the republican political and economic system, which relegated black Cubans to greater poverty and marginalization in the decades after independence. For the framers of this program, these economic and health demands were simply reparations or, in their words, a demand that the state "compensate for this historical disparity and confront the grave problems faced by the race of color and fundamentally resolve them."[95] As these debates highlight, by the 1930s, the idea that the state had a fundamental responsibility to meet the health demands of the Cuban poor had moved beyond the medical nationalist writings of Cuban physicians, nurses, and public health officials, becoming a widespread political discourse rooted in a growing concept of a fundamental right to health. Despite this growing consensus, however, most of the far-reaching proposals articulated in the 1936 program would fail to materialize. The radical hopefulness that flowered with the 1933 revolution gradually faltered in light of continuing repression, deepening corruption, and growing authoritarianism. Black poverty grew unabated, leaving its mark on the many lives cut short by tuberculosis.

## "OUR DUTY AS SANITARIANS IS TO POINT OUT THE PROBLEM"

While they often ignored the racial dimension, nurses, journalists, public health officials, and reformers spent the first decades after independence regularly calling attention to the relationship between poverty, housing, and disease in the Cuban capital and urging greater government action to protect the health and lives of the Cuban poor. Certainly, some progress was made. The city's tuberculosis dispensary diagnosed the disease, and visiting nurses helped the sick and their families understand how to manage it and avoid infection. The national sanatorium provided six months of rest, sun, and nutritious food to those fortunate enough to secure a spot. And the clinic for advanced cases gave the very sick what limited treatment options were available in the decades before antibiotics finally gave physicians a way to cure the disease. But as a drumbeat of conference speeches, reports, radio addresses, and newspaper articles indicated, these efforts were profoundly insufficient, given the enormity of the problem. Urban health services needed vastly more funding, with more hospital and sanatorium beds, and health codes needed enforcement. Beyond enforcing existing laws and expanding institutions, most health advocates understood that extensive economic reforms were needed to reduce urban poverty and improve worker housing. Despite vocal support for these measures from top officials at the Ministry of Health, next to nothing was done to address these root causes of tuberculosis mortality in Havana.

In his scathing 1925 speech on urban health in the Cuban capital, the sanitary engineer José A. Cosculluela divided the history of post-Spanish urban health into two phases. The first, from 1900 to 1915, represented "the victorious process of life over death," with the extirpation of yellow fever, robust public health action, and improving health statistics. The second period was one of sanitary decline, represented by corruption and fraud at all levels of government. Cosculluela decried rampant corruption in the Ministry of Health that made a mockery of health regulations that, if enforced, could have worked to improve the living conditions of the poor and reduce the city's high mortality rates. Politically connected but unqualified individuals were put in key positions, "and today we must watch how venal and corrupt functionaries, devoid of any technical or sanitary understanding, shamelessly misspend funds dedicated to the efficient functioning of public services."[96] There is much truth to Cosculluela's critique. By the 1910s and 1920s, corruption was endemic across the government, and ostensibly technical positions were often given out to political supporters. Health codes were selectively enforced, allowing for the deterioration of conditions in the city's poorest *solares*. Together, this amounted to an abdication of government responsibility for the health of the city's poorest residents.

As an increasingly broad set of voices made clear, however, tuberculosis did not pose a technical or scientific challenge so much as a political one. Officials from within the Ministry of Health were increasingly clear about the need for aggressive action to rein in the cost of living in the capital and improve the quality of housing. In speeches, reports, and essays, they called attention to how the lack of government funding hobbled tuberculosis efforts and therefore led to unnecessary deaths. They spoke of the nationalist promise of a healthy republic and harkened back to the success of the yellow fever campaign as a model for a national medical campaign based on a firm commitment to extirpate a disease from the island. They advocated for government-controlled rents, the building of workers' housing, state-run food stores for the poor, and improved wages for workers, all of which would have addressed the root causes of tuberculosis mortality. But these proposals required political will to confront the entrenched economic power of landlords and merchants—all to protect the health of the city's most marginalized: the poor, Cubans of color, and *solar* residents. Despite the growing support for such action, political commitment to tackle the tuberculosis crisis would not be forthcoming.

By the early 1930s, however, advocates of robust state responsibility for the health of the poor would gain a powerful new ally. Once again, the island's neocolonial economy proved a decisive influence in the direction of Cuban health politics, as a dearth of clients able to pay for medical services seemed to threaten the livelihood of Cuban physicians. In response, the Cuban Medical Federation—the main organizational body of the island's physicians whose main goal had traditionally been protecting the interests of private practitioners—became an unlikely voice calling for the vast expansion of public medical services in order to meet both the employment needs of physicians and the medical needs of the poor.

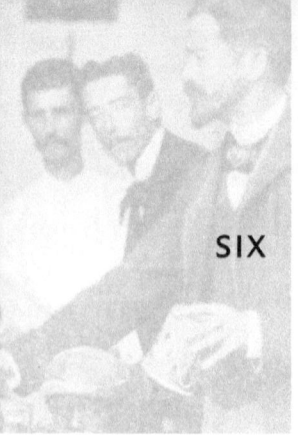

## SIX  To Fight These Powerful Trusts and Free the Medical Profession

Spanish Mutualism, Medicine, and Revolution, 1925–1935

ON THE WARM, rainy afternoon of September 27, 1933, one of the largest demonstrations in the history of the Cuban Republic took place in the streets of Havana. Despite the inclement weather, "a well-dressed throng" of over 40,000 men and women, a mix of Spanish immigrants and Cubans, marched from Havana's Parque Central, along the tree-lined Paseo del Prado, and up to the presidential palace.[1] They met there to protest a recent decree by the new president, Ramón Grau San Martín, requiring all physicians wishing to practice medicine in Cuba to be members in good standing of the new National Medical College. On the Paseo del Prado, crowds shouted, "Down with the Medical Federation!" while Spanish merchants across the island closed their shops in protest against the presidential decree.[2]

Why would a law governing private medical practice create such public discord? On the face of it, the decree was not unusual. National medical colleges were official bodies that regulated the practice of medicine, set standards for medical education, and organized against unlicensed medical practice. International medical organizations such as the Association Professionnelle Internationale des Médecins, the precursor to the World Medical Association, had for years been pushing for physicians' mandatory membership in national medical colleges. Countries such as Spain, Holland, Bulgaria, and Czechoslovakia had passed similar laws in recent decades.[3]

Yet in Cuba these measures touched off a series of sometimes violent conflicts that would shape Cuban medicine for decades. The Medical College Law was passed in the immediate wake of the 1933 revolution that ousted the dictatorship of President Gerardo Machado, as part of a flurry of nationalist reforms passed by the short-lived government of President Grau San Martín between September 1933 and January 1934. The law had the overwhelming support of Cuban physicians but ran directly against the interests of Havana's

Spanish-immigrant-run private hospital system. In the midst of political tumult and a resurgence of Cuban nationalism, the measure exacerbated long-standing hostility between Cuban physicians and Spanish immigrant institutions. At issue was not just the regulation of medical practice, but whether the powerful *centros regionales*, the Spanish immigrant societies that controlled these private hospitals, would accede to the labor demands of the Cuban Medical Federation (Federación Médica de Cuba, or FMC). On a more fundamental level, physicians argued, this was a struggle over the future of Cuban medicine.

The *conflicto médico*, as it became known, combined medical labor struggles with nationalist politics and anti-Spanish sentiment, a combustible mix during a time of political and economic instability. By early January 1934, tensions exploded. In the midst of the continuing medical labor conflict, the Cuban military was ordered to occupy Spanish-run hospitals. Pitched battles broke out between police and supporters of the Spanish hospital system. Government support for the physicians wavered: under pressure from the powerful Spanish immigrant sector, the Grau government stopped enforcing the Medical College Law. In response, medical workers from across the country staged the most extensive medical strike in Cuban history. On the morning of January 19, 1934, 25,000 doctors, nurses, pharmacists, midwives, and hospital workers walked off the job. Hospitals, clinics, dispensaries, and pharmacies across the island stopped caring for the sick. The strike caused enormous chaos: according to one American observer, "Critically ill patients were abandoned, equipment was destroyed, general panic ensued. Relatives and friends flocked to the hospitals to care for suffering and dying patients. Surgeons were kidnapped at gun point by frantic husbands and fathers, forced to attend patients."[4] In retaliation for the strike, medical offices and pharmacies were bombed, pharmacists were attacked, and a physician was assassinated in broad daylight.

Throughout these conflicts, and in the wake of the medical strike, Cuban physicians debated the politics, the organization, and the meaning of medical practice. What kind of labor was doctoring? Were physicians like other workers, who should organize for better wages and work conditions, or more akin to "medical priests" for whom labor struggles sullied their professional reputations and threatened their class standing? What was the social role of medicine, and what was the proper role of the state in regulating medical practice or expanding access to medical care? While physicians were never a unified body, their answers to these questions changed over time, in response to their worsening economic situation, the failure of labor mediation efforts, and a growing consensus that the problems of Cuban medicine required radical solutions.

Having examined the development of Cuban health politics through the emergence of medical nationalism and the creation of the new health ministry, in relation to campaigns to address new outbreaks and endemic health problems, and from the perspective of health officials, nurses, reformers, and urban residents, in this final chapter I turn our attention to the city's physicians. It explores the politics of medical labor in early-twentieth-century Cuba, tracing the changing meanings of medical practice in times of political, professional, and economic crisis. In the early decades of the twentieth century, even as laboratory discoveries and new medical therapies gave biomedicine greater prestige, medical practice was transforming in ways that physicians believed threatened their autonomy, social standing, and class status. In the wake of the 1929 economic crash, Cuban physicians found themselves in an increasingly precarious position: with most of Havana's residents receiving care between the substandard but free public hospital system and the system of low-cost Spanish immigrant mutual aid hospitals, Cuban physicians found their standard of living dropping dramatically, as competition in the medical marketplace forced down earnings. Organized under the FMC, Cuban physicians targeted the *centros regionales* both for the low wages they paid their medical staffs and for extending low-cost medical care to those who could afford to pay for medical services at market rate. Long-standing medical nationalist politics shaped this conflict, as Cuban physicians argued that once again, Spanish mercantile interests blocked the progress of Cuban medicine and endangered the health and future of the Cuban people.[5] As these professional struggles intersected with the growing popular demand for health care, however, physicians became unlikely advocates for the expansion of the state medical sector.

Medical politics was also shaped by the revolution that toppled the dictatorship of General Gerardo Machado (1925–33). The ouster of Machado both exacerbated political tensions within the medical sector and presented new opportunities for physicians to advance their sectoral concerns. Revolutionary politics influenced a new generation of leftist young doctors and medical students, who organized into the Ala Izquierda Médica, or Medical Left Wing, and pushed the Medical Federation to link its class interests to the broader political and social problems of the Cuban people. As the Ala Izquierda argued, the same conditions of neocolonial development that facilitated the illness of so many Cubans—an economy largely in the hands of North Americans and Spaniards, entrenched and deepening poverty, and insufficient public medical services—also prevented most Cuban physicians from making a decent living. After a painful medical strike, the failure of international mediation efforts, and the increased government hostility to the demands of Cuban doctors, the medical sector seemed to have exhausted the possibilities for change within the system. Cuban physicians increasingly believed that the private medical system itself was fundamentally broken. The social forces unleashed with the fall of Machado transformed the Cuban medical class, leading to increased support for the radical reconfiguring of medical practice on the island. More and more, physicians began linking their professional interests to the health needs of the Cuban people and insisting that the answer to both was the vast expansion of public medical services.

## SPANISH MUTUALISM AND THE FORMATION OF THE CUBAN MEDICAL FEDERATION

In a 1930 editorial for the *Tribuna Médica*, the official organ of the FMC, Cuban internist Félix Hurtado Galtés described the professional, economic, and cultural trends that had transformed the practice of medicine in postindependence Cuba.[6] According to Hurtado, what had traditionally been a respectful and friendly relationship between doctors and their patients had been upended by a series of transformations on both sides of the doctor/patient dyad. First, the class makeup of the medical profession had changed dramatically in the decades after independence. In early-twentieth-century Cuba, medical education expanded dramatically, as lowered university tuition and the promise of economic mobility increasingly brought students "from the most humble classes" into medical school.[7] Unlike previous generations of medical practitioners, who largely came from Cuba's elite families, newer physicians viewed medicine not just as a prestigious and socially useful practice but as an important route to economic advancement.[8] In the years after independence, both the number and percentage of students studying medicine at the University of Havana increased substantially, with over 70 percent of the university's students studying medicine by 1915.[9] By the 1929–1930 academic year, just as Cuba was descending into its deepest post-independence economic crisis, there were over 1,500 medical students at the University of Havana.[10] For Hurtado, himself of "humble background," the shifting class makeup of Cuban medicine was "one of the determining factors of the current crisis," for the rise of medicine as a path to material progress coincided with the disappearance of medicine as an altruistic "priestly mission."[11] In earlier times, he argued, the physician was a valued counselor to the family; "his influence within the heart of the home was decisive." Now, however, "that dignified representative of the Hippocratic science, who wore a top hat and a frock coat, has disappeared," replaced, he argued, by a less-qualified physician more interested in economic gain.[12]

But if the Cuban physician had changed since independence, so had the patient. Powerful Spanish immigrant mutual aid health care organizations, rooted in the late nineteenth century but transformed after independence, dramatically altered the doctor/patient relationship in Havana. Initially founded as mutual aid organizations for working-class peninsular immigrants, the centros regionales brought together immigrants from particular regions of Spain: the Centro Gallego was a Galician organization, the Centro Canario brought together Canary Islanders, etc.[13] At the height of their membership, the three largest and oldest centros, the Centro de Dependientes, Centro Asturiano, and Centro Gallego, together had 176,000 members, drawn largely from Havana's residents.[14] By far their most important service was the medical care that members received.[15] Their hospitals were among the best equipped in the country, and members would come from across the island for treatment at the Centro Asturiano's Covadonga Hospital or the Centro Gallego's hospital, La Benéfica. All of these benefits were available for a very modest monthly fee, generally within reach of most Spanish immigrant workers. But while the centros were originally mutual aid organizations for the urban immigrant working class—providing a form of insurance against poverty and illness—their membership increasingly included Cubans of Spanish descent (with Cubans of color explicitly denied membership), as well as growing numbers of bankers, merchants, and other elite sectors of Spanish immigrant society. Indeed, the central conflict between the centros and the FMC was the issue of whether the centros should allow wealthy residents to become members and receive the same access to low-cost medical care as the working-class membership.

For the FMC, the loss of professional authority was rooted firmly in the rise of the centros regionales. According to Hurtado, the centros helped transform the Cuban doctor from a respected figure of scientific and moral authority to a common paid employee. The earlier personalistic relationship between doctors and patients, predicated on the scientific and moral authority of the physician and the deference of the patient, was transformed by the shifting economics of medical practice in the capital, the narrowing of class differences between doctors and their patients, and the rise of the "medical trusts" of the centros regionales. The result, according to Hurtado, was a galling loss of respect and professional authority. Rather than respectfully heed the physician's counsel, patients now "raise[d] themselves to be relentless judges of the actions of the doctor, within the strictest technical terrain. Now family members dispute the diagnosis of the doctor, he is not believed, [another doctor] is brought in behind his back, and finally he is dismissed like a servant."[16]

While many factors led to the formation of the Cuban Medical Federation, the most important was the increasingly precarious economic position of Cuban physicians by the 1920s. Within months of the 1925 founding of the FMC, members of its executive committee approached the *centros regionales* with a list of demands, including labor contracts for physicians, improved medical facilities and equipment, and an agreement on income or class limits on membership in the *centros*. They were initially confident that their demands would be met, as the federation already had within its membership the overwhelming majority of Cuban physicians and seemed to have the backing of the country's political elite, but relations with the Spanish societies were fraught from the start. Brief work stoppages and threats of medical strikes led to improved working conditions at several *centros*, but the larger concern over the limitation of benefits to working-class and middle-class members was not achieved and would remain a major source of conflict.[17]

For Cuban physicians, the main problem with the *centros regionales* was the distorting effects of their health services on the medical marketplace of the capital. According to the FMC, the *centros* drove down wages for physicians who faced increasing competition in the already crowded medical marketplace of Havana. Cuba, like other countries in the region, had a very unequal geographical distribution of physicians.[18] With high rates of rural poverty, relatively few physicians were able to find enough paying clients to make a living outside the capital. According to a 1934 report from the International Labour Office, almost half of the country's physicians practiced within the city limits of Havana.[19] But a large percentage of the city's residents either were covered by public medical services or were members of the *centros regionales*. Approximately 40 percent received low-cost health care through the *centros* while another 37 percent of the city's population was eligible, due to poverty, for free medical care in one of the city's public clinics.[20] This left the 1,200 physicians practicing in the capital competing for less than a quarter of the urban population who purchased medical services on the open market. What made the situation especially untenable for the federation's doctors was the fact that the *centros regionales* allowed their wealthiest members access to the same low-cost medical care, thereby denying Cuban physicians access to them as paying clients. The result was the increased underemployment of Cuban doctors and a decline in physicians' incomes.

This issue was at the forefront of Cuban ophthalmologist J. M. Penichet's address before the 1927 annual meeting of the American Medical Association. Penichet argued that unless the Cuban medical community could come to an accord with the *centros*, "the practice of our noble profession in Cuba will be almost impossible." Penichet stressed the unfair competition Cuban practitioners faced from the Spanish *centros*: while originally created to serve the needs of the Spanish working class, now "the rich, the very rich, belong just as well to these societies. The highest representatives of the banking business, commerce, industry, government, and politics are the principal associates of these institutions." While the highest echelons of the Spanish immigrant elite took advantage of the *centros'* low-cost medical care, the *centros'* largely Cuban medical staff "work[ed] day and night" for a "ridiculous" salary. "That is why," he noted, "we have founded the Cuban Federation of Physicians, to fight these powerful trusts and free the medical profession."[21]

In the years after the 1914 bubonic plague outbreak, lingering resentment of Spanish immigrant merchants dovetailed with these economic pressures and fed into a nationalist repudiation of the Spanish *centros*. For Cuban physicians trying to make ends meet in early-twentieth-century Havana, Spanish domination of the medical marketplace seemed a galling colonial vestige. From early on, the Federation's newspaper *La Tribuna Médica* tapped into this nationalist sentiment, repudiating lingering Spanish colonialist attitudes and questioning the meaning of Cuban independence if "now, the enemies of yesterday have more power in the republic than those who were the victors."[22] In contrast to the island's weak Hispanophilic political class, that refused to confront Spanish economic power, the FMC declared it would "struggle with all its might so that Cuba [would] be for Cubans."[23]

## ECONOMIC CRISIS AND MEDICAL PRACTICE UNDER MACHADO

Already suffering from the twin problems of medical competition in Havana and the dominance of the *centros regionales* in the capital's medical market, Cuban physicians were dealt a massive blow by the post-1929 economic depression. The economic crisis brought mass unemployment, the growth of shantytowns on the city's outskirts, food lines, and hunger marches. Already by 1930, a quarter of the Cuban population was unemployed, while those urban workers lucky enough to have jobs found their wages drop by half.[24] In scenes reminiscent of postreconcentration conditions in 1899, the streets of Havana were filled with the hungry and the homeless. As hunger grew, health conditions worsened. Infant mortality rates almost tripled during the worst years of the crisis, and tuberculosis mortality rates spiked.[25] Worsening health indices were exacerbated by deteriorating conditions in the city's public hospitals, which suffered severely as the result of budgets cuts.[26] Likewise, the city's Spanish mutual aid medical system was hit hard by tumbling enrollments, as many workers could no longer afford the monthly fees.[27] With unemployment high and wages dropping, the market for private medical services contracted sharply. Urban residents, in other words, could no longer afford to pay for medical care. By the early 1930s, the Cuban medical profession was in a state of profound crisis. According to a 1935 Commission on Cuban Affairs report, "Since the depression, physicians have suffered perhaps more than any other group."[28]

Throughout the economic crisis, the FMC continued its struggle with the *centros regionales*, but to little effect. To resolve the stalemate, the FMC held two conventions on Spanish mutualism, each outlining proposals for limiting the medical benefits of the *centros* to their working- and middle-class membership. The federation hoped that the move would force wealthy *centro* members to purchase medical services on the open market, thereby relieving some of the economic pressure on the medical sector. But although several *centros* agreed to study the proposals, but no changes were made.[29] In the summer of 1932, with the *centros* continuing to refuse their demands, the FMC declared a strike against all of them. But the strike failed when some federated physicians continued working in the *centros*' clinics and hospitals; in response, the federation expelled the strikebreaking doctors. In a sign of the violence to come, the home of a prominent FMC physician, Ricardo Núñez Portuondo, was bombed.[30]

The Cuban Medical Federation demanded the unity of its members in its struggles against the Spanish regional societies. But unity was hard to come by, as is evidenced by the growing list of strikebreakers expelled from the federation whose names appeared in the *Tribuna Médica* in the early 1930s. But if unity was difficult to achieve on important labor actions, political unity was impossible. According to the largely conservative executive committee of the early 1930s, the FMC was an apolitical professional organization; if it nurtured close ties to the Machado government, it was only in order to advance the professional cause of Cuban physicians. As the Machado dictatorship wore on, however, the close ties the FMC leadership sought with the regime became increasingly intolerable to the many critics of the regime within the organization, who accused the executive committee of "transform[ing] the Federation into an instrument of the Dictatorship."[31] These tensions underscored a central and largely unspoken fact about the federation: it held within its ranks physicians from wildly different economic backgrounds and political perspectives. But with the economic collapse and the growing political crisis, these tensions threatened to rend the organization's fragile consensus.

As Robert Whitney has argued, the late 1920s in Cuba were marked precisely by the increased mobilization of groups that had traditionally been outside the political process, such as students, professors, urban and rural workers, and lower-rank soldiers.[32] Channeling a growing opposition to Machado, disaffection with corrupt republican political institutions, and resistance to U.S. political and economic control, these emerging groups transformed Cuban politics. While originally organized around ostensibly apolitical professional and economic issues, Cuban physicians grew frustrated with what they saw as government complicity with the deterioration of medical practice on the island, and they increasingly made political demands and pushed the federation to tackle political questions.

But there would be costs to distancing the FMC from the government. In reality, Cuban physicians were, and had been for decades, heavily reliant on the political favors that came from cultivating close links with Cuban politicians at all levels. The politicization of medicine had been a problem since independence, as both jobs and medical care in Havana's public hospitals and clinics were subject to the city's patronage system. According to former national director of *beneficencia* Félix García Rodríguez, corruption was endemic in Cuban public health institutions: politicians distributed hospital posts, positions within the Ministry of Health, and even hospital beds to political supporters and their families.[33] As Félix Hurtado Galtés complained, it was common for Cuban families to seek out a "political friend and influential person" to solicit employment in public hospitals for their young medical school graduates.[34] The collapse of the Cuban economy made public sector jobs increasingly sought-after, almost certainly exacerbating the problem of medical patronage as political connections became increasingly essential for securing employment in the public medical sector.[35] This situation undoubtedly tempered many physicians' criticism of the Machado regime.[36] Further, by cultivating close ties with the regime, the FMC had been able to secure some favorable measures, such as a 1932 decree more strictly limiting medical attention in public hospitals to the poor, as well as "special treatment" for the growing number of physicians imprisoned by Machado for antigovernment activity.[37]

But as the anti-Machado movement grew, so did physicians' disaffection with the political closeness of the FMC to the Machado regime, and the medical sector began to splinter along political lines. As protests against the dictatorship increased, large numbers of medical students and physicians allied with the anti-Machado movement were imprisoned. But now physicians within the federation, led by Ángel Arturo Aballí and Alfredo Recio, began to directly take the executive committee to task.[38] During the 1932 national assembly of the FMC, an earlier rule requiring that delegates be at least five years beyond medical school was overturned, opening the federation to a new and increasingly radical group of young physicians. This greatly increased the power and presence of the anti-Machado Left within the internal politics of the FMC. Rejecting calls to remain apolitical, new "tendencies" emerged within the FMC, openly articulating medical and federative questions from clear political perspectives. These included the Ala Izquierda Médica (Medical Left Wing), which favored the linking of patient and physician demands and the radical expansion of public medical services, led by Gustavo Alderguía, a former political prisoner and member of the radical student organization Ala Izquierda Estudiantil (Student Left Wing).

The emergence of the Ala Izquierda Médica in late 1932 marks a key moment in the history of the FMC and, indeed, in the history of Cuban medicine. While Cuban physicians had for years been pushing for government reform and decrying the effects of Cuba's neocolonial position on medical practice, the Ala Izquierda framed these concerns within a broadly socialist anti-imperialist politics and pushed for a sweeping transformation of both the Cuban medical and political systems. For the Ala Izquierda, the medical crisis of the 1930s resulted from both Cuban neocolonial dependency and the organization of medicine under capitalism, with medical services "respond[ing] to the economic and political interests of the dominant classes" rather than the needs of patients or the economic interests of medical workers.[39] Criticizing the lack of government investment in public hospital and medical services, the Ala Izquierda envisioned a radical expansion of government health services, including the growth of the hospital sector in the capital and the provinces, the creation of new dispensaries for tuberculosis and other "social diseases," and the establishment of public disability, health, and unemployment insurance.[40] The Ala Izquierda saw a clear link between the interests of physicians and patients and fought for both improved wages for medical workers and increased medical care for the Cuban poor, thereby opening up space for patient/physician alliances that would become important in the following years.

In stark contrast to the executive committee's calls for broad unity among federated physicians, the Ala Izquierda highlighted the class cleavages and lack of common interest among Cuban physicians. It shot back at accusations of "politicizing" laid on it by elite and conservative sectors of the FMC by arguing that the elite sectors of the federation used calls for unity and apoliticism to paper over important class differences among Cuban doctors. Rather than "fracture or split the forces of the medical sector," as more conservative factions within the FMC alleged, Ala Izquierda physicians hoped "to lead the defense of the interests of the poor and middle-class physicians who constitute the majority" of Cuban doctors. In the tumultuous period that began in the summer and fall of 1933, the Ala Izquierda began to take a leading position within the federation and pushed for increasingly aggressive tactics to further the cause of the medical majority.

## THE REVOLUTION OF 1933

The emergence of the Ala Izquierda Médica coincided with a broader radicalization of Cuban politics in the early 1930s. As the Machado regime increasingly suppressed strikes and marches, imprisoned political opponents, and assassinated enemies, a broad opposition movement crystallized and became increasingly radicalized. The cycle of protest, repression, and radicalization quickened during the first half of 1933, as bombings, assassinations, and the bloody repression against protesters and labor leaders occurred with increasing regularity. By the summer, the situation in Havana was slipping out of Machado's control. In late July, a transportation workers' strike paralyzed the city, and by early August, other sectors joined what became, under the leadership of the Cuban Communist Party and the Confederación Nacional Obrera de Cuba (National Confederation of Cuban Workers), a general strike. On August 7, a violent clash between demonstrators and police led to scores of deaths. (The FMC, which had been planning a small medical strike that day, canceled the action so that physicians could attend to the wounded.) In the aftermath of the August 7 massacre, Havana exploded in popular mobilization. As Louis A. Pérez Jr. writes, "The general strike had acquired the full proportions of a revolutionary offensive."[41] Facing a revolution from below and under pressure from Washington to step down, President Gerardo Machado y Morales quietly resigned on August 12, fleeing the country under the cover of darkness.

With the fall of Machado, the policies of rapprochement followed by the executive committee of the FMC proved costly. The forty-seven physicians held in Machado's prisons—and the numerous others forced into exile—served as a clear indictment of the FMC's leaders.[42] Several members of the executive committee, including president Ricardo Núñez Portuondo, were forced to resign. The new executive committee was strongly aligned with the revolutionary anti-Machado sector of the federation, which quickly came into new prominence in the fall and winter of 1933.[43]

On September 10, the Cuban Provisional Revolutionary Government, made up of an unstable coalition of radical students and low-level military officers, came into power under the presidency of Ramón Grau San Martín, a physician and popular university professor. Buoyed by the popular mobilizations, the Grau government quickly instituted a series of far-reaching progressive reforms: the Platt Amendment, which had formalized Cuba's political dependence on Washington, was unilaterally abrogated; women gained the right to vote; an eight-hour workday was established; agrarian reforms, including a minimum wage for sugarcane workers, were instituted; the Ministry of Labor was established; and the "nationalization of labor" law, which required 50 percent of all workers in agriculture, commerce, and industry to be Cuban citizens, was passed. This last law was aimed specifically at the capital's Spanish commercial elite, who tended to hire only Spanish workers in their warehouses, bodegas, and cafés.

Cuban physicians were delighted to have one of their own in the presidency. In many ways, Ramón Grau San Martín seemed to be the embodiment of Cuba's medical nationalist tradition. A longtime professor of physiology and dean of the medical school, Grau had been an active member of the FMC. A third of his new cabinet were medical men: he appointed Carlos E. Finlay as his secretary of health, the revolutionary pharmacist Antonio Guiteras as his secretary of the interior, and the surgeon and professor of medicine Manuel Costales Latatu as his secretary of education. His social policies, such as improving wages and mandating safe and healthy work conditions, instituting worker accident insurance, and reducing utility rates, worked toward improving the health of Cuban workers. Finally, in abrogating the Platt Amendment, his government eliminated the long-standing mechanism of U.S. sanitary control over the island. Cuban physicians were therefore hopeful that the Grau government would find a resolution to the *conflicto médico*. Their hopes were well founded, for one of the first decrees passed by the new government was the Ley de Colegiación Médica Obligatoria, which required all practicing physicians to be members of the new Colegio Médico Nacional, or National Medical College.

In passing the Ley de Colegiación Médica Obligatoria, President Grau finally gave the FMC the tool it would need to force the *centros regionales* to concede to its demands. The law put the Cuban Medical Federation in charge of the new National Medical College and required that all practicing physicians solicit membership in the National Medical College within ten days of the law taking effect (September 20).[44] Physicians who continued to practice medicine in violation of the law would have their medical licenses revoked. The new National Medical College could therefore force the *centros regionales* into accord, or else the *centros* would risk the medical college barring its members from practicing medicine in these institutions. Since practically all of the physicians who continued to practice medicine in the main *centro* hospitals were expelled former members of the FMC, this gave the National Medical College enormous leverage. This was precisely the critique of the Spanish ambassador, who in a carefully worded letter to the Cuban secretary of state asked that the decree be revoked.[45] The ambassador argued that he "would have no objection to the forced membership in the College, if the National Medical College . . . were an independent and impartial organism constituted by all of the physicians of the republic," but entrusting the functioning of the National Medical College to the FMC exclusively, "was the equivalent of granting an illegal and unjust privilege in favor of the Medical Federation." Indeed, now that the FMC had sole control over the new medical college, the scores of physicians who had been expelled from its ranks were in a perilous situation.

Given the new scenario, the *centros regionales* understood that their best chance to avoid giving in to the federation's demands was to have the law overturned. They waged a massive effort to rally their tens of thousands of members against the new law and to discredit the FMC. Five of the capital's main Spanish immigrant institutions quickly organized the massive march and demonstration of September 27 (which opened this chapter) as a public show of force.[46] Flyers handed out in the days before the demonstration exhorted members of the city's Spanish mutual aid organizations, "whether workers, students, bankers, industrialists, shopkeepers, clerks or professionals in general," to come out and support their "noble and altruistic cause." In a sign of a rapidly shifting political discourse—given the general conservative bent of the *centros regionales*—flyers for the march proclaimed these medical institutions "the representation *por excelencia* of Socialist Cooperatives in Cuba."[47] On the day of the protests, Spanish commerce displayed its power as Spanish-run shops across the country shut their doors in solidarity with the *centros*. As the *New York Times* correspondent in Havana noted, "Many merchants believe a general lockout [of Spanish-run businesses] will result if the government does not take steps to modify this decree."[48] The *Times* also reported that a general lockout among commercial houses would "completely paralyz[e] industry and commerce" on the island.[49] Indeed, the one-day lockout was enough to transform the urban landscape. According to one observer, with "almost all of the commerce of the capital" controlled by the Spanish, "the closing of their establishments was enough to make our city look like it was a holiday."[50]

The Spanish protests in late September were just one of the many problems the new government faced. The worker mobilization that had helped bring down Machado threatened the fragile Grau coalition as well. New waves of strikes continued into the fall, as unions took advantage of the revolutionary moment to push for more radical changes.[51] Meanwhile, the reformist government was under attack from the Right. The United States refused to recognize the Grau government. Business associations and merchants refused to pay taxes to it, and Spanish import houses kept their warehouses full of unloaded goods, refusing to release food.[52] The Spanish demonstration, rightly described as "an impressive manifestation and protest by the professional, industrial and business classes and property owners," portended the potential costs of supporting Cuban physicians over the powerful Spanish immigrant sector.[53] In response to Spanish pressure, the government briefly suspended the Ley de Colegiación Médica, pending possible modification.[54] While the law was reinstated after five days, key provisions of it were never enforced. It seems that the Grau government that this strategy would both neutralize attacks from the Spanish sector and assuage the Cuban Medical Federation. But, as we will see, this middle path was unsustainable, as the new National Medical College pushed forward with its plans to force the *centros regionales* to accede to its demands. With government support for the new medical college wavering, federated physicians organized the first general medical strike in Cuban history.

## MEDICAL STRIKES

In late December 1933, the FMC held its annual national assembly in Havana. Although, there was much dissension over the many issues before the assembly, delegates were united in their frustration with the government. After seven years of pushing for a Ley de Colegiación Médica, the Grau government finally passed the decree but had refused to fully enforce it. In an atmosphere of labor mobilization across the country, the National Medical College voted unanimously to hold a general medical strike on January 19. Over the next weeks, members of the Ala Izquierda Médica took the lead in organizing the strike. One of the main goals of the Ala Izquierda was to "break the isolation of the physicians" and link the struggles of doctors to those of other medical workers in a broad "unified front" of the medical sector.[55] Over the following weeks, this broad-based national alliance of physicians, nurses, medical students, midwives, veterinarians, pharmacists, medical laboratory workers, and the employees of the municipal health services was organized under the aegis of the National Confederation of Cuban Workers, the radical labor confederation that had helped organize the general strikes that precipitated the fall of Machado.[56]

The following weeks were eventful. While this broad medical alliance was being organized, Cuban courts ruled in favor of the National Medical College in its attempt to suspend the medical licenses of the strikebreaking doctors who continued working in the *centros*' hospitals. When these doctors refused to abide by the ruling, Ministry of Health officials, accompanied by officers from the national police, shut down the city's Spanish-run hospitals. Battles erupted at the Quinta de Dependientes hospital and at the Centro Gallego's La Benéfica hospital, as "patients, even the disabled . . . armed themselves with sticks to throw them out," preventing their closure.[57] At the rest of the city's Spanish hospitals, patients who could walk were sent home, "most of the patients [still] in their night clothes," while the most severe cases were placed together under the care of Ministry of Health physicians.[58] The following day, crowds gathered at the Quinta de Dependientes hospital and prevented Ministry of Health officials from entering.[59] Reflecting the coming breakdown of the Grau government coalition, Colonel Fulgencio Batista, the Cuban army chief, sent military troops to guard and reopen the hospitals, letting the suspended physicians back in, in violation of the court's ruling.[60] Two days later, Batista moved against the president in a bloodless coup and installed Carlos Mendieta as the new president of the republic.

On January 19, just as Mendieta was putting together his new cabinet, over 25,000 medical workers, including the overwhelming majority of Cuba's 2,542 licensed physicians, went on strike.[61] Every Cuban hospital, clinic, and pharmacy was shuttered, and federated physicians refused to treat private patients. Professional nurses joined the strike, demanding higher pay and better work conditions, as did midwives, pharmacists, and hospital staff. Workers from the Ministry of Health walked off in solidarity.[62] Organized under the "Unified Front," medical workers presented the Mendieta government a common list of demands, including an eight-hour day and higher minimum wage for all medical workers, the rehiring of striking doctors at Spanish hospitals, and the official recognition of the union.[63]

The medical strike was incredibly disruptive. For the duration of the strike, neither medical care nor medicine would be available. Midwives refused to attend births, and doctors refused to perform autopsies or sign death certificates, leaving bodies slowly piling up in city morgues.[64] Although the National Medical College promised that it would provide "emergency services in all of [the island's] centers of population, so as not to abandon those in immediate danger of death," it seems that emergency medical services were not provided in any systematic way.[65] One police officer, hoping to find medical attention for a wounded fellow officer, reported having "checked all the hospitals and clinics, observing a total absence of doctors and nurses."[66] According to the conservative Havana daily *Diario de la Marina*, "Not even seriously ill patients and urgent cases are being given aid, as the Colegio Medico offered."[67]

Those with the resources to do so could seek medical attention outside the country, such as Antonio Mendoza, from a prominent Cuban banking family, who took his eleven-year-old son to Miami by airplane to be operated on for acute appendicitis.[68] Cubans without this kind of wealth were less lucky. City residents, for lack of better options, brought the wounded to police stations, where they were "treated by laymen."[69] One woman, unable to find any doctors or midwives, was driven to a police station in search of medical help, "having given birth in the middle of the transport which brought her."[70] According to *Diario de la Marina*, "Great numbers of people showed up at the Ministry of Health ... in search of medicine for their sick relatives and doctors which could attend them," but they "obtained nothing."[71] The newspaper named more than fifteen patients in Havana who died without medical attention, including a twenty-three-year-old man who died of the flu, "the elderly Quintin Jauloreana, [who] died without medical attention in the Las Animas Hospital," and "a boy of six or seven months" who died at the Nuestra Señora de Mercedes Hospital.[72]

Many city residents were understandably furious with the strikers. *Diario de la Marina* railed against a medical strike "decreed in neglect of the laws of humanity." According to the conservative paper, the strike "provided in Havana and in all the cities of the Republic the painful spectacle of the sick cast out of the hospitals and the clinics abandoned without mercy for the wounded, while the pharmacies remain closed, refusing to sell medicine to the public."[73] Most strikes, the editors argued, were organized against "el patrón," but in the case of the medical strike, those harmed by the strike "had taken no part in the argument."[74] Indeed, it seems that the majority of the city's residents blamed the physicians for the strike, and soon newspapers started reporting threats of violence against the city's doctors. One article reported on a Havana resident who went to the Ministry of Health in search of medicines for his daughter who was critically ill from diphtheria. He could not find medical help for his daughter, "although in the most pathetic terms he pled for mercy for the little sick girl. 'If she dies,' he said, 'some doctor will pay for this crime.'"[75] On the evening of January 21, "a commission of residents, representing all of the neighborhoods of the city" visited the editorial offices of *Diario de la Marina* to "express the indignation with which the people of Havana see the attitude of the pharmacists and doctors who refuse to lend the slightest aid to the sick. 'We are sure,' said the visitors, 'that the hour is very close to when the people rise against the pharmacies.'"[76] One letter to President Mendieta from an angry resident described the "popular desire, without class distinction, to attack the doctors and exterminate them, killing them if necessary. If this strike continues," he wrote, "we will see many dead physicians."[77]

Indeed, violence did break out in response to the strike. On the morning of January 20, a group of physicians on the medical college's strike committee heard that a pharmacy in central Havana had opened in violation of the strike agreement. Four physicians, including the young socialist doctor José Elias Borges, armed themselves with revolvers and went to the pharmacy to demand it remain closed for the duration of the strike. An argument broke out between the four doctors and the pharmacist and his employees, as "other individuals attacked the pharmacy, breaking some windows." As the physicians turned to leave, the pharmacist shot and killed Borges. Hours later, a group of young men broke into the pharmacy and set it on fire.[78] Meanwhile, across the island, buildings associated with the FMC and its members were attacked: in the town of Caibaguán, Sancti Spiritus, the local medical clinic was bombed on the morning of January 21; that night, the Havana home of Dr. Cosme de la Torriente was bombed; two days later, the headquarters of the medical college of Cienfuegos was also bombed.[79] In Matanzas, neighbors attempted to burn down a pharmacy closed under strike orders, but the conflict ended when the local military forced the pharmacist to open his store in exchange for giving him protection.[80]

But the medical college had support as well. On January 20, a group of patients mobilized in support of the medical workers' demands. According to the Associated Press, "Several hundred patients crowded around the presidential palace all morning shouting 'Down with the strike breakers!'"[81] Leftist students also held demonstrations in support of the strikers in Havana's Parque Central.[82] Meanwhile, rumors began circulating that the city's Spanish merchants were planning a general commercial lockout in solidarity with the *centros regionales*. The National Confederation of Cuban Workers, for its part, "threatened a general strike in support of the doctors" if the medical strike was not soon resolved.[83]

Finally, on the night of January 23, the government and representatives from the Unified Front of medical workers negotiated to end the strike. The broad agreement granted medical workers many of their core demands, including the "strict enforcement of the Medical College Law, without outside interference"; an eight-hour workday for medical workers; the removal of strikebreaking doctors from private hospitals and clinics; and raises for all public medical workers, including nurses, doctors, midwives, and subordinate hospital staff, with equal pay for equal work for women and youth.[84] The government rejected the medical college's demand that it pass a law denying the wealthy membership in the *centros regionales*' medical programs; instead, the Mendieta government agreed to submit the matter to arbitration by the International Labour Office, promising to immediately abide by its rulings.

While the agreement ended the strike, tensions remained high over the following weeks. On February 4, a group of federated physicians from the health ministry were performing a routine medical inspection of the Spanish-run Quinta de Dependientes hospital, which was still under military occupation. As they were leaving, the physicians were attacked by a large crowd of the hospital's workers and other members of the Spanish Centro de Dependientes, who threw stones at the physicians' automobile. In response, soldiers fired into the crowd, killing two and injuring four.[85] Two weeks later, as the new Mendieta-Batista government gained stronger footing and began "taking a firmer hand with labor," the government dissolved the National Medical College and suspended all its decrees, including the key requirement that physicians be required to be members in good standing in order to practice medicine in Cuba.[86] The FMC had lost its main weapon against the *centros regionales*.

## PROLETARIANIZATION AND RADICALIZATION

The 1934 medical strike brought to the fore the central questions that had been plaguing the Cuban Medical Federation since the late 1920s: was the FMC essentially an apolitical professional organization or more akin to a labor union for physicians? Were physicians essentially medical laborers who performed a technical service in exchange for a wage, and whose natural allies were other sectors of the Cuban working class? Or should medicine be seen more like a scientific priesthood, ostensibly apolitical but naturally aligned with the "better classes" of the island? If professional healing granted physicians certain social privileges—respect, authority—what were the responsibilities that this social position entailed? These were not theoretical questions but would shape the organizing work of Cuban physicians as they worked out the implications of the strike. As observers noted, changing economic conditions were leading to what contemporaries referred to as the "proletarianization" of Cuban medicine—Cuban physicians could no longer count on the autonomy of private practice but were now increasingly salaried employees of public or private hospitals and clinics—but would this be embraced or rejected? In a changing Cuba, would physicians cling to an older vision of individual private practice advocated by some sectors of the FMC, or should the organization of medicine itself be radically transformed, as the Ala Izquierda advocated? In the months that followed the 1934 strike, this debate simmered within the medical community, as the suppression of the medical college and the failure of the International Labour Office's mediation efforts led physicians to increasingly embrace more radical alternatives for Cuban medicine.

The question of whether Cuban physicians were "really" workers was at the center of several scathing critiques of the January medical strike. According to the *Diario de la Marina*, physicians served a necessary social function and therefore had no right to strike. Unlike industrial workers, the editors warned, "the priest, the soldier and the doctor must always be prepared to combat the devil, the enemy, and the microbe."[87] In his letter to President Mendieta on the strike, G. R. Martoreli struck a similar note. Martoreli was incensed that physicians were "playing the role of the oppressed worker," falsely putting themselves "in the place of the working classes that unionize to defend themselves against the capital which oppresses and exploits them."[88] For Martoreli, who seems to have been a member of one of the Spanish *centros regionales*, Cuban physicians, not the *centros*, were earning money off the backs of the people and charging exorbitant fees for private care, while the *centros* provided low-cost quality health care for the city's working and middle classes. For *Diario de la Marina*, both the status of the medical profession and the particular work of doctoring made the unionization of physicians a ridiculous proposition. Masons, the editors argued, could ask for three pesos for a day's work and unionize so that all masons received the same pay for the same work. But was a mason's labor analogous to a physician's? For *Diario de la Marina*, the answer was a clear "no": the FMC's doctors wanted "all of the benefits of proletarianization without any of its inconveniences."[89]

But this vision of the physician as a wealthy and respected man of science was a thing of the past. According to the federation, changing economic conditions, the exploitation of medical labor by the *centros regionales*, and the government's indifference or hostility to the physicians' demands now required more combative tactics: "The wealthy physician who lived with great comforts has been substituted by the poor doctor who drags his scientific treasure through an impoverished home, who suffers the exploitation of hunger wages, when not a humiliating unemployment. The social concept of the doctor has changed. The ministry [priesthood, *sacerdocio*] is the pretext for exploitation. Poverty is the goad for rebellion."[90] The strike was incredibly unpopular, *La Tribuna Médica* acknowledged, but in the end, "we physicians should not aspire to be loved more, but to be respected more."

In June, the International Labour Office investigators Cyrille Dechamp and Moisés Poblete Troncoso submitted their report on "the medical problem and medico-mutualist healthcare in Cuba."[91] The authors largely agreed with the Cuban Medical Federation's critique that the medical crisis was caused, in part, by the "insufficient opportunities for the practice of medicine" due to the *centros regionales*' dominance of the capital's medical market, and advocated for a law limiting medical care at the *centros* to the poor and middle classes.[92] But for Dechamp and Troncoso, the root of the problem was not the *centros regionales* but, rather, the "economic situation of the country and the plethora of doctors" practicing in Cuba.[93] In other words, there were simply too many doctors in Cuba, and Cubans were currently too poor to pay for their services. While the report noted that a national maternal insurance program, which was then being organized, could provide new opportunities for medical practice, they found the *problema médico* to be essentially a market-based problem that would require a market-based solution: reduce the supply of physicians by cutting back on medical education or increase demand for medical services by improving the national economy.

While the ILO report was lauded by the leadership of the Cuban Medical Federation, the Ala Izquierda Médica rejected its findings.[94] They refuted the idea that Cuba had too many doctors, when so many poor and rural Cubans continued to lack access to basic medical services. For the Ala Izquierda, the roots of the medical crisis lay not in an excess number of physicians, but rather in the neocolonial economy itself, in the decades of elite and governmental indifference to public medical care, and in Cuba's "extraordinary lack of hospitals and other medical services . . . a state of affairs that faithfully reflects the economic and political interests of the dominant classes."[95] Rejecting the essentially market-based solutions of the ILO report, the Ala Izquierda pointed out that the health problems of the Cuban people and the economic problems of the medical sector could both be solved by a radical reorganization of medical practice on the island, with a massive public investment in urban and rural health services. With most rural workers unable to access medical services, new government-run rural hospitals and clinics could solve the medical labor crisis and finally ensure that all Cubans had access to quality health care.

But to achieve these reforms, Cuban physicians would need to shed the idea that they were not part of the exploited working mass and join forces with the broader Cuban working class to fight together for their common goals. If Dechamp and Poblete Troncoso warned of the potential "dangers entailed by the proletarianization of a particularly cultured sector of society," the Ala Izquierda embraced "proletarianization" as an opportunity for the medical workforce to unite with the broader Cuban working class.[96] "Doctors should see in the struggle with the other sectors related to medicine and with all the laboring masses of the country the only [struggle] capable of satisfying their demands," announced an editorial in the fall of 1934.[97]

Over the coming months, the FMC began openly debating the merits of a radical reconfiguration of medical practice. In November, La Tribuna Médica published "The Socialization of Medical Services and Related Services" by the Ala Izquierda Médica's Eduardo Odio Pérez.[98] The article was the clearest articulation yet of the Cuban medical Left's vision for a transformed medical system that would meet the needs of both physicians and the greater Cuban population. As Odio Pérez notes, while there was an elite segment of the FMC that had a large enough private clientele that allowed them to "live in abundance," the great majority of physicians either earned a small but stable salary in public or private hospitals or worked for themselves and earned little. Meanwhile, due to a lack of hospital services, "close to 70% of the Cuban population does not receive adequate medical care."[99] "After many years of bloody struggle and long debates within and outside of the Cuban Medical Federation," Odio Pérez argued, "the only and definitive solution has to be the socialization of medical services." The plan that Odio Pérez outlines is fascinating, not least because it describes precisely the kind of health care system that was put in place by the Cuban Revolution after 1959. Under the plan he put forth, "all medical services, dental services, midwifery services, etc., [would] be controlled and underwritten by the State," and all hospitals, clinics, and pharmacies would be converted to state institutions. All health services and medicines would be administered free of charge by the state. Preventative medical care would be radically expanded, and physicians and medical services would be "distributed throughout the territory in such a way that all citizens have easy access to them." Medical education would be free, but the number of medical professionals would be regulated according to the needs of the country.[100] In the one key difference from the post-1959 Cuban system, "those professionals that do not want to join the state organization [would] be free to have a private practice."[101] While the program would be costly, Odio Pérez argues that a simple 5 percent tax on public and private salaries would be more than enough to cover the costs of creating this extensive public health care system.

While the plan seems radical from the perspective of the FMC—in which the Ala Izquierda still represented a small, if influential, minority—new space had opened up for this kind of critique in the wake of the 1934 strike. After the suppression of the National Medical College, with the medical economy still in disarray, with the government increasingly hostile to the demands of Cuban doctors, and with the power of the *centros regionales* intact, Cuban physicians were increasingly open to new ideas. As they almost universally acknowledged, the Cuban medical system was bad for both doctors and patients. This conjecture created an opening for the Ala Izquierda and its allies within the broader Cuban Left to link the struggles of Cuban physicians to those of their patients and to consider the benefits of a state-run health care system.[102] The continuing revolutionary situation in the country, with worker occupations, bombings, strikes, and marches continuing throughout the year, surely added to the sense of possibilities and certainly gave impetus to the medical Left.

That fall, the Cuban daily *Ahora* published an article by Dr. Edelmiro A. Félix in favor of a state-run medical system that received letters of support from other physicians in the country.[103] Other articles in *La Tribuna Médica* offered sympathetic assessments of socialized medicine or pushed Cuban physicians to link their struggles to the broader Cuban working class.[104] Even the archconservative *Diario de la Marina* printed a translation of George W. Aspinwall's "A Plea for Socialized Medicine," originally published in the *American Mercury*.[105] For Aspinwall, medical care was a social "right, . . . not a private or public charity," and should therefore be provided free of charge by the state, with medical practice organized by the state in a system very similar to what Odio Pérez described in *La Tribuna Médica*.[106] In another sign of the times, the Cuban medical journal *Cirugía Ortopédica* published a sympathetic assessment of the Soviet medical system written by the elite Cuban orthopedist Alberto Inclán. Inclán praised the rapid advances in the organization of medical services and education in the USSR, although he stopped short of advocating a state-run medical system in Cuba, arguing "such a beautiful system can only develop integrally within a Soviet state."[107] Nevertheless, the fact that the aristocratic Inclán, a champion horse breeder and hardly a radical, would write a sympathetic account of the Soviet health system speaks volumes about space for radical critiques of the Cuban medical system that were created through the medical struggles of 1933 and 1934.[108]

Over the course of 1934, Cuban medical politics underwent a broad shift. The violence of the medical strike and the government suppression of the medical college, the failure of mediation efforts, and the continuing economic crisis for Cuban physicians all led the FMC's members to rethink their single-minded focus on the Spanish regional societies as the cause of their woes. Physicians increasingly linked their economic interests to the health interests of their patients and pressed the government to ensure that all Cubans had access to health care. Public medical workers took the lead, taking the government to task for terrible conditions in public hospitals, clinics, and sanatoriums, which suffered from official neglect and poor funding. As obstetrician José Chelala Aguilera argued, the Mendieta-Batista government was prioritizing the military and foreign debts over the health of the Cuban people, "allocating excessive funds to the Army, creating multiple new positions in the police, [and] paying the foreign debts owed to Speyer and [J. P.] Morgan, while the *pueblo* is plunged in misery and practically no funds are allocated to the hospitals."[109] In the fall, the physicians employed at the government antituberculosis sanatorium La Esperanza organized and presented a list of demands to the Ministry of Health, asking for increased public funding for the hospital, both to improve the conditions of care for the sanatorium's patients and improve the "starvation wages" of the hospital's medical staff.[110] Physicians organized similar movements at several other state and municipal medical institutions, all linking the interests of patients and doctors.[111] The federation supported all of these movements and was increasingly vocal in its criticism of government for the "state of abandon" of Havana's public hospitals.[112]

As we have seen, by the 1920s and 1930s, a growing chorus of Cubans were calling for greater state investment in the health of the Cuban people. Nurses, health officials, feminists, journalists, and black fraternal organizations all rejected the idea that health should be the privilege of the wealthy, while low wages, terrible living conditions, and underfunded public medical services condemned so many to disease and early death. Invoking Jose Martí's call for a nation "with all, and for the good of all," they called upon the state to guarantee the basic requirements of health—decent housing, affordable food, and free quality health care to those that needed it. But while Cuban doctors often urged greater state investment in public health, the traditional ideal of a private medical practice still held enormous sway, and many were leery of the implications of a government guaranteed right to medical care. The strike and its aftermath, however, transformed this calculus. While most physicians continued to reject the goal of an entirely state-run medical system, a growing number demanded a radical expansion of public health care to meet both the health needs of the Cuban people and the employment needs of the medical sector. In a January 1935 interview published in the newspaper *Acción*, FMC president José Bisbé echoed many of these arguments, which had consistently been voiced by the Ala Izquierda.[113] When asked whether he believed that there was an "overproduction" of physicians in the university, as the ILO report argued, Bisbé replied that there was not. Rather, "what is necessary is to open up new horizons to the doctor.... The state needs to multiply medical services. There is a lack of hospitals. There are health department chiefs in charge of huge territories that they cannot possibly attend to. Where they cannot even vaccinate [everyone]. [Medical services] need to be brought to the countryside. And this, naturally, requires doctors and demands money to pay these doctors."[114]

In the coming years there would be a push to expand public medical services and move health care more firmly into the countryside. But the FMC would be sidelined from these processes. Tensions between the FMC and the Mendieta-Batista government came to a head during the first three months of 1935. In January, Havana's municipal medical workers struck, calling for the removal of political influence from hiring and firing of medical personnel and for the better funding of city clinics and hospitals.[115] In response, police rounded up known strike organizers, two emergency clinics were occupied by the national police, and medical students and physicians were arrested at the FMC's social club.[116] Meanwhile, popular opposition to the Mendieta-Batista government continued to grow in the face of state repression and the suppression of civil liberties. In early March, workers hoping to force the removal of the Mendieta-Batista government organized the largest general strike in Cuban history, with over 500,000 Cubans participating.[117] With government officials believing that the university was a center of opposition organizing, the military was ordered to occupy the university and its Calixto García Hospital.[118] In solidarity with both the occupied hospital's medical staff and the broader strike movement, physicians and other medical workers in public sector hospitals and clinics across the city joined the general strike. At this point, the Mendieta-Batista government had had enough of the Cuban Medical Federation: the federation's offices were sacked by the military, and striking physicians at the Mazorra Hospital, the Asilo de Ancianos, La Esperanza sanatorium, the municipal hospital, and others were fired. Just as other labor unions across the country were violently suppressed by the military, the FMC was declared an illegal organization and forcibly dissolved.[119] For aligning itself too closely with the broader labor movement, the federation was finally caught up in the government's violent suppression of dissent.

During the January 1934 strike, El Diario de la Marina warned that the unionization of the medical class held the seeds of socialism, asking what would be the end result of unionization if not the "bureaucratization [of medicine] by the state."[120] Sectors of the medical class certainly did look forward to a future revolutionary state that would take health care as a central task and organize a national system beneficial to both physicians and patients. And indeed, the 1934 medical strike and subsequent political realignment of the FMC highlights a moment where the economic interests of physicians aligned with the health interests of the poorest Cubans, creating the conditions for an unusual alliance for the expansion of public medical services. Yet most of the federation's doctors did not consider themselves revolutionaries and did not seek a state-run medical system. Rather, most hoped for a mixed medical system that had a significant public sector, providing needed medical care to the Cuban poor both in the cities and in the underserved countryside, but that had room for private practice and even some mutual aid health services.

But this balance would be difficult to strike. The public medical sector remained chronically underfunded, the *centros regionales* remained impervious to the efforts of Cuban physicians to rein in their practices, and medical fees remained out of reach for much of the city's population. While conditions for Cuban physicians would generally improve in the coming decades, as the economy recovered from the effects of the depression, medical services would still be overwhelmingly limited to the capital, leaving the countryside reliant on a few private practitioners or unlicensed healers. Nevertheless, Cuban medical politics was transformed during this period, as both patients and doctors increasingly claimed health care as a right to be ensured by the state. In 1940, these demands would be partly met by a far-reaching new social democratic constitution whose provisions would improve the living and labor conditions of the working class and enshrine the right to medical care for those too poor to pay for it.

# Conclusion
The Right to Live in Health in Postcolonial Havana

In his 1936 report to Cuban president Miguel Mariano Gómez, Secretary of Health Manuel Mencía pulled no punches in describing the dismal state of Cuban health institutions. After years of "government indifference," Mencía admitted, Cuba's hospital and public health infrastructure was falling apart.[1] Hospitals across the country were in terrible condition, with many in desperate need of repairs. Suffering from a lack of funding that "could not be more egregious," public hospitals could barely afford such basics as surgical equipment, X-ray film, intravenous equipment, proper food for patients, or even essential medicines.[2] Insufficient funding for public health work led to regular outbreaks of epidemic disease and left endemic illness untreated.[3] In the cities, lack of access to clean water and utterly insufficient sewerage led to epidemics of typhoid, while inattention to rural and suburban drainage led to exploding mosquito populations, feeding an out-of-control malaria problem. Polio, intestinal parasites, typhoid, syphilis, malaria, leprosy—these were all significant problems that a lack of funding prevented the Ministry of Health from properly addressing. Félix García Rodríguez, the former director of Beneficencia for the health ministry, concurred, excoriating Cuban politicians for the nation's state of sanitary abandon: "While the Congress is one of the costliest in the world and the Army and Navy are excellently and overabundantly equipped," he wrote, the amount of money spent per capita on public health had suffered "a criminal decline," falling by a third since 1909.[4] Corruption in hospital and health ministry appointments and the creation of sinecures in local health departments added to the chaos and disorder in Cuba's sanitary institutions.[5]

This situation was all the more frustrating given the hopeful beginnings of Cuban public health. As García Rodríguez reminded his readers, Carlos J. Finlay had hailed the birth of the republic as coming "at the dawn of an age of enlightenment, in the midst of a sparkling atmosphere of scientific discovery, so that its first breaths have been of progress and noble aspirations."[6] Cuba's transition from colony to republic had been shaped by a generation of medical nationalist luminaries, including such figures "of singular scientific prominence" as Carlos J. Finlay, Juan Guiteras, Joaquín Jacobsen, and Jorge Le-Roy y Cassá.[7] At the turn of the century, this generation of physicians and scientists had sought to guide Cuba away from the suffering, disease, and death that marked the recent colonial past and harness the benefits of science and medicine to create a modern, healthy, and independent republic. In response to both U.S. imperial sanitary oversight and the reality of urban poverty and disease, they created innovative health institutions, spearheaded far-reaching sanitary campaigns, and worked to transform a people "ignorant of modern hygiene" into a healthy and modern citizenry. But by the late 1930s, health officials like Manuel Mencía observed with obvious bitterness that "Cuban public health, which had attained the greatest heights [in] banishing diseases as serious as yellow fever . . . has since steadily declined."[8]

For those familiar with twentieth-century Cuban history, this narrative of rising hopes and dashed dreams, of promising starts and steady declines, is an all-too-common trope. Certainly, there is much truth to it, as this book has shown, and there are enough examples of dashed dreams to have filled countless books of history and political commentary over the past century.[9] But while Mencía and García Rodríguez had ample evidence for their dim view of Cuban public health institutions in the late 1930s, this perspective occludes as much as it reveals, for even in its failures we can see the transformation of Cuban medicine, the growing popular demands and changing politics that would have such a lasting impact on Cuban health.

As this book has demonstrated, in the decades after the end of Spanish rule a series of political, economic, cultural, and social factors converged in sometimes surprising ways to give medicine outsized importance in postindependence Cuban politics and, conversely, to give the state outsized importance in the development of Cuban medicine. Cuba's international sanitary obligations under the Platt Amendment converged with and helped fuel a discourse of medical nationalism that tied the colonial past to disease, suffering, and backwardness. In its place, medical nationalists dreamed of a modern, healthy republic, and while they disagreed in its implementation, they shared the conviction that they had both the ability and the responsibility to build medical institutions that would meet the people's health needs and also be an example of scientific excellence on par with any other. But if both nationalism and the need to maintain sovereignty required extra attention to public health, the neocolonial economy imposed its own legacies, and together these material and political realities prevented the full realization of the medical nationalist vision. In the cases of the plague, infant mortality, tuberculosis, and even the organization of the medical profession, medical nationalist hopes crashed against the rocks of economic instability, lack of government funding, endemic corruption, and most importantly, the high cost of living and depressed wages that relegated huge swaths of the urban population to an early grave.

But rather than tamp down popular expectations, this process was transformative for both medical workers and the Cuban public. This book is about the emergence of a new politics, but it has identified its locus less in the better-known mass movements and revolutionary politics of the era than in the much more intimate everyday interactions between urban residents and medical practitioners. When families brought their children, husbands, or parents to the clinic or hospital, or welcomed into their homes the health department's visiting nurses, they entrusted these public institutions and agents of the state with the health of their loved ones. For the doctors, nurses, and health officials tasked with this profound responsibility, each interaction was an opportunity to use their acquired expertise and experience to improve the lives of their patients. These interactions were often fraught, of course, and popular-class women and men often rejected the elitism and intrusiveness of medical reformers who hoped to "modernize" their personal habits, their forms of childcare, or their ways of living. But cumulatively, these quotidian interactions became opportunities to learn. Urban residents increasingly took up the "gospel of hygiene" and integrated the lessons of the laboratory into their home lives. And nurses, doctors, and health officials increasingly learned about the lives of the urban poor, as they heard from mothers the difficulties they encountered making ends meet in an exorbitantly expensive city, and saw with their own eyes the effects of poor housing and lack of affordable childcare on their fellow urban residents.

As became increasingly clear to health officials, nurses, physicians, and other reformers, the best way to address major urban health problems was to alleviate the underlying economic conditions that facilitated ill health, through reforms that would lower the cost of living, improve housing conditions, and provide healthy childcare options and inexpensive or free medical services to the poor. While some public and private programs attempted to do just that, they were consistently hobbled by a lack of funding that itself reflected underlying economic relations and inconsistent political will among the nation's elected officials. But over time, new health campaigns, projects, and institutions helped generate new popular expectations for a healthy republic and for a government that took seriously the health conditions of the people. A growing chorus of Cubans began demanding health services not as a privilege for the wealthy or well-connected but as a fundamental right of all citizens. These demands converged in complex ways with national economic realities: with little domestic wealth to fund the kinds of private health charities that were a staple of North American health practice, medical practitioners and the Cuban people alike increasingly turned to the state to meet the island's pressing health needs. And with the national economy providing few employment opportunities for Cuban physicians, they became unlikely allies in the push for state medicine. By the late 1930s, these rising popular expectations joined with growing demands for structural economic changes that would improve the health of the Cuban people, leaving their imprint in the island's new foundational charter.

ON JULY 1, 1940, members of the Cuban Constitutional Assembly met in the small town of Guaímaro in the central province of Camaguey to sign a new constitution. The location was symbolic, for it was there, in April 1869, that Carlos Manuel de Céspedes and other rebel leaders signed Cuba's first constitution during the Ten Years War against Spain. At the same long wooden table used by their nineteenth-century counterparts, the men and women of the Constitutional Assembly signed one of the most progressive legal documents of its time. The 1940 constitution redefined state-citizen relations, vastly increasing the role of the state in the economy and establishing an array of new legal protections for workers. Physicians were well-represented in the assembly—their number was second only to that of lawyers—and many of the constitution's provisions reflected long-standing medical nationalist proposals to improve health by reducing economic inequality and vastly expanding the role of the state in the nation's health landscape. The constitution set minimum wages and mandated an eight-hour workday, a forty-four-hour workweek, and a one-month paid vacation. It enshrined women's voting rights and outlawed discrimination on the basis of gender, race, color, and class. It mandated robust social security provisions, including old age, disability, and unemployment protections as well as maternity benefits such as paid three-month maternity leave and employment protections that prohibited dismissal during pregnancy. Incorporating demands at the center of the campaign to reduce infant mortality, the constitution required employers to give nursing mothers two half-hour breaks each day to nurse their infants.

The constitution replaced the old Secretaría de Sanidad y Beneficencia with a new Ministry of Health and Social Assistance (Ministerio de Salubridad y Asistencia Social), and incorporated the National Advisory Board on

Tuberculosis (Consejo Nacional de Tuberculosis) into the ministry, giving antituberculosis work an expanded reach and national stature. Reflecting long-standing concerns of the FMC over the influence of politicians over public health and hospital personnel, the new Ministry of Health and Social Assistance would be an "exclusively technical" institution.[10] State medical institutions were to remain "above politics," with personnel chosen on the basis of technical capacity rather than political affiliation. The constitution also stipulated that each municipality would have a public clinic or dispensary, which would both expand public health care in the interior of the island and employ more Cuban physicians in the state medical sector.

But the provision with the most far-reaching implications for health was included under Article 10 of the constitution, which enshrined—for the first time in Cuban history—the fundamental right of all Cuban citizens to medical care. Among the five fundamental rights of Cuban citizens under Article 10 was the right "to receive social assistance and public benefits with, in the former case, prior affirmation of need." During the republic, public benefits were largely limited to the provision of free medical care in public hospitals, clinics, and dispensaries. But Cuba's *beneficencia* tradition had long shied away from acknowledging a "right" to aid. As we have seen, the term itself, close in meaning to "state charity," implied that such aid represented government largesse rather than any intrinsic citizen right. That Cubans might come to think of state aid as a right was, in fact, a major concern of American Department of Public Charities officials during the first U.S. occupation. The new constitution turned this relationship on its head, however, and redefined the meaning of state support for the health of the poor.

According to the physician, former national director of Beneficencia, and member of the 1940 Constitutional Assembly Félix García Rodríguez, by the 1930s, state support for the poor had everywhere become a "primordial obligation of the State." Indeed, it was increasingly recognized as such by governments from across the political spectrum, from post-Revolutionary Mexico to fascist Italy and the New Deal United States.[11] For García Rodríguez, the colonial concept of *beneficencia*, "with its always humiliating implication of charity, of a gift, or favor or alms," was now being replaced with the more modern concept of "public assistance" based on a clear sense of social rights and state responsibility. This modern model of social assistance was based not on charity but on social solidarity, as "reparations for secular injustices" based on an understanding that poverty arose not out of laziness but "from the defects of a poorly organized economic system."[12] Implicit in this vision of citizen rights and state responsibility was the understanding that the unfettered capitalist economy was malformed, that it was—as so many nurses, doctors, and social reformers had been arguing for decades—a fundamental cause of illness in postcolonial Cuba. The obligation of the state was therefore to do what it could to meet the health needs of those whose suffering emerged out of the neocolonial economy itself. As García Rodríguez made clear, this "health right," finally formalized by the 1940 constitution, "obliges the State to protect all citizens against all risk from disease."[13]

This robust conception of state responsibility, however, was not a foreign imposition but, rather, was deeply rooted in postcolonial Cuban medical nationalism. It was present in the 1903 speech that Pedro Albarrán Domínguez gave before the Cuban House of Representatives in support of the Ministry of Health, when he declared that the "right to exist, the right to live, necessarily comes before all other rights of man. The State has the obligation to guarantee these rights before all others." But Albarrán shared the confidence of his generation of medical nationalists that hygiene and basic public health action alone could protect citizens from disease.[14] The reality, which would only become clearer with time, was that without substantive measures to reduce poverty, the efficacy of Cuban health campaigns to reduce mortality would be critically compromised. As Sebastián Beltrán Moreno wrote in a 1937 editorial reflecting on the failures of Cuban antituberculosis work, "Poverty is the cause of failure for all health policy."[15] But by the late 1930s, these two threads finally came together: the robust ideal of state responsibility for health was increasingly interpreted as *requiring* economic interventions to address the central role that poverty played in creating the conditions for disease and death.

When we look at the history of health in early-twentieth-century Cuba, the lives of those often left out of the historical narrative come into clearer focus: the nursing students orphaned by the War of Independence that transformed Cuban hospitals, the country doctor that emerged from humble roots to tackle disease and poverty in the capital, and the *solar* resident whose powerful book forced Cubans to confront realities most wished to ignore. Filtered through the fragmented republican archive we also get a glimpse of the innumerable urban residents that demanded public medical services—a hospital bed for a tubercular spouse or milk for their child. As their actions remind us, before being enshrined in national charters, "rights" are the claims that people make, reflecting their lived realities and material needs. The health rights formalized in the 1940 Constitution reflected and emerged out of popular health demands, which, over time, forced nurses, physicians, and health officials to confront the chasm between their medical nationalist ideals and the reality of disease and death that were the natural product of entrenched poverty and medical neglect.

Of course, it is one thing to establish a legal right and another thing entirely to provide the institutional framework to make that right a reality. While the 1940 constitution vastly expanded the role of the state in providing health and social services, these provisions were only haltingly and partially implemented. Medical services remained overwhelmingly limited to the capital, while wide swaths of the countryside remained without key medical services. Rural hunger and disease continued largely unabated, and national public health services remained underfunded. Public health services continued to be plagued by political influence. Nevertheless, even while statistical data on rural health for this period is partial (given the inadequate reach of public health institutions), it seems that overall health indices in 1950s Cuba were relatively good. Life expectancy in 1960 was the second highest in Latin America, while the infant mortality rate was the lowest in Latin America and lower than that of some European countries.[16] As McGuire and Frankel argue in their study of mortality decline in prerevolutionary Cuba, the availability of free or low-cost medical services in the larger cities, especially Havana, was largely responsible for the island's relatively low mortality rate in 1958.[17] Throughout this period, a significant portion of the population had access to low-cost health services through the *centros regionales* or newer medical cooperatives, while poor urban residents could access free medical care through the public hospital system.

While the history of health and medical care in the republic remains understudied, much better known is the impressive attention given to health care in Cuba in the wake of the 1959 Cuban Revolution.[18] Universal access to quality health care has become a signature achievement of the Cuban Revolution. In the early 1960s, the new revolutionary government nationalized health services. It began expanding access to medical care in the countryside with the creation of the Rural Health Service and created a national system of comprehensive polyclinics. Emphasizing health screening and preventative care, while providing free medical care to all Cuban citizens, these reforms were both popular and successful and led to significant improvements in overall Cuban health indices. Today the island boasts a lower infant mortality rate than the United States and has among the highest life expectancy rates and doctor-to-patient ratios in the world. That these reforms were organized in the context of a crippling embargo and the emigration of almost half of the country's physicians in the early years of the revolution is impressive and speaks to the great importance that Cuban officials attached to expanded access to medical care.

Within Cuban revolutionary discourse, this expansion in health services represented a sharp break with the past. The prerevolutionary period, the story goes, was marked by disease, starvation, and poverty, by a state that neglected the health of the people. The revolutionary government, by contrast, would correct this historical failure, making public health a matter of highest state concern. This is the story that is usually told, both in Cuba and abroad, as Cuban officials and supporters of the revolution have regularly touted the expansion of rural health services and overall improvements in public health as proof of the revolution's legitimacy. Indeed, after the success of the 1959 revolution, Fidel Castro regularly pointed to the disease, hunger, and poverty of the countryside as a sign of the central failings and illegitimacy of the Batista government, the health impacts of empire, and the failed legacy of the "neocolonial republic" as a whole.[19]

Strikingly, however, critics of the Cuban Revolution also often point to health care under the revolution, but as a sign of the fundamental illegitimacy of the revolutionary government. According to critics, the island already had excellent official health indicators in the prerevolutionary period, and the supposed "health miracle" since the 1960s is based on falsified health statistics.[20] In either case, however, the health of the Cuban people is tied to the legitimacy of the Cuban government. But as we have seen, this discourse linking political independence and government legitimacy to the health conditions of the Cuban people did not begin with the Cuban Revolution but was a central element of turn-of-the-century Cuban medical nationalism. In the decades that followed independence, this discourse would be taken up at different times to shape a variety of health campaigns and conflicts, to highlight the failure of the government to care for its citizens, to target immigrants and the poor, and to make powerful claims for state intervention in the economy to preserve the health of the most vulnerable. Throughout these conflicts and debates, and through the daily contact between the urban sick and the men and women trained to care for them, new ideas emerged, unlikely alliances were forged, and consensus was achieved that health and access to medical care are the birthright of every Cuban.

# NOTES

## ABBREVIATIONS

ANC     Archivo Nacional de Cuba, La Habana, Havana, Cuba
AH     Audencia de la Habana
CPRC     Citizens' Permanent Relief Committee Records
FE     Fondo Especial
HFP     Homer Folks Papers, Columbia University Archives, New York, N.Y.
HSP     Historical Society of Pennsylvania, Philadelphia
LOC     Library of Congress, Manuscripts Division, Washington, D.C.
MGC     Records of the Military Government of Cuba, 1898–1903
RA     Registro de Asociaciones
SP     Secretaría de la Presidencia
USNA     National Archives of the United States of America, College Park, Md.
UVA-SP     Library of the University of Virginia, Special Collections Library, Papers of Jefferson Randolph Kean

## INTRODUCTION

1. Congreso de la República de Cuba, *Diario de sesiones del Congreso*.
2. Congreso de la República de Cuba, *Diario de sesiones del Congreso*, 90.
3. Congreso de la República de Cuba, *Diario de sesiones del Congreso*, 91.
4. Congreso de la República de Cuba, *Diario de sesiones del Congreso*, 92.
5. Departamento de Sanidad de la Habana, *Manual de práctica sanitaria*, iii.
6. Tomes, *Gospel of Germs*; Wangensteen and Wangensteen, *Rise of Surgery*; Rosner, *A Once Charitable Enterprise*; Starr, *Social Transformation of American Medicine*; Rosenberg, *Care of Strangers*; Worboys, *Spreading Germs*.
7. See Ferrer, *Insurgent Cuba*; Fischer, *Modernity Disavowed*; Ferrer, *Freedom's Mirror*; Finch, *Rethinking Slave Rebellion in Cuba*; and Childs, *1812 Aponte Rebellion*.
8. See Tone, *War and Genocide in Cuba*, and Barcia Zequeira, *Una sociedad en crisis*.
9. Espinosa, *Epidemic Invasions*; Stepan, "Interplay between Socio-Economic Factors and Medical Science." On the colonial politics of U.S. public health work abroad, see also Anderson, *Colonial Pathologies*; Birn, *Marriage of Convenience*; Laveaga, *Jungle Laboratories*; Palmer, *Launching Global Health*; and McCoy and Scarano, *Colonial Crucible*, 273–326.
10. On postindependence Cuban medicine, see Funes Monzote, *El despertar del asociacionismo científico en Cuba*; Naranjo Orovio and García González, *Medicina y racismo en Cuba*;

García González and Álvarez Peláez, *En busca de la raza perfecta*; Palmer, "Beginnings of Cuban Bacteriology"; Gutiérrez, "Disease, Empire, and Modernity in the Caribbean"; Lambe, *Madhouse*; Urban, "The Sick Republic" and "The 'Black Plague'"; and Rodríguez Expósito, "La Primera Secretaría de Sanidad," *Carlos J. Finlay, and Dr. Juan N. Dávalos*. See also the work of Gregorio Delgado García, editor and major contributor of Cuba's *Cuadernos de la Historia de la Salud Pública*.

11. Indeed, these circuits have been at the center of both the Atlantic and Caribbean history fields. See, for example, Scott, *Common Wind*; Ferreira, *Cross Cultural Exchange in the Atlantic World*; Rodgers, *Atlantic Crossings*; Putnam, *Radical Moves*; and Ferrer, *Freedom's Mirror*.

12. On the disease implications of these Atlantic and circum-Caribbean interconnections, see Espinosa, *Epidemic Invasions*; Markel, *Quarantine!*; Echenberg, *Plague Ports*; Palmer, *Launching Global Health*; Kraut, *Silent Travelers*; De Barros, Palmer, and Wright, *Health and Medicine in the Circum-Caribbean*; and McNeill, *Mosquito Empires*.

13. Among the very few works on Spanish immigrants in Cuba, see Iturria, *Españoles en la cultura cubana*; Maluquer de Motes Bernet, *Nación e inmigración*; and Naranjo Orovio and García González, *Medicina y racismo en Cuba*.

14. On nineteenth- and twentieth-century urban growth, housing, and poverty in Havana, see Bay y Sevilla, *La vivienda del pobre*; Chailloux Cardona, *Síntesis histórica de la vivienda popular*; Scarpaci, Segre, and Coyula, *Havana*; García, *Beyond the Walled City*; and Horst, "Sleeping on the Ashes."

15. Scarpaci, Segre, and Coyula, *Havana*, 43–45.

16. "Sanitation Files Ruined by Flames Started by Arson," *Havana Post*, February 7, 1933; "Spain Acts to Help Youth Seized in Cuba," *New York Times*, February 7, 1933.

17. "Bomb Blast at Havana Laboratory," *New York Times*, December 18, 1932.

18. Antoinette Burton, "Archive Fever, Archive Stories," in Burton, *Archive Stories*, 6. See also Trouillot, *Silencing the Past*, and Stoler, *Along the Archival Grain*.

19. See, for example, Thomas, *Cuba*; Ruiz, *Cuba*; Suchlicki, *Cuba, from Columbus to Castro*; Pérez, *Cuba under the Platt Amendment*; and Helg, *Our Rightful Share*.

20. Palmer, Piqueras, and Sánchez Cobos, *State of Ambiguity*; Pappademos, *Black Political Activism and the Cuban Republic*; Riaño San Marful, *Gallos y toros en Cuba*; Joseph and Nugent, *Everyday Forms of State Formation*; Sanders, *Vanguard of the Atlantic World*; Thurner and Guerrero, *After Spanish Rule*; Thurner, *From Two Republics to One Divided*; Adelman, *Colonial Legacies*; Mallon, *Peasant and Nation*.

21. Foucault, *Birth of the Clinic*; Tomes, *Gospel of Germs*; Anderson, *Colonial Pathologies*; Rogaski, *Hygienic Modernity*; Meade, *Civilizing Rio*; McKiernan-González, *Fevered Measures*; Markel, *Quarantine!*

22. This book is in close conversation with recent scholarship that looks at struggles over social rights in twentieth-century Latin America, such as Grandin, *Last Colonial Massacre*; Fischer, *Poverty of Rights*; Caulfield, *In Defense of Honor*; Suárez Findlay, *Imposing Decency*; Adair, *In Search of the "Lost Decade"*; Romero Sanchez, *The Building State*; and McDonald, "Peripheral Citizenship." This work is also indebted to recent scholarship on postcolonial states that looks at how rights were negotiated and contested. See Chambers, *From Subjects to Citizens*; Ahlman, *Living with Nkrumahism*; Ahmed, *Afghanistan Rising*; and Mitchell, *Rule of Experts*.

23. Brotherton, *Revolutionary Medicine*.

CHAPTER ONE

1. Parker, *Cubans of To-day*, 487.
2. Delfín, *Treinta años de médico*, 7–12.
3. Cuba's third and final War of Independence from Spanish rule began in early 1895. The initial War of Independence, known as the Ten Years' War, was fought between 1868 and 1878 and was followed by the short-lived Guerra Chiquita, or Little War (1879–80).
4. "Dispensario La Caridad," *Diario de la Marina*, November 15, 1899.
5. On the difficulty of assessing the numbers of those killed or displaced by the final War of Independence, see Tone, *War and Genocide in Cuba*, 209–17.
6. See Tone, *War and Genocide in Cuba*, 223.
7. See Tyrell, *Reforming the World*.
8. "Doomed to Die of Starvation," *San Francisco Chronicle*, April 26, 1897.
9. "Grim Death in Awful Form," *San Francisco Chronicle*, May 3, 1897.
10. Of course, early commentators and historians wrote celebratory assessments of U.S. relief, social welfare, and health reforms in Cuba. See, for example, Bangs, *Uncle Sam Trustee*, and Chapman, *History of the Cuban Republic*.
11. Tone, *War and Genocide in Cuba*, 193.
12. Tone, *War and Genocide in Cuba*, 213.
13. Pérez, *Cuba between Empires*, 152.
14. "Distress in Cuba," *The Sun* (Baltimore), January 12, 1898.
15. "Report of Brigadier General William Ludlow," in U.S. War Department, *Annual Reports of the War Department for the Fiscal Year Ended June 30, 1900*, vol. 1, pt. 4, p. 9.
16. "Report of Brigadier General William Ludlow," in U.S. War Department, *Annual Reports of the War Department for the Fiscal Year Ended June 30, 1900*, vol. 1, pt. 4, p. 9.
17. See Tone, *War and Genocide in Cuba*, chap. 14.
18. López, "Ambliopía por desnutrición," 237.
19. Tone, *War and Genocide in Cuba*, 213.
20. "Starvation of Reconcentrados in Cuba."
21. "Awful in Havana: The Reconcentrados Are All About Starved," *Minneapolis Journal*, May 15, 1898, 2.
22. "Dispensario La Caridad," *Diario de la Marina*, November 15, 1899.
23. An 1899 "Special Hygiene Commission" report shows that the vast majority of commercial sex workers were orphaned girls with few other means of survival. See Alfonso y García, *La prostitución en Cuba*, 20.
24. "Dispensario La Caridad," *Diario de la Marina*, November 15, 1899.
25. Kean, "Needs of the Department of Charities," 538.
26. Kean, "Needs of the Department of Charities," 537–38; letter from E. S. J. Greble to the Governor of Havana, May 27, 1899, Greble Papers, LOC.
27. Kean, "Hospitals and Charities in Cuba," 141.
28. The institution had its roots in the Real Casa de Maternidad, or Royal House of Maternity, dating from 1687, and the Real Casa de Beneficencia, or the Royal House of Public Charities, which was formed in 1792. In 1852, they combined to form a single institution.
29. The inmates of the asylum were distributed to other institutions in the city. The

Junta de Patronos, the governing board of the Casa de Beneficencia, protested the conditions at the Santa Clara convent where girls and toddlers were held, citing their "very bad hygienic conditions," but to no effect. Many later died in their new institutions. See Cabrera, *La Casa de Beneficencia y la Sociedad Económica*, 106, 46.

30. Delfín, *Treinta años de médico*, 109.

31. Delfín, *Treinta años de médico*, 64.

32. Delfín, *Treinta años de médico*, 104–5.

33. Barcia Zequeira, *Una sociedad en crisis*, 119–237.

34. The geologist Robert T. Hill, writing in 1898, suggested that this combination of black poverty and disproportionate black population in the provinces hardest hit by the reconcentration led to a disproportionate black mortality. See Hill, *Cuba and Porto Rico*, 106–7. Indeed, the 1899 census shows a disproportionate decrease in the population of Cubans of color. See Helg, *Our Rightful Share*, 271–72n161.

35. Nevertheless, Spanish regional societies struggled during the war to maintain their membership and continue providing services. See *El libro del Centro Asturiano*, 61–62.

36. See, for example, the Asilo San Vicente de Paul, in Havana's Cerro neighborhood. See "Report of Maj. E. St. Greble, Superintendent, Department of Charities, Department of Havana," in U.S. War Department, *Annual Reports of the War Department for the Fiscal Year Ended June 30, 1900*, pt. 11, *Report of the Military Governor of Cuba on Civil Affairs*, vol. 1, pt. 2, p. 398.

37. Hoganson, *Fighting for American Manhood*.

38. "Appeal for Food and Money: President McKinley Asks That Charity Be Extended Cuban Sufferers," *Omaha World Herald*, December 25, 1897.

39. Box 3, folder 1, CPRC, HSP.

40. Box 3, CPRC, HSP.

41. Caroline H. Pemberton to the Citizens' Permanent Relief Committee, box 3, folder 1, CPRC, HSP.

42. Juan Guiteras to Citizens' Permanent Relief Committee, box 3, folder 1, CPRC, HSP.

43. "Report of E. Winfield Egan, M.D.," in Barton, *Red Cross in Peace and War*, 642.

44. See "Corrected Consolidated Record of Deaths for the Years 1890 to 1900 for the City of Havana," series 2, box 19, Brooke Papers, HSP.

45. Carl Schurz, "The Philanthropic Policy," *Harper's Weekly*, April 9, 1898.

46. See box 9, CPRC, HSP.

47. See "Corrected Consolidated Record of Deaths for the Years 1890 to 1900 for the City of Havana," series 2, box 19, Brooke Papers, HSP.

48. George Kennan, "The Regeneration of Cuba," *Outlook*, June 10, 1899, 334–40.

49. See G. W. Hyatt to Clara Barton, September 24, 1898, and G. W. Wyatt to Stephen Barton, November 11, 1898, Red Cross File, American National Red Cross, 1878 to 1957, Relief Operations, Spanish-American War, Correspondence, Special, Hyatt, George W., 1898 to 1899, Barton Papers, LOC.

50. G. W. Hyatt to Stephen Barton, October 17, 1898, Red Cross File, American National Red Cross, 1878 to 1957, Relief Operations, Spanish-American War, Correspondence, Special, Hyatt, George W., 1898 to 1899, Barton Papers, LOC. Emphasis in the original.

51. Letter to Clara Barton on September 24, 1898, Red Cross File, American National

Red Cross, 1878 to 1957, Relief Operations, Spanish-American War, Correspondence, Special, Hyatt, George W., 1898 to 1899, Barton Papers, LOC.

52. G. W. Wyatt to Stephen Barton, October 17, 1898, Red Cross File, American National Red Cross, 1878 to 1957, Relief Operations, Spanish-American War, Correspondence, Special, Hyatt, George W., 1898 to 1899, Barton Papers, LOC.

53. G. W. Hyatt to Clara Barton, September 24, 1898, Red Cross File, American National Red Cross, 1878 to 1957, Relief Operations, Spanish-American War, Correspondence, Special, Hyatt, George W., 1898 to 1899, Barton Papers, LOC.

54. Suárez, "Notes from Cuban Relief Department," 375.

55. See "General Orders, No. 4, Headquarters Department of Havana," in "Report of Brigadier General William Ludlow, Commanding Department of Havana and Military Governor of the City of Havana, Cuba," in U.S. War Department, *Annual Reports of the War Department for the Fiscal Year Ended June 30, 1899, Report of the Major-General Commanding the Army*, January 7, 1899, 294–96.

56. "Report of Brigadier General William Ludlow, Military Governor of Habana and Commanding Department of Habana," in U.S. War Department, *Annual Reports of the War Department for the Fiscal Year Ended June 30, 1899, Report of the Major-General Commanding the Army*, pt. 1, p. 223; "Report of Brigadier General William Ludlow, Military Governor of Habana and Commanding Department of Habana," in U.S. War Department, *Annual Reports of the War Department for the Fiscal Year Ended June 30, 1900*, vol. 1, pt. 4, pp. 22–23.

57. "Report of Brigadier General William Ludlow, Military Governor of Habana and Commanding Department of Habana," in U.S. War Department, *Annual Reports of the War Department for the Fiscal Year Ended June 30, 1899, Report of the Major-General Commanding the Army*, pt. 1, p. 223.

58. "Report of Brigadier General William Ludlow, Military Governor of Habana and Commanding Department of Habana," in U.S. War Department, *Annual Reports of the War Department, Department for the Fiscal Year Ended June 30, 1900*, vol. 1, pt. 4, p. 22.

59. "Lazy Element in Cuba," reprinted in *Washington Post*, March 24, 1899.

60. January 28, 1899, confidential letter from J. R. Brooke to Gen. H. C. Corbin, series 2, box 16, Brooke Papers, HSP.

61. "Providing for Weyler's Victims," *Chicago Daily Tribune*, March 25, 1899.

62. "American Charity Abused," *Washington Post*, February 25, 1899. See also "Cuban Frauds: Rich People Fed by the United States," *Los Angeles Times*, January 1, 1899, and "Indiscreet Giving of Charity," *Baltimore Sun*, September 11, 1899.

63. See Ferrer, *Insurgent Cuba*; Pérez, *Cuba between Empires*; and Hoganson, *Fighting for American Manhood*.

64. Pérez, *Cuba between Empires*, 212.

65. See Ferrer, *Insurgent Cuba*, chap. 7.

66. For an excellent overview of the history of welfare in the United States, see Katz, *In the Shadow of the Poorhouse*.

67. Barton, *Red Cross in Peace and War*, 643.

68. Suárez, "Notes from Cuban Relief Department," 377.

69. Suárez, "Notes from Cuban Relief Department," 377.

70. Suárez, "Notes from Cuban Relief Department," 378.

71. Suárez, "Notes from Cuban Relief Department," 378.

72. Suárez, "Notes from Cuban Relief Department," 378.

73. Report from M. R. Suárez to the Adjutant-General Department of Habana, April 30, 1900, in "Report of Brigadier General William Ludlow, Military Governor of Habana," in U.S. War Department, *Annual Reports of the War Department for the Fiscal Year Ended June 30, 1900, Report of the Lieutenant-General Commanding the Army*, pt. 1, p. 29.

74. Report from M. R. Suárez, General-Superintendent, Cuban Relief Department, to the Adjutant-General Department of Habana, in "Report of Brigadier General William Ludlow, Military Governor of Habana," in U.S. War Department, *Annual Reports of the War Department for the Fiscal Year Ended June 30, 1900*.

75. See Chap. 4.

76. Kean, "Hospitals and Charities in Cuba," 142.

77. Wood, "Military Government of Cuba," 173.

78. Letter from [Laura Drake] Gill to Folks, February 9, 1900, box 19, HFP.

79. Katz, *In the Shadow of the Poorhouse*, chap. 3.

80. Kean, "Hospitals and Charities in Cuba," 140.

81. The law drew clear boundaries for what kinds of institutions the state would directly fund, making municipalities officially responsible for maintaining local hospitals and dispensaries for the destitute sick and asylums for the destitute or chronically ill elderly. To private institutions fell all charities not provided for by the state or municipalities.

82. According to Civil Order 271, a "destitute child" was defined as "one not possessed of sufficient means for self-support, and who has neither parents nor grandparents, or whose parents or grandparents, if living, are unable to provide for the support of said child, or have abandoned it, or have habitually and grossly neglected to provide for its physical well-being, or are habitual drunkards, or are of notoriously immoral character, or are confined in a prison, or in a hospital for the insane" (J. R. Kean, "Report of the Department of Charities for the Period from July 1 to December 31, 1901," in Kean, *Report of Major J. R. Kean*, 5:63).

83. The new training schools for nurses are discussed in Chapter 2.

84. Homer Folks, "Havana—July 25, 1900," 2, box 19, HFP.

85. "General Wood and Cuban Charities," *Chicago Daily Tribune*, June 8, 1902.

86. See Gillette, "Military Occupation of Cuba."

87. See Klein, *Shock Doctrine*.

88. Kean, "Needs of the Department of Charities," 538–39.

89. For example, Major E. St. John Greble criticized them as being "little better than refuges where the sick and destitute children were herded and cared for in the most primitive manner" ("Report of Maj. E. St. J. Greble, Superintendent, Department of Charities, January 2, 1901," in U.S. War Department, *Annual Reports of the War Department for the Fiscal Year Ended June 30, 1900*, pt. 11, *Report of the Military Governor of Cuba on Civil Affairs*, vol. 1, pt. 2, p. 322).

90. Letter from Clara Barton to Leonard Wood, March 4, 1900, Letters Received, File 1900: 1775, 4, USNA/MGC. Emphasis added.

91. Homer Folks, "Charity Administration in Cuba," July 1900, box 19, HFP.

92. Report from M. R. Suárez to the Adjutant-General Department of Habana, April 30, 1900, in "Report of Brigadier General William Ludlow, Military Governor of

Habana," in U.S. War Department, *Annual Reports of the War Department for the Fiscal Year Ended June 30, 1900, Report of the Lieutenant-General Commanding the Army*, pt. 1, p. 29.

93. Homer Folks, "Charity Administration in Cuba," July 1900, box 19, HFP.

94. Undated, Letters Received, File 1900: 3112, USNA/MGC.

95. Report from M. R. Suárez to the Adjutant-General Department of Habana, April 30, 1900, in "Report of Brigadier General William Ludlow, Military Governor of Habana," in U.S. War Department, *Annual Reports of the War Department for the Fiscal Year Ended June 30, 1900, Report of the Lieutenant-General Commanding the Army*, pt. 1, p. 29. See also Suárez, "Notes from Cuban Relief Department," 378.

96. While many of the *reconcentrados* who survived their stay in the shelter had moved on, by May 1900, around 250 remained. See Homer Folks, "Charity Administration in Cuba," July 1900, box 19, HFP, 2.

97. "Notes of Inquiry Made into Circumstances of Inmates at Los Fosos," n.d., box 19, HFP.

98. Knowllys E. Nevins, report to "Headquarters Division of Cuba, Office of Superintendent Charities and Hospitals," August 17, 1900, reprinted as Appendix IX in "January 2, 1901 Report of Major W. C. Gorgas, Chief Sanitary Officer, City of Havana," in U.S. War Department, *Annual Reports of the War Department for the Fiscal Year Ended June 30, 1900*, pt. 11, *Report of the Military Governor of Cuba on Civil Affairs*, vol. 1, pt. 2, p. 385.

99. Suárez, "Notes from Cuban Relief Department," 378.

100. See, for example, letters between Elsa Trotzig and Clara Barton in the Barton Papers, LOC, and the letters in HFP. Once their tours in Cuba were over, many American *beneficencia* workers cycled back into reform work at home.

101. Civil Order 271, in J. R. Kean, "Report of the Department of Charities for the Period from July 1 to December 31, 1901," in Kean, *Report of Major J. R. Kean*, 5:77.

102. "Report of Brigadier General William Ludlow, Commanding Department of Havana and Military Governor of the City of Havana, Cuba," in U.S. War Department, *Annual Reports of the War Department for the Fiscal Year Ended June 30, 1899, Report of the Major-General Commanding the Army*, January 7, 1899, 217.

103. "Report to the Adjutant General of the Department of Cuba, Havana, August 26, 1901," in Kean, *Report of Major J. R. Kean*, 5:4–5.

104. "Report to the Adjutant General of the Department of Cuba, Havana, August 26, 1901," in Kean, *Report of Major J. R. Kean, Civil Report*, 5:4.

105. "Report to the Adjutant General of the Department of Cuba, Havana, August 26, 1901," in Kean, *Report of Major J. R. Kean*, 5:4.

106. "Report to the Adjutant General of the Department of Cuba, Havana, August 26, 1901," in Kean, *Report of Major J. R. Kean*, 5:12.

107. Cuba, Departamento de Beneficencia, *El Nuevo Departamento de Beneficencia*, 10.

108. Kean, "Report of the Department of Charities for the Period from July 1 to December 31, 1901," in Kean, *Report of Major J. R. Kean*, 5:12.

109. "Report to the Adjutant General of the Department of Cuba, Havana, August 26, 1901," in Kean, *Report of Major J. R. Kean*, 5:8.

110. H. L. Scott, "Correspondence from Adjutant General HL Scott to Superintendent of the Department of Charities," June 28, 1901, Letters Received, 1899–1902: 1901, 200, USNA/MGC.

111. Kean, "Report to the Adjutant General of the Department of Cuba, Havana, August 26, 1901," in Kean, *Report of Major J. R. Kean*, 5:8.
112. Dehogues, "Condiciones que deben exigirse a los enfermos," 407–9.
113. Martínez, "La asistencia médica a domicilio," 125.
114. Bangs, *Uncle Sam Trustee*, 207.
115. "General Wood and Cuban Charities," *Chicago Daily Tribune*, June 8, 1902.
116. Finlay, "Algunos problemas respecto a las escuelas de enfermeras," 79.

CHAPTER TWO

1. "Academia de Ciencias," *Diario de la Marina*, May 16, 1902.
2. Barnet, *Concepto actual de la medicina*, 4.
3. Santos Fernández, "Discurso leído," 8–9. A few years later, Jorge Le-Roy y Cassá made the same point, that the new public health practices had proven wrong the old belief "that Cuba is a country with a tropical climate, it has to be *perforce* a most unhealthy and deadly region" (Le-Roy y Cassá, "La sanidad en Cuba," 47–48).
4. Barnet, *Concepto actual de la medicina*, 16.
5. Barnet, *Concepto actual de la medicina*, 13.
6. Barnet, *Concepto actual de la medicina*, 14.
7. Santos Fernández, "Discurso leído," 10.
8. Espinosa, *Epidemic Invasions*; Stepan, "Interplay between Socio-Economic Factors and Medical Science." See also Iglesias Utset, *Las metáforas del cambio*, 41–44.
9. "Gen. Greene's Report," *New York Times*, January 1, 1899.
10. According to K. D. Patterson, the disease killed at least 100,000 to 150,000 in the United States between the first recorded outbreak in 1693 and the final New Orleans outbreak in 1905. See Patterson, "Yellow Fever Epidemics and Mortality in the United States," 855.
11. Yellow fever outbreaks in the U.S. South were regularly traced back to Havana, the most recent outbreak paralyzing New Orleans in late 1897. See Espinosa, *Epidemic Invasions*, 27–28.
12. All of these come from the 1899 and 1900 yellow fever case books, box 25, Gorgas Papers, LOC.
13. See Matthews, *New-Born Cuba*, 119–20; "Brief Report of Sanitary Dept. on its Organization," Records of Other Offices, Correspondence and Related Documents of the Dept. of Havana, 1899–1900, box 2, entry 102, file 3318, USNA/MGC; "Report of Brigadier-General William Ludlow, Military Governor of Habana," in U.S. War Department, *Annual Reports of the War Department for the Fiscal Year Ended June 30, 1900, Report of the Lieutenant-General Commanding the Army*, pt. 2, p. 18.
14. "Report of Major W. C. Gorgas, Chief Sanitary Officer of Havana, February 5, 1901," in U.S. War Department, *Annual Reports of the War Department for the Fiscal Year Ended June 30, 1900*, pt. 11, *Report of the Military Governor of Cuba on Civil Affairs*, vol. 1, pt. 2, p. 227.
15. "Report of Major W. C. Gorgas, Chief Sanitary Officer of Havana, February 5, 1901," in U.S. War Department, *Annual Reports of the War Department for the Fiscal Year Ended June 30, 1900*.
16. Howard Crutcher, "Freedom from Filth," *New York Times*, April 27, 1898. On the slow

and messy process of scientific change, Kuhn's *Structure of Scientific Revolutions* is perhaps the most famous example, but see Tomes, *Gospel of Germs*, for an excellent overview of how germ theory was slowly adopted during the late nineteenth and early twentieth centuries, often coexisting with earlier environmental explanations for disease causation.

17. On early reactions to Finlay's mosquito theory of yellow fever, see Espinosa, *Epidemic Invasions*, 58.

18. Matthews, *New-Born Cuba*, 95; "Havana as It Is: Present Conditions in the Cuban Capital," *New York Times*, January 1, 1899.

19. Indeed, in 1890, Diego Tamayo excoriated Spanish neglect of sanitary services, which left the city a "dunghill under a *plétora excrementicia*" (qtd. in Delfín, *Nociones de higiene*, vii). See also Cuadrado, "Necesidad de higiene pública," and Wilson, *El problema urgente*.

20. Iglesias Utset, *Las metáforas del cambio*, chap. 1. Anderson, in his *Colonial Pathologies*, makes an analogous case for the U.S. occupation of the Philippines.

21. "Ludlow's Views on Cuba: He Speaks of Natives as a Race of Orphans," *New York Tribune*, November 17, 1899.

22. "Report of Major W.C. Gorgas, Chief Sanitary Officer of Havana, February 5, 1901," in U.S. War Department, *Annual Reports of the War Department for the Fiscal Year Ended June 30, 1900*, 232.

23. Matthews, *New-Born Cuba*, 116.

24. "Cleaning up Havana," *Washington Post*, April 4, 1899.

25. Manuel Delfín, "Algo de higiene," *La Higiene*, March 1900, 102.

26. With 21.02 physicians for every 10,000 residents, the city of Havana had proportionally more doctors than Paris (14.73) or New York City (15.83). At the national level, the disparities are even more striking. Cuba had 777.6 physicians per million residents, just over twice the United States, at 388.7 per million, and significantly more than any European nation. The United Kingdom, for example, had 578 per million; Spain, 305; France, 380; and Germany, 355. See U.S. War Department, Office of the Census of Cuba, *Report of the Census of Cuba*; "Statistics of Physicians of Paris"; New York State Medical Association, *Medical Directory*, 7; U.S. Census Office, *Census Reports*, ccxlv; and Mulhall, *Dictionary of Statistics*, 387. The national data comparing Cuba and Europe was cited by Adrian López Denis in his excellent "Disease and Society in Colonial Cuba," 67.

27. See Pruna, *La Real Academia de Ciencias*.

28. Palmer, "Beginnings of Cuban Bacteriology."

29. These included *Crónica Médico Quirúrgica de la Habana* (Medical and Surgical Chronicle of Havana); *Anales de la Academia de Ciencias Médicas, Físicas y Naturales de la Habana* (Annals of the Royal Academy of Medical, Physical and Natural Sciences of Havana); *La Higiene* (Hygiene); *El Progreso Médico* (The Progress of Medicine); *Revista de Ciencias Médicas* (Journal of Medical Sciences); and *La Habana Médica* (Medical Havana). For more on the history of these journals, see Funes Monzote, *El despertar del asociacionismo científico en Cuba*.

30. It was Malberty who first proposed the creation of the Cuban Ministry of Health. See Teuma, *La secretaría de sanidad y beneficencia*, 26–28.

31. Alonso García, "Diego Tamayo Figueredo," 198.

32. For example, Juan Guiteras Gener, whose family was forced into exile, earned acclaim for his cutting-edge pathology research in Philadelphia and Charleston and

became known as a leading expert on yellow fever. Eusebio Hernández and Diego Tamayo both studied in Paris. Hernández worked alongside the famous Parisian obstetrician Adolph Pinard, and Tamayo spent time working at Pasteur's laboratories, where he learned new serological and vaccination techniques and brought the new anti-rabies vaccine to Cuba in 1887.

33. De Quesada y Miranda, Anecdotario martiano, 70

34. Ubieta, Efemérides de la revolución cubana, 364; Rubens, Liberty, 212.

35. Called El Club Profesional Oscar Primelles, in honor of a young physician who died on the battlefield of the independence struggle in 1895. See Constitution and By-laws of the Professional Club Oscar Primelles, 1. New York was a center of revolutionary exile activity, and physicians like Tamayo were among the leadership of the Partido Revolucionario Cubano.

36. In his memoirs, Delfín writes that in early 1898, a man visited his practice every day feigning sickness, only to inevitably try to engage Delfín in conversation about the independence struggle. Delfín later found out that the man was a spy working for the Spanish government. See Delfín, Treinta años de médico, 101–3.

37. Delgado García, "Dr. Enrique Núñez de Villavicencio y Palomino," 44.

38. As he wrote in the preface to his 1902 study on prostitution and venereal disease in Cuba, "We are the inheritors of a Revolution, which not only operated in the fields of combat, but also in field of ideas; which was not limited to the overthrow of a Government, but to put in its place a system, making rise from the breast of a Colony plagued with impurities, a more perfect society" (Alfonso y García, La prostitución en Cuba, ii). This discourse of an "impure" or diseased colony is a constant in the Cuban medical literature of the period. See, for example, "Higiene pública," La Habana Médica, December 1899, and Edelmann, "Desinfección urbana."

39. Edelmann, "Desinfección urbana," 339.

40. "Nuevos horizontes," La Habana Médica, January 1900.

41. Cuadrado, "Necesidad de higiene pública," 253; Delfín, Nociones de higiene, xiv.

42. Delfín, Treinta años de médico, 108–10.

43. "Sesión pública ordinaria de 11 de Marzo de 1900," Anales de la Academia de Ciencias Médicas, Físicas y Naturales de la Habana 36 (1900): 333. The sanitarian Miguel Barnet concurred, arguing that "the laws of health have not yet penetrated among the great popular masses, and are, therefore, very rarely observed" (Barnet, Concepto actual de la medicina, 13).

44. Even among medical professionals and educated elites, environmental understandings of disease causation lingered well into the twentieth century, often overlapping with bacteriological understandings of disease. This can be seen all over U.S. military reports from the occupation. See, for example, "Report of Brigadier General William Ludlow, Military Governor of Habana," in U.S. War Department, Annual Reports of the War Department for the Fiscal Year Ended June 30, 1900, 15–16.

45. For an excellent work on the popularization of hygienic precepts in the late-nineteenth- and early-twentieth-century United States, see Tomes, Gospel of Germs.

46. Manuel Delfín, "Dispensario La Caridad: Quinto año de su fundación," La Higiene, November 30, 1901, 842–43.

47. Manuel Delfín, "Los servicios sanitarios," La Higiene, May 1901, 597.

48. Manuel Delfín, "Por qué mueren tantos niños," La Higiene, June 1900, 205.

49. Tamayo y Figueredo, *Discurso leído*, 16. See also Guiteras, "La inmigración china," and McLeod, "We Cubans Are Obligated Like Cats to Have a Clean Face."

50. Delfín, "Un frase de Gen. Wood." *La Higiene*, July 1905, 679.

51. Le-Roy y Cassá, "La sanidad en Cuba," 43.

52. Pons, "La tuberculosis en el porvenir." The use of evangelical language to describe the proselytizing of hygienic precepts was quite common in early-twentieth-century Cuba. José López del Valle described how Havana's physicians eagerly "brought to every home the 'good news' of the coming 'new epoch' and the evangelism and teachings of hygiene" (López del Valle, "Desenvolvimiento de la sanidad y de la beneficencia en Cuba," 704). On the evangelism of hygiene in the United States during this period, see Tomes's excellent *Gospel of Germs*.

53. Enrique Acosta, "Profilaxis de la tuberculosis en la Isla de Cuba," *Boletín Mensual de la Liga Contra la Tuberculosis de Cuba*, January 1903, 95–98.

54. "Persistencia en la propaganda," *Boletín Mensual de la Liga Contra la Tuberculosis de Cuba*, August 1902, 16–17. On the early years of the Cuban Anti-Tuberculosis League, see Gutiérrez, "'An Earnest Pledge to Fight Tuberculosis,'" 280–96.

55. "Propaganda de la liga: Cajas de fósforos," *Boletín Mensual de la Liga Contra la Tuberculosis de Cuba*, January 1903, 100; "Abanicos: Propaganda de la liga," *Boletín Mensual de la Liga Contra la Tuberculosis de Cuba*, February 1903, 113.

56. Pérez, *On Becoming Cuban*; Iglesias Utset, *Las metáforas del cambio*.

57. This transnational exchange of policy ideas was a mainstay of the Progressive Era in the United States. For a great discussion of North Atlantic transnational social policy debates, see Rodgers, *Atlantic Crossings*.

58. See, for example, "Discurso del Dr. Juan Guiteras," *Boletín Oficial de la Secretaría de Sanidad y Beneficencia* 1 (1909): 148–49.

59. This was particularly the case with efforts to confront infant mortality in Cuba. See Chap. 4.

60. The journal regularly pushed for political and institutional reforms, from the need for the state regulation of milk safety to asking churches to sanitize holy water basins to prevent the spread of disease. See Enrique Acosta, "Revista de higiene," *La Higiene*, June 1900, 174.

61. Manuel Delfín, "Bañar al niño," *La Higiene*, June 1900, 206; Manuel Delfín, "Por qué mueren tantos niños," *La Higiene*, June 1900, 205; H. de Rothschild, "El amamantamiento: Elección de una nodriza," *La Higiene*, January 1902, 1044.

62. Subjects tackled in "Mañanas científicas" ranged from the basics of germ theory and microscopic evidence of bacteria and the need for cleanliness and hygiene to ward off disease, to the dangers of alcohol to the immune system.

63. Manuel Delfín, "Marimacho," *La Higiene*, April 10, 1900, 109.

64. De la Guardia, *Higiene pública*, 3.

65. "Sesión pública ordinaria de 11 de Marzo de 1900," *Anales de la Academia de Ciencias Médicas, Físicas y Naturales de la Habana* 36 (1900): 333; Edelmann, "Desinfección urbana," 339. De la Guardia quotes a similar critique published in *El Progreso Médico* in late 1899. See de la Guardia, *Higiene pública*, 3.

66. "Sesión pública ordinaria de 11 de Marzo de 1900," *Anales de la Academia de Ciencias Médicas, Físicas y Naturales de la Habana* 36 (1900): 333–36.

67. Delfín, letter to John G. Davis, in "Brief Report of Sanitary Dept. on its Organization," Records of Other Offices, Correspondence and Related Documents of the Dept. of Havana, 1899–1900, box 2, entry 102, file 3318, USNA/MGC.

68. Glanders is a disease common to horses that is deadly to humans, and it accounted for a small but regular portion of the city's death rate from infectious diseases.

69. Manuel Delfín, "El muermo y la intervención," La Higiene, February 1901, 490. What's worse, from the perspective of Cuban medical reformers, was the fact that glanders was first transmitted to the island via a glanderous horse from the United States, where the disease was endemic, in 1872. See G. P. P., "El muermo y la historia," La Higiene, November 1901, 839.

70. The commission was composed of Cuban physicians Juan Guiteras, Carlos J. Finlay, and Antonio Albertini, alongside American military scientists. See "Report of Major W. C. Gorgas, Chief Sanitary Officer of Havana, February 5, 1901," in U.S. War Department, Annual Reports of the War Department for the Fiscal Year Ended June 30, 1900, 229.

71. De la Guardia, Higiene pública, 3.

72. De la Guardia, Higiene pública, 7. On the required reporting of infectious disease, see "Report of Major W.C. Gorgas, Chief Sanitary Officer of Havana, February 5, 1901," in U.S. War Department, Annual Reports of the War Department for the Fiscal Year Ended June 30, 1900, 229. The diseases required to be reported to the Sanitary Department were tuberculosis, leprosy, glanders, yellow fever, diphtheria, smallpox, and typhoid fever.

73. Letters Received, File 1900: 1466, USNA/MGC.

74. De la Guardia, Higiene pública, 3.

75. As Abrisqueta complained, "Has the bay been cleaned? No." "Have the sewers been built? No." Rather, "money has been wasted" (Luis de Abrisqueta, "El fantasma americano," La Higiene, August 1900, 279–80).

76. "Report of Major W.C. Gorgas, Chief Sanitary Officer of Havana, February 5, 1901," in U.S. War Department, Annual Reports of the War Department for the Fiscal Year Ended June 30, 1900, 305.

77. In Havana, tuberculosis alone was responsible for almost ten times as many deaths as yellow fever in 1899. See "Report of Major W.C. Gorgas, Chief Sanitary Officer of Havana, February 5, 1901," in U.S. War Department, Annual Reports of the War Department for the Fiscal Year Ended June 30, 1900, 297. Since tuberculosis affected natives and nonnatives at largely the same rate, the proportion of Cubans killed by tuberculosis compared with yellow fever was much, much higher.

78. "Unclimatized" was a term common in the nineteenth century to describe those who had not gained immunity to yellow fever through previous exposure. Manuel Delfín, "El muermo y la intervención," La Higiene, February 1901, 490.

79. "The Failure of the Feather Duster," Washington Post, August 12, 1900.

80. For an excellent discussion of the Yellow Fever Commission's experiments to prove Finlay's theory, one of which led to the death of Jesse Lazear, see Espinosa, Epidemic Invasions, chap. 4.

81. As Espinosa notes, two-thirds of the health department's work crews were reassigned to this mosquito work. See Espinosa, Epidemic Invasions, 64.

82. Gorgas, "Short Account of the Results of Mosquito Work," 134; Gorgas, Work of the Sanitary Department, 14.

83. Gorgas, *Work of the Sanitary Department*, 15.
84. Espinosa, *Epidemic Invasions*, 67.
85. Letter to HR Carter (a friend) from Gorgas, October 8, 1901, box 3, Gorgas Papers, LOC.
86. G. P. P., "El muermo y la historia," *La Higiene*, November 1901, 839.
87. Letters Received, 1899–1902, File 1902: 224, USNA/MGC.
88. Leonard Wood to Secretary of War, February 19, 1901, General Correspondence, 1901, box 30, Wood Papers, LOC.
89. See Leonard Wood to Secretary of War, February 23, 1900, General Correspondence, 1900, box 28, Wood Papers, LOC.
90. Leonard Wood to Secretary of War, February 19, 1901, General Correspondence, 1901, box 30, Wood Papers, LOC.
91. See Elihu Root to Wood, February 21, 1901, and Elihu Root cable to Wood, February 25, 1901, both in General Correspondence, 1901, box 30, Wood Papers, LOC.
92. Duque, "Sanidad y beneficencia."
93. Manuel Delfín, "Los cubanos y el saneamiento," *La Higiene*, May 1902, 1043.
94. Manuel Delfín, "Los cubanos y el saneamiento," *La Higiene*, May 1902, 1043.
95. Manuel Delfín, "Los cubanos y el saneamiento," *La Higiene*, May 1902, 1043.
96. Gandarilla, *Contra el yanqui*, 77.
97. "Las primeras enfermeras cubanas," *La Lucha*, November 11, 1902; "Escuela de enfermeras de la república de Cuba," 292.
98. *Trained Nurse and Hospital Review* 30, no.1 (January 1903): 46; "Las primeras enfermeras cubanas," *La Lucha*, November 11, 1902.
99. "Las primeras enfermeras cubanas," *La Lucha*, November 11, 1902; "Escuela de enfermeras de la república de Cuba," 286.
100. Cantero, "Escuela de enfermeras," 384.
101. Quintard, "Nursing in Cuba," 396.
102. Kean, "Hospitals and Charities in Cuba," 43.
103. Nuñez, "Asistencia hospitalaria y asistencia a domicilio," 271. G. W. Hyatt described the same repulsion toward the hospital among reconcentrado families in 1898. See G. W. Hyatt to Stephen E. Barton, November 25, 1898, Red Cross File 1957, American National Red Cross, 1878 to 1957, Relief operations, Spanish-American War, Correspondence, Special, Hyatt, George W., 1898 to 1899, Barton Papers, LOC.
104. Nuñez, "Asistencia hospitalaria y asistencia a domicilio," 271; Quintard, "Nursing in Cuba," 396.
105. Quintard, "Nursing in Cuba," 396; Martínez Moreno, "Algunas consideraciones sobre la manera de ser de nuestros hospitales," 57; Finlay, "Escuelas de enfermeras," 359.
106. Nuñez, "Asistencia hospitalaria y asistencia a domicilio," 271; "Escuela de enfermeras de la república de Cuba," 292.
107. See letter from JR Kean to Adjutant General, July 17, 1901, Letters Received, 1899–1902, File 1901: 200, USNA/MGC, and Hibbard, "Establishment of Schools for Nurses in Cuba," 986. Also see Martínez Moreno, "Algunas consideraciones sobre la manera de ser de nuestros hospitales," 57–58.
108. Martínez Moreno, "Algunas consideraciones sobre la manera de ser de nuestros hospitales."

109. See Vogel, *Invention of the Modern Hospital*; Rosner, *A Once Charitable Enterprise*; Starr, *Social Transformation of American Medicine*, esp. chap. 4.

110. Letters Received, File 1900: 1466, USNA/MGC. It seems that Cubans of all classes shared the understanding that hospitals were dangerous, male spaces, to be avoided by women and children if possible. Speaking before the 1901 National Conference of Charities in Washington, D.C., the Cuban physician Emilio Martínez noted the preference women had for the dispensary over the hospital. "I do not know if it is so in other countries," he told his audience, "but with us women and children have a repulsion to going to hospitals." Indeed, the gendered contrast between dispensary and hospital patients is striking, with women making up 61 percent of the patients at the Tamayo Dispensary, while over three-quarters of patients at Hospital No. 1 were (also mostly poor) men. See *Proceedings of the Twenty-Eighth National Conference of Charities and Correction*, 387–88.

111. "Escuela de enfermeras de la república de Cuba," 288; Hibbard, "Establishment of Schools for Nurses in Cuba," 987.

112. Hibbard, "Cuba: A Sketch," 841. Also see Hibbard, "Establishment of Schools for Nurses in Cuba."

113. Finlay, "Escuelas de enfermeras," 357. In an effort to build public support for the work of Cuban nursing, this conference had nine speakers, including nurses, physicians, and an American Catholic priest, speaking in favor of the nursing schools.

114. Kean, *Report of Major J. R. Kean*, 5:57. See also Rodríguez de Tío, "Asilo huérfanos de la patria," 63.

115. Indeed, the word *desagradable* is repeatedly used by nurses and their supporters to describe the daily labor of professional nursing. See Finlay, "Escuelas de enfermeras," 358, and O'Donnell, "Dificultades con que se tropieza," 374.

116. On the maintenance of class/race hierarchy in Latin America through controlling the contact elite women had with non-elite men, see Martinez-Alier, *Marriage, Class, and Colour in Nineteenth-Century Cuba*; Suárez Findlay, *Imposing Decency*; Caulfield, *In Defense of Honor*; and Caulfield, Chambers, and Putnam, *Honor, Status, and Law in Modern Latin America*.

117. O'Donnell, "Dificultades con que se tropieza," 373–74. Another American nurse, Lucy Quintard, was equally sensitive to the factors that led Cubans to oppose the schools of nursing, including "the ill repute of hospitals and their employees," the "rigid rules governing the lives" of Cuban women, and the "strong prejudices against a woman occupying positions which would take her from the shelter of her own home, especially when it meant that she must live entirely away from home" during her three years of nurse training. See Quintard, "Nursing in Cuba," 399.

118. "Escuela de enfermeras de la república de Cuba," 286.

119. Quintard, "Nursing in Cuba," 397.

120. Quintard, "Nursing in Cuba," 399.

121. Jover, "La institución de la enfermera cubana y la caridad," 386. Carlos E. Finlay also took pains to describe the "so essentially feminine qualities" of the Cuban nurse; see Finlay, "Escuelas de enfermeras," 856.

122. Cantero, "Escuela de enfermeras," 284.

123. Cantero, "Escuela de enfermeras," 283.

124. Jover, "La institución de la enfermera cubana y la caridad," 386; Ortiz y Coffigny,

"Algunas consideraciones sobre las escuelas de enfermeras," 85; "Escuela de enfermeras de la república de Cuba," 293; "Las enfermeras cubanas," *Boletín Oficial de la Secretaría de Sanidad y Beneficencia* 1 (1909): 147.

125. Quintard, "Nursing in Cuba."

126. On the effort to ensure that prostitutes and nursing students be kept separate, see letter from José A. Frias to J. R. Kean, September 18, 1901, Letters Received, 18991902, File 1901: 2363, USNA/MGC.

127. "Las escuelas de enfermeras," *Cuba y América* 6, no. 42 (December 14, 1902): 558.

128. Finlay, "Algunos problemas respecto a las escuelas de enfermeras," 81.

129. "Las enfermeras," *Diario de la Marina*, April 24, 1904.

130. "Las enfermeras," *Diario de la Marina*, April 24, 1904.

131. Cantero, "La enfermera," 302.

132. Fernández, "Escuela central de enfermeras cubanas," 382.

133. Cantero, "La enfermera," 302.

134. Fernández, "Escuela central de enfermeras cubanas," 282.

135. Fernández, "Escuela central de enfermeras cubanas," 282.

136. *Contra la tísis; Fiebre amarilla; Instrucciones populares para evitar el contagio y la propagacion de la escarlatina*; Barnet, *La peste bubónica*; Barnet, *La sanidad en Cuba*; López del Valle, *El Departamento de Sanidad de la Habana*.

137. Charles Magoon to Secretary of War, June 8, 1907, box 989, no. 7, 2, Records of the Provisional Government of Cuba, USNA.

138. López del Valle, "Nationalization of Sanitary Services," 87.

139. Juan Manuel Plá to Provisional Governor of Cuba, October 8, 1906, Deposit of R. H. Kean, box 2, 1902–19, UVA-SP.

140. López del Valle, "Desenvolvimiento de la sanidad y de la beneficencia en Cuba," 710.

141. J. R. Kean to Provisional Governor Magoon, August 10, 1908, box 989, no. 17, 2, Records of the Provisional Government of Cuba, USNA.

142. López del Valle, "Nationalization of Sanitary Services," 86.

143. According to Delfín, these bribes were rare at first, "but it appears that this evil has become worse day by day" (*Treinta años de médico*, 109–10).

144. January 11, 1908, letter from Kean to the National Sanitary Board, Deposit of R. H. Kean, box 2, 1902–19, #8857, UVA-SP.

145. López del Valle, "Nationalization of Sanitary Services," 105.

146. López del Valle, "Nationalization of Sanitary Services," 3.

147. "Havana Reported Unclean," *Washington Post*, November 7, 1905.

148. Congreso de la República de Cuba, *Diario de Sesiones del Congreso*, 92–93.

149. Congreso de la República de Cuba, *Diario de Sesiones del Congreso*, 94.

150. J. R. Kean to Provisional Governor Magoon, August 10, 1908, box 989, no. 17, 16, Records of the Provisional Government of Cuba, USNA.

151. See "J. R. Kean to Major Meritte W. Ireland (12/26/07)," Additional Papers of Jefferson Randolph Kean, Accession #1331-b, box 1, UVA-SP. Also see "J. R. Kean to 'My Dear Mentor' (2/09/09)," Additional Papers of Jefferson Randolph Kean, Accession #1331-b, series III: Bound Letterpress Copy Book No. 4, 1909 Feb–1910, UVA-SP.

152. Le-Roy y Cassá, "La sanidad en Cuba," 45.

153. Duque, "Sanidad y beneficencia."

154. "Sanitary Work in Cuba under the Provisional Government of Intervention," Additional Papers of Jefferson Randolph Kean, Accession #1331-b, series III: Bound Letterpress Copy Book No. 4, 1909 Feb–1910, UVA-SP.

155. Teuma, La secretaría de sanidad y beneficencia, 21.

156. "La secretaría de sanidad y beneficencia," Vida Nueva, February 1909, 7–9.

CHAPTER THREE

1. "Testimony of Asunción Flores," legajo 677, expediente 2, folio 43, ANC/AH.

2. Unless otherwise noted, all details of the Gumersindo Pérez case are from legajo 677, expediente 2, ANC/AH.

3. "Otra víctima más de la peste bubónica," La Discusión, April 30, 1914; "Ayer por la tarde falleció un nuevo bubónico," El Mundo, April 30, 1914.

4. Echenberg, Plague Ports, 435–36.

5. "La peste," Vida Nueva, April 1914, 73; "Cumpliendo un deber," La Lucha, March 27, 1914, morning ed.

6. Meza, "Nuestra inmigración util," 305.

7. Tamayo y Figueredo, Discurso leído, 14; Santos Fernández, "La inmigración," 5; Tamayo y Figueredo, "Necesidad de asociaciones particulares de carácter filantrópico," 336.

8. The 1906 Law of Immigration and Colonization set aside almost a million dollars to support white immigration. See López, Chinese Cubans, 147.

9. See, for example, McNeill, Mosquito Empires; Cañizares Esguerra, "New World, New Stars"; Stepan, Picturing Tropical Nature; Bell, "'Pestilence That Walketh in Darkness'"; and Peard, "Tropical Disorders and the Forging of a Brazilian Medical Identity."

10. Gorgas, "Conquest of the Tropics for the White Race," 767.

11. Tamayo y Figueredo, Discurso leído, 17.

12. U.S. War Department, Office of the Census of Cuba, Report on the Census of Cuba, 1899; Cuba, Oficina Nacional del Censo, Censo de la República de Cuba, 1907; Dirección General del Censo, Census of the Republic of Cuba, 1919.

13. Santos Fernández, "La inmigración," 13.

14. Dirección General del Censo, Census of the Republic of Cuba, 1919, 677; Pérez, Cuba under the Platt Amendment, 82–83.

15. Dirección General del Censo, Census of the Republic of Cuba, 1919, 677; de la Fuente, "Two Dangers, One Solution," 33.

16. De la Fuente, "Two Dangers, One Solution," 37.

17. Wright, Cuba, 135–36.

18. These would go on to engender a growing series of conflicts with Cuban physicians, culminating in a 1934 medical strike. See Chap. 6.

19. See López, Chinese Cubans, chap. 5.

20. Legajo 12, 83, ANC/SP; Guiteras, "La inmigración china"; Ortiz, "Consideraciones criminológicas acerca de la inmigración en Cuba," 344–45; Meza, "Nuestra inmigración útil," 320–24.

21. Guiteras, "La inmigración china," 561.

22. Legajo 121, 83, ANC/SP. Emphasis in original.

23. Plague outbreaks hit Bombay in 1896; Alexandria, Oporto, and Honolulu in 1899; and Sydney, Buenos Aires, Rio de Janeiro, San Francisco, and Glasgow in 1900. See Echenberg, *Plague Ports*.

24. Barnet, *La peste bubónica*, 4. The text of Barnet's presentation was later published in a pamphlet by the Junta Superior de Sanidad and distributed for free; it included maps of the outbreaks in Asia and Mexico, as well as illustrations of *Yersinia pestis* under the microscope.

25. "Un brote de peste bubónica," *La Discusión*, March 6, 1914. La Asociación de Dependientes, or the Employees' Association, was one of the most important Spanish immigrant mutual aid organizations in the city, with a membership in the thousands.

26. "Un brote de peste bubónica," *La Discusión*, March 6, 1914.

27. "Un brote de peste bubónica," *La Discusión*, March 6, 1914.

28. "Nuevo triunfo de la sanidad cubana," *La Discusión*, March 10, 1914.

29. "Ridículo pánico por la peste bubónica," *El Triunfo*, March 8, 1914.

30. "Un brote de peste bubónica," *La Discusión*, March 8, 1914.

31. Under the provisions of the International Sanitary Convention that Cuba signed during the Segunda Convención Sanitaria Internacional de las Repúblicas Americas in Washington, D.C., in 1905, signatories were required to immediately report cases of yellow fever, cholera, and the bubonic plague. See "Poder ejecutivo," *Gaceta Oficial de la República de Cuba* 4, no. 109 (1905): 3359.

32. "Alarmas imprudentes," *El Diario Español*, March 10, 1914.

33. Duque, "Al 'Medical Record,'" 345.

34. "An Article from the 'Army and Navy Journal' and Reply to the Director of Public Health," *Sanidad y Beneficencia*, January 1911, 79.

35. Guiteras, "La sanidad cubana y la opinión extranjera," 5.

36. Guiteras, "An Open Letter," 679.

37. Guiteras, "An Open Letter," 680.

38. "El tráfico marítimo quebrantado por la peste bubónica," *La Discusión*, March 8, 1914.

39. *La Política Cómica* 9, no. 435 (March 1914).

40. "Nuevo triunfo de la sanidad cubana," *La Discusión*, March 10, 1914.

41. "El tráfico marítimo quebrantado por la peste bubónica," *La Discusión*, March 8, 1914.

42. "La bubónica," *El Triunfo*, March 7, 1914.

43. See, for example, "La bubónica," from March 7, 1914, and "La sanidad y la peste," from March 12, 1914.

44. "Alarmas imprudentes," *El Diario Español*, March 10, 1914.

45. See, for example, "Un brote de peste bubónica," *La Discusión*, March 6, 1914; "No Doubt Now That It Is Plague," *La Lucha*, March 10, 1914; and Guiteras, "La peste bubónica en Cuba."

46. "No Doubt Now That It Is Plague," *La Lucha*, March 10, 1914.

47. "Cerramos la puerta," *La Discusión*, March 6, 1914.

48. The language used, repeated indignantly by *El Diario Español* over the coming weeks, was "porque sabemos que de allí existe y que ese Gobierno ha mentido repetidas

veces y de una manera descarada sobre el particular" ("Así hablan las autoridades!," *El Diario Español*, March 20, 1914).

49. "Así hablan las autoridades!," *El Diario Español*, March 20, 1914.
50. "Así hablan las autoridades!," *El Diario Español*, March 20, 1914.
51. "¿Peste o berrenchín?," *El Triunfo*, March 10, 1914.
52. "La peste bubónica y las autoridades sanitarias," *El Diario Español*, March 24, 1914.
53. "La peste bubónica y las autoridades sanitarias," *El Diario Español*, March 24, 1914.
54. "Cumpliendo un deber," *La Lucha*, March 27, 1914, morning ed.
55. "Contra la peste," *El Mundo*, April 16, 1914.
56. "Duro con ellos!," *La Lucha*, March 18, 1914, morning ed.
57. "Conversaciones del Doctor" was a regular column that ran throughout 1914 on topics from tuberculosis to nutrition, childcare to public health administration. Aimed primarily at women readers, the columns often took the form of dialogues between "the doctor" and women who came to his medical office for advice. The series was reproduced by *El Figaro* and distributed as free pamphlets. See Barnet, *Conversaciones del Doctor*.
58. Enrique Barnet, "Conversaciones del Doctor," from *El Figaro*, March 3, 1914.
59. "Alrededor de la peste: Optimismo de las autoridades sanitarias—hablando con los Dres Núñez, Guiteras, y López del Valle," *La Lucha*, March 30, 1914.
60. "Alrededor de la peste: Optimismo de las autoridades sanitarias—hablando con los Dres Núñez, Guiteras, y López del Valle," *La Lucha*, 30 March 1914.
61. "La peste pubónica avanzando," *La Lucha*, April 14, 1914, morning ed.
62. "Siguiendo el curso la bubónica," *La Lucha*, April 13, 1914.
63. "Siguiendo el curso la bubónica," *La Lucha*, April 13, 1914.
64. "Otra víctima de la terrible bubónica," *La Discusión*, April 14, 1914.
65. "Otra víctima de la terrible bubónica," *La Discusión*, April 14, 1914.
66. "Otra víctima de la terrible bubónica," *La Discusión*, April 14, 1914.
67. "El brote de peste bubónica," *La Discusión*, April 15, 1914.
68. "La Habana aterrada ante el azote de La Sanidad," *El Triunfo*, April 15, 1914.
69. "Otra víctima de la terrible bubónica," *La Discusión*, April 14, 1914.
70. "Otra víctima de la terrible bubónica," *La Discusión*, April 14, 1914.
71. "Otra víctima de la terrible bubónica," *La Discusión*, April 14, 1914.
72. "El brote de peste bubónica," *La Discusión*, April 15, 1914.
73. "El brote de peste bubónica," *La Discusión*, April 15, 1914.
74. "La peste pubónica avanzando," *La Lucha*, April 14, 1914, morning ed.
75. "La Habana aterrada ante el azote de La Sanidad," *El Triunfo*, April 15, 1914.
76. "La peste pubónica avanzando," *La Lucha*, April 14, 1914, morning ed.
77. See "La Habana aterrada ante el azote de La Sanidad," *El Triunfo*, April 15, 1914, and "La peste bubónica avanzando," *La Lucha*, April 14, 1914, morning ed.
78. "El brote de peste bubónica," *La Discusión*, April 15, 1914.
79. "Sobre la peste bubónica: Los perjuicios de las medidas sanitarias," *El Diario Español*, April 14, 1914.
80. "Sobre la peste bubónica," *El Diario Español*, April 14, 1914.
81. "Sobre las indemnizaciones: El mejor justo medio, el derecho," *El Diario Español*, April 16, 1914.
82. See "El cubano Rodelgo, bubónico," *La Discusión*, April 18, 1914; "Otro caso más

de peste," *La Discusión*, April 23, 1914; and "El brote de peste bubónica: Las mercancías de baratillo número 1," *La Discusión*, May 2, 1914.

83. Guiteras, "La peste bubónica en Cuba," 318.
84. "Pequeñeces," *El Diario Español*, April 15, 1914.
85. "Los dos azotes: La Sanidad y la peste," *El Triunfo*, April 18, 1914.
86. "La peste," *Vida Nueva*, April 1914, 74.
87. "Igual para todos," *La Lucha*, April 17, 1914.
88. "Principios de reacción," *El Diario Español*, April 19, 1914.
89. Wright, *Cuba*, 166. See also Thomas, *Cuba*, 501.
90. "Pequeñeces," *El Diario Español*, April 15, 1914.
91. See Pérez, *On Becoming Cuban*.
92. See Chap 2.
93. See McLeod's excellent discussion of the racial politics of malaria control in McLeod, "We Cubans are Obligated Like Cats to Have a Clean Face."
94. Galarreta, "La inmigración haitiana, jamaiquina y china"; Le-Roy y Cassá, *Inmigración anti-sanitaria*; "Los peligros de la inmigración china," *Diario de la Marina*, November 23, 1922.
95. "En los últimos cuatro años . . . ," *Heraldo de Cuba*, December 1922, cited in Le-Roy y Cassá, *Inmigración anti-sanitaria*, 19.
96. "El decreto sobre inmigración de antillanos," *Diario de la Marina*, October 5, 1922.
97. Kraut, *Silent Travelers*, 2–4.
98. Echenberg, *Plague Ports*; Zulawski, "Environment, Urbanization, and Public Health."
99. Gómez, *Compilación sanitaria de Cuba*, 59.

## CHAPTER FOUR

1. "Registro Civil," *El Mundo*, April 20, 1912.
2. Le-Roy y Cassá, *La mortalidad infantil en Cuba*, 28; Guiteras, "Mortalidad de los niño en la república," 661.
3. Rothstein, "Trends in Mortality in the Twentieth Century," 77.
4. Between 1904 and 1913, the total number of infants who died during the summer months (May–August) was 56 percent higher than during the colder fall and winter months of October–January. See Le-Roy y Cassá, *La mortalidad infantil en Cuba*, 23–24.
5. Hernández and Ramos, *Homicultura*, 117.
6. Examples from the 1910s of Cuban physicians and scientists linking the island's infant mortality rate to its status as civilized include Fosalba, "La mortinatalidad y mortalidad infantil," and de la Portilla, "Contribución al estudio y tratamiento de las gastro-enteritis en los niños." For post–Cuban Revolution analogues, see Andaya, *Conceiving Cuba*, 48–50.
7. Quoted in de la Cruz y Ugarte, *Obligaciones del estado en relación con la beneficencia infantil*, 4.
8. Legajo 12263: 420, folio 8, ANC/RA.
9. For a clear example of the former, see Manuel Delfín, "Por que mueren tantos niños," *La Higiene*, June 1900.
10. Cuba, Oficina Nacional del Censo, *Censo de la República de Cuba*, 1907; Stubbs, "Gender Constructs of Labour in Prerevolutionary Cuban Tobacco."

11. Cuba, Oficina Nacional del Censo, *Censo de la República de Cuba*, 1907.
12. Hicks, "Hierarchies at Home."
13. Pérez, *Cuba under the Platt Amendment*, 82. On the city's housing market, see Chap. 5.
14. "Mujeres en miseria," *La Higiene*, December 1906, 824.
15. Delfín, *La Casa del Pobre*, 10.
16. See data for infant mortality in Havana in Fosalba, "La mortinatalidad y mortalidad infantil," 404.
17. Fosalba, "La mortinatalidad y mortalidad infantil," 42–145.
18. Fosalba, "La mortinatalidad y mortalidad infantil," 175.
19. Delfín, *La Casa del Pobre*, 26.
20. Delfín, *La Casa del Pobre*, 5.
21. Legajo 6, no. 36, ANC/SP.
22. Legajo 6, no. 36, ANC/SP. On American fears of "institutional pauperization," see Chap. 1.
23. The number of Havana families that signed up for aid grew steadily every year. In its first year, 108 families approached the organization for support, but by 1912–13, over 950 families, representing 1,581 women and 1,598 children, petitioned the organization for support. See Delfín, *La casa del pobre*, 11–14.
24. Delfín, *La Casa del Pobre*, 22.
25. In 1908 the organization could give out an average of $68 in aid per family per year, but with need rising and income dropping, in 1913 the organization could only give families an average of 7.35 per year. See Delfín, *La Casa del Pobre*, 11–13.
26. Delfín, *La Casa del Pobre*, 21.
27. "Protecting the Health of Cuban Babies," *The Survey*, September 18, 1915, 552.
28. Cepeda, *Eusebio Hernández*, 38–39.
29. Hernández and Ramos, *Homicultura*, 105. As Nancy Stepan notes, puericulture responded to late-nineteenth-century French concerns over France's low birthrate relative to its industrial and imperial competitors, England and Germany, providing a framework for pronatalist government policies. See Stepan, *Hour of Eugenics*, 77–78.
30. Cepeda, *Eusebio Hernández*, 60.
31. Hernández and Ramos, *Homicultura*.
32. Hernández and Ramos, *Homicultura*, 52–54.
33. On how many of these institutions gained root in the United States and shaped Progressive Era child welfare policies, see Meckel, *Save the Babies*.
34. For homiculture's relationship to Latin American eugenics, see Stepan, *Hour of Eugenics*, 76–84. On the relationship between homiculture, eugenics, and Cuban social science, see Bronfman, *Measures of Equality*, 107–34. See also García González and Álvarez Peláez, *En busca de la raza perfecta*, and Turda and Gillette, *Latin Eugenics in Comparative Perspective*.
35. Hernández and Ramos, *Homicultura*, 106.
36. Hernández and Ramos, *Homicultura*, 107.
37. Varona Suárez, "Homicultura," 7; Hernández and Ramos, *Homicultura*, 102.
38. Varona Suárez, "Homicultura," 3.
39. Hernández and Ramos, *Homicultura*, 107.
40. Legajo 106: 20, ANC/SP.

41. Taboadela, *Report of the Work*, 5.
42. Taboadela, *Report of the Work*, 13–14.
43. Taboadela, *Report of the Work*, 6.
44. Taboadela, *Report of the Work*, 19.
45. Taboadela, *Report of the Work*, 22.
46. "Protección a la infancia," *Boletín Oficial de la Secretaría de Sanidad y Beneficencia* 12 (1914): 628.
47. See the regular reports on the Servicio de Higiene Infantil published in the *Boletín Oficial de la Secretaría de Sanidad y Beneficencia*.
48. Taboadela, *Report of the Work*, 7.
49. Ramos, "Servicio de Higiene Infantil," 212.
50. See Fosalba, "La mortinatalidad y mortalidad infantil"; Le-Roy y Cassá, *La mortalidad infantil en Cuba*; Guiteras, "Mortalidad de niños en la república."
51. Plasiencia, "La leche que se consume en la Habana," 241.
52. Barnet, *Conversaciones del doctor*, 22.
53. Taboadela, *Report of the Work*, 20.
54. Taboadela, *Report of the Work*, 21.
55. Taboadela, *Report of the Work*, 22.
56. Barnet, *Conversaciones del doctor*, 22.
57. Barnet, *Conversaciones del doctor*, 23.
58. Barnet, *Conversaciones del doctor*, 31.
59. Legajo 563, no. 3, ANC/AH.
60. Barnet, *Conversaciones del doctor*, 22.
61. Barnet, *Conversaciones del doctor*, 23.
62. Barnet, *Conversaciones del doctor*, 40.
63. "Higiene infantil," *Vida Nueva*, November 1913, 246.
64. Barnet, *Conversaciones del doctor*, 40.
65. "Higiene infantil," *Vida Nueva*, November 1913, 246.
66. See Meckel, *Save the Babies*; De Barros, *Reproducing the British Caribbean*; Blum, *Domestic Economies*, 71–102; and Barney, "Maternalism and the Promotion of Scientific Mothering."
67. Valdés, "Mortalidad infantil," 104.
68. Ramos, "Servicio de Higiene Infantil," 213.
69. "Concurso Nacional de Maternidad," *Diario de la Marina*, January 2, 1918; Cuba, Secretaría de Sanidad y Beneficencia, *Servicio de Higiene Infantil*, 7.
70. For Better Baby Contests abroad, see Meckel, *Save the Babies*, 151, and Stern, "Making Better Babies."
71. Aragón, "El Concurso Nacional de Maternidad de 1918." See also debate on funding the *concurso* from the November 28, 1918, Havana City Council meeting, tomo 37, p. 26, Actas Capitulares del Ayuntamiento de la Habana, Libro de Borradores, Archivo de la Oficina del Historiador de la Ciudad de la Habana.
72. The term was from José Antonio López del Valle, quoted in Aragón, "El Concurso Nacional de Maternidad de 1918," 170.
73. Cuba, Secretaría de Sanidad y Beneficencia, *Servicio de Higiene Infanti1*, 8.
74. Aragón, "El Concurso Nacional de Maternidad de 1918," 171–72.

75. Aragón, "El Concurso Nacional de Maternidad de 1918," 171.

76. Lebredo, "La mortalidad infantil," 219.

77. Lebredo, "La mortalidad infantil," 225.

78. On the emerging Cuban women's movement, see Stoner, *From the House to the Streets*, and González Pagés, *En busca de un espacio*.

79. At its inaugural meeting in 1913, Mariana Seva de Menocal, the wife of the Cuban president, was named president of honor; Concepción Escardo de Freyre, wife of the Havana mayor, was named president; and the "seven vice-presidents were chosen from among the leading ladies of Cuba" ("National Congress of Mothers of the Republic of Cuba," *Child Welfare Magazine*, December 1913, 108).

80. Alfonso "La beneficencia en Cuba," 477.

81. As the organization's bylaws make clear, the group's founders believed that "everything that is done to reduce [infant mortality rates] is necessary and patriotic work; therefore, this Committee will have as its primordial goal the struggle against the excessive mortality of children in early childhood" ("Comite de Señoras Para la Protección de la Infancia en el Distrito de la Habana Nueva," legajo 1187, no. 30737, folios 7 and 2, ANC/RA).

82. Legajo 1187, no. 30737, folio 2, ANC/RA.

83. Legajo 1187, no. 30737, folio 13, ANC/RA.

84. Legajo 1187, no. 30737, folios 13 and 14, ANC/RA. The Bando de Piedad, or Band of Piety, was also known as the Sociedad Protectora de Niños, Animales y Plantas (Protective Society for Children, Animals, and Plants) and was formed in 1905 by Jeannette Ryder, a Wisconsin-born philanthropist who had come to Cuba during the first U.S. occupation with her physician husband.

85. "Visitas e inspecciones practicadas por la doctora mestre en la creches y casa de beneficencia y maternidad durante el mes de Julio," *Boletín Oficial de la Secretaría de Sanidad y Beneficencia de la Isla de Cuba* 18 (1917): 506.

86. Legajo 1187, no. 30737, folio 15, ANC/RA.

87. Alfonso "La beneficencia en Cuba," 414.

88. Alfonso "La beneficencia en Cuba," 419.

89. Health concerns were central to the demands articulated at both National Women's Congresses—the second was held in 1925—which emerged from the work of organizations such as the Congreso Nacional de Madres and the women of the Creche Habana Nueva. In addition to seeking voting rights for women, the "Conclusions of the First National Women's Congress" included calls for increased attention to eugenics and puericulture in public education and a call for the government to enforce existing protective legislation for children (which included health provisions). See *Memoria del Primer Congreso Nacional de Mujeres* and *Memoria del Segundo Congreso Nacional de Mujeres*.

90. Mederos de Fernández, "Protección a la niñez," 317.

91. López del Valle, *Los adelantos sanitarios*.

92. See, for example, Eusebio Hernández's 1912 "Manifiesto del General Eusebio Hernández a los Liberales y al país," reprinted in Hernández and Cepeda, *Ciencia y patria*, 117–26. Hernández later spoke publicly of his support for the young Soviet Union

and even declared himself a "Bolshevik." On Hernández's support for the USSR, see Hernández and Cepeda *Ciencia y patria*, 52–56.

93. See Bronfman, *Measures of Equality*, 121–23. On the development of eugenics in Latin America, see Stepan, *Hour of Eugenics*. For the development of Cuban eugenics, see García González and Álvarez Pérez, *En busca de la raza perfecta*; García González, "El desarrollo de la eugenesia en Cuba"; and Arvey, "Sex and the Ordinary Cuban."

94. *Actas de la Segunda Conferencia Panamericana*, 154–56.

95. *Actas de la Segunda Conferencia Panamericana*, 154.

96. *Actas de la Primera Conferencia Panamericana*, 54.

97. See López del Valle, *Los certificados médicos pre-nupciales*, 11. While no sterilization measures were ever passed in Cuba, a eugenic marriage certificate law did make it into law in 1929. But, as Alejandra Bronfman notes, it lacked any implementation measures, so its passage was purely formal.

98. See Fosalba, "La mortinatalidad y mortalidad infantil"; Le-Roy y Cassá, *La mortalidad infantil en Cuba*.

99. Ramírez Ros, "La tuberculosis en la raza negra."

100. See, for example, figure 4–2, above, as well as the images on pp. 9, 15, and 37 of Cuba, Secretaría de Sanidad y Beneficencia, *Servicio de Higiene Infantil*, and "Concurso Nacional de Maternidad y Exposición de Niños—1920," *Boletín Oficial de la Secretaría de Sanidad y Beneficencia* 23 (1920): 312.

## CHAPTER FIVE

1. Ramírez Ros, "La tuberculosis en la raza negra."

2. Ramírez Ros, "La tuberculosis en la raza negra." Emphasis in the original.

3. Ramírez Ros, "La tuberculosis en la raza negra." Emphasis in the original.

4. On the romanticism of consumption in nineteenth-century Europe and North America, see Lawlor, *Consumption and Literature*.

5. In 1927, for example, half of the city's tuberculosis deaths occurred among residents between the ages of 20 and 39, 15 percent were 19 years old or younger, and less than 30 percent were between ages 40 and 59. These numbers are consistent with Havana's tuberculosis mortality statistics throughout the early decades of the republic. For the 1927 statistics, see Jorge Le-Roy, "Informe anual sanitario y demográfico del término municipal de la Habana, correspondiente al año 1927," *Sanidad y Beneficencia: Boletín Oficial* 33, nos. 3–6 (March–June 1928): 69–133.

6. "Informe anual sanitario y demográfico del término municipal de la Habana, correspondiente al año 1929," *Boletín Oficial de la Secretaría de Sanidad y Beneficencia*, 35, nos. 1–6 (January–June 1930): 23–24.

7. Qtd. in Bay y Sevilla, *La vivienda del pobre*, 18.

8. Roberts, *Infectious Fear*, 4.

9. This estimate is repeated throughout the early republic. See Tamayo y Figueredo, "La vivienda en procomún," 239, and Chailloux Cardona, *Síntesis histórica de la vivienda popular*, 162. Chailloux argues that around 200,000, or about a third of the city's population, lived in these kinds of conditions.

10. Ultraviolet radiation from sunlight, on the other hand, kills *Mycobacterium tuberculosis* and can reduce the risk of transmission. See *Core Curriculum on Tuberculosis*, 21–25, and U.S. Agency for International Development, *Nutrition and Tuberculosis*.

11. Tamayo y Figueredo, "La vivienda en procomún," 236.

12. López del Valle, "Casas de vecindad," 266.

13. According to the 1919 Secretaría de Sanidad census of *casas de vecindad*, there were 1,548 in the city center (Habana Vieja and Centro Habana), 188 in the Cerro neighborhood, 217 in Jesus del Monte, 81 in Vedado, and 14 in Casa Blanca. See Bay y Sevilla, *La vivienda del pobre*, 106.

14. See, for example, Chailloux Cardona, *Síntesis histórica de la vivienda popular*, 101, and "Arreglando el mundo: Viviendas," El Mundo, February 28, 1924.

15. Chailloux Cardona, *Síntesis histórica de la vivienda popular*, 108.

16. See Chailloux Cardona, *Síntesis histórica de la vivienda popular*, 124.

17. Pérez, "La vivienda de nuestra clase pobre," 14.

18. Chailloux Cardona, *Síntesis histórica de la vivienda popular*, 139, 141. In his 1950 study of one Cuban solar, David W. Ames found that 69.5 percent of the inhabitants were black or mestizo. See Ames, "Negro Family Types in a Cuban Solar," 160.

19. Chailloux Cardona, *Síntesis histórica de la vivienda popular*, 139–40. See also de la Fuente, *Nation for All*, 114–15.

20. Chailloux Cardona, *Síntesis histórica de la vivienda popular*, 141.

21. See, for example, George Duroy, "Machacando en hierro frío," Labor Nueva, May 14, 1916, 6; Ramírez Ros, "Sobre el mismo tema de la tuberculosis"; Gustavo E. Urrutia, "Armonias: El busilis," Diario de la Marina, September 1, 1929; "Por el mejoramiento de la vivienda," Adelante, September 1937, 1; and "Hasta cuando los alquileres," Mediodía, January 17, 1938, 14.

22. De la Fuente, *Nation for All*, 117. See also Chaps. 3 and 6.

23. Cuba, Dirección Nacional del Censo, *Census of the Republic of Cuba: 1919*, 677–79.

24. Catalina Pozo Gato, "Con su permiso, amigo," La Mujer, November 15, 1930, 4.

25. "Discurso del Dr. Juan Santos Fernández," Boletín Oficial de la Secretaría de Sanidad y Beneficencia 1 (1909): 635; "La vida de nuestra clase pobre descrita por el Dr. Tamayo," El Mundo, January 16, 1915; "Casas de vecindad," Vida Nueva, February 1915, 25.

26. De la Fuente, *Nation for All*, 114.

27. Mariblanca Sabas Alomá, "La mujer de solar," Carteles, March 17, 1929, 16.

28. Mariblanca Sabas Alomá, "La mujer de solar," Carteles, March 17, 1929, 16.

29. Ferrer, *Insurgent Cuba*.

30. García Mendoza, "Las viviendas de los pobres y la tuberculosis," 331.

31. See Bronfman, *Measures of Equality*.

32. Fernando Méndez Capote, "Medio social de las ciudadelas," Anales de la Academia de Ciencias Medicas, Físicas y Naturales de la Habana 51 (1915): 623.

33. Tamayo y Figueredo, "La vivienda en procomún," 240; Bay y Sevilla, *La vivienda del pobre*, 104, 106.

34. Chailloux Cardona, *Síntesis histórica de la vivienda popular*, 142.

35. Fuentes, "Casas de vecindad," 841; the second study is cited in Chailloux Cardona, *Síntesis histórica de la vivienda popular*, 143.

36. Tamayo y Figueredo, "La vivienda en procomún," 240.

37. Sánchez de Fuentes, "Profilaxis de la tuberculosis en Cuba," 542.
38. Sánchez de Fuentes, "Profilaxis de la tuberculosis en Cuba," 543.
39. Gómez, Compilación sanitaria de Cuba, 14–15.
40. López del Valle, "Casas de vecindad," 266–67.
41. Sánchez Martínez, Guía del policía cubano, 159.
42. López del Valle, "Casas de vecindad," 267.
43. López del Valle, "Casas de vecindad," 266.
44. Cosculluela, La salubridad urbana, 20.
45. Hibbard, "Trabajos sobre la tuberculosis en Cuba," 285.
46. Hibbard, "Trabajos sobre la tuberculosis en Cuba"; López del Valle, Lecciones populares sobre la tuberculosis, 5–6.
47. Deulofeu, "Aire puro en el tratamiento de la tuberculosis," 130.
48. See, for example, Hibbard, "Trabajos sobre la tuberculosis en Cuba"; Hibbard, "Como viven nuestros pobres"; Merelles, "Reposo"; and Deulofeu, "Aire puro en el tratamiento de la tuberculosis."
49. Bay y Sevilla, La vivienda del pobre, 67.
50. Urban, "The Sick Republic," 94.
51. But in a in a 1911 paper given before the Second National Medical Congress of Cuba, Dr. José Aleman suggested that this gender disparity might also be attributable to the daytime hours of the tuberculosis dispensary, which prevented persons with less flexible working hours from attending a consultation. See "Relación de los trabajos realizados por la Secretaría de Sanidad, mayo, junio, y julio de 1918," Boletín Oficial de la Secretaría de Sanidad y Beneficencia 20 (1918): 222–23, and Aleman, "Consideraciones sobre 444 enfermos examinados," 26.
52. "Relación de los trabajos realizados por la Secretaría de Sanidad, mayo, junio, y julio de 1918," Boletín Oficial de la Secretaría de Sanidad y Beneficencia 20 (1918): 222–23.
53. Merelles, "Reposo."
54. Merelles, "Reposo," 129.
55. Merelles, "Reposo," 128, 129.
56. Deulofeu, "Aire puro en el tratamiento de la tuberculosis," 130–31.
57. "Flagelo social," Carteles, August 25, 1929.
58. Aldereguía, "La tuberculosis en la raza negra."
59. Aldereguía, "La tuberculosis en la raza negra."
60. De la Fuente, Nation for All.
61. See Helg, Our Rightful Share.
62. Gustavo E. Urrutia, "Armonias: El busilis," Diario de la Marina, September 1, 1929; Aldereguía, "La tuberculosis en la raza negra."
63. Ramírez Ros, "Sobre el mismo tema de la tuberculosis."
64. Robaina, El Negro en Cuba, 124–33; Cook, "Urrutia."
65. Ramírez Ros, "La tuberculosis en la raza negra."
66. See Chap. 6.
67. Ramírez Ros, "Sobre el mismo tema de la tuberculosis."
68. Morillo de Govantes, "La tuberculosis en la raza negra: Contestando al Sr. Primitivo Ramírez Ros," Diario de la Marina, August 25, 1929.
69. Ramírez Ros, "Sobre el mismo tema de la tuberculosis."

70. Ramírez Ros, "La tuberculosis en la raza negra."
71. Mederos de Fernández, "Las Isabelinas," in *La mujer en el frente social de Cuba*, 181.
72. Gustavo E. Urrutia, "Armonías: El busilis," *Diario de la Marina*, September 1, 1929.
73. Jacobsen, "Problem of Tuberculosis in Cuba," 118.
74. Jacobsen, "Problem of Tuberculosis in Cuba," 118.
75. Jacobsen, "Problem of Tuberculosis in Cuba," 118.
76. Cosculluela, *La salubridad urbana*, 20.
77. See Chap. 4.
78. Sánchez de Fuentes, "Profilaxis de la tuberculosis en Cuba," 550.
79. Bay y Sevilla, *La vivienda del pobre*, 67.
80. Fuentes, "Como puede intervenir?," 359.
81. Jacobsen, "Problem of Tuberculosis in Cuba," 123–24. Others echoed this language of the yellow fever success as a model for fighting tuberculosis. See, for example, "Flagelo social," *Carteles*, August 25, 1929, and Pons, "La tuberculosis en el porvenir."
82. Jacobsen, "Problem of Tuberculosis in Cuba," 123–24.
83. See Hibbard, "Como viven nuestros pobres," and Hibbard, "Trabajos sobre la tuberculosis en Cuba."
84. Pons, "La tuberculosis en el porvenir," 31.
85. Ramírez Ros, "La tuberculosis en la raza negra."
86. Aldereguía, "La tuberculosis en la raza negra."
87. Mariblanca Sabas Alomá, "La mujer de solar," *Carteles*, March 17, 1929, 16.
88. Ramírez Ros, "Sobre el mismo tema de la tuberculosis."
89. Ramírez Ros, "La tuberculosis en la raza negra."
90. Ramírez Ros, "Sobre el mismo tema de la tuberculosis."
91. *Programa*.
92. See Pappademos, *Black Political Activism and the Cuban Republic*, and de la Fuente, *Nation for All*, 161–71, 200–209.
93. *Programa*, 3–4.
94. *Programa*, 6–12.
95. *Programa*, 4.
96. Cosculluela, *La salubridad urbana*, 24.

**CHAPTER SIX**

1. "40,000 in Parade of Protest in Cuba," *New York Times*, September 28, 1933.
2. J. D. Phillips, "Cuban Reds Urge Rule by Workers," *New York Times*, September 27, 1933; "Recognition Bid by Cuba Seen," *Daily Boston Globe*, September 28, 1933.
3. See "Comentarios referente a la colegiación medical obligatoria," *Tribuna Médica*, October 1933, 341.
4. "Cuba: Health-Insurance Test-Tube," *California and Western Medicine* 46, no. 6 (June 1937): 446. Physicians in the United States closely followed the deteriorating situation of Cuban doctors in the 1920s and 1930s. For U.S. medical perspectives on the Cuban medical conflicts, see "Medical Practice in Cuba," 1890; "Health Insurance Societies of Cuba—Psuedo State Medicine and with a Vengeance," *California and Western Medicine*, February 1932, 116; "Cuban Doctors on Strike," *California and Western Medicine*, September

1932, 200; and R. G. Leland, "The Practice of Medicine in Cuba," AMA Bulletin, June 1933, 95.

5. See Chaps. 2 and 3.
6. Hurtado Galtés, "Editorial."
7. Hurtado Galtés, "Editorial," 3.
8. Hurtado Galtés, "Editorial," 3.
9. Danielson, Cuban Medicine, 122n2.
10. Buell et al., Problems of the New Cuba, 116.
11. Hurtado Galtés, "Editorial," 3.
12. Hurtado Galtés, "Editorial," 4
13. The exception was the Centro de Dependientes, or Clerks' Club, which originally served the city's Spanish immigrant employees but, like other centros, eventually expanded to accept merchants, bankers, professionals, etc.
14. Buell et al., Problems of the New Cuba, 38. This number includes the many Cubans who were eventually allowed to join the associations, as well as Cubans and Spaniards from other Cuban provinces, who would travel to the capital to receive the low-cost, quality medical care that was increasingly difficult to find outside Havana. This researcher had two great uncles who were among those who made the trek from the eastern town of Las Tunas to receive medical care at the Centro Asturiano's Covadonga Hospital in Havana in the early 1930s.
15. According to a 1935 report, about 75 percent of centros' fee income went into medical care. See Buell et al., Problems of the New Cuba, 38–39.
16. Buell et al., Problems of the New Cuba, 4. This sense of a declining respect for physicians among Cuban patients is a common theme in the pages of Tribuna Médica. See, for example, "Una carta interesante del Doctor Oscar Montero," Tribuna Médica, August 20, 1927, and "El problema económico de la clase médica," Tribuna Médica, June 15, 1930.
17. Fernández Conde, Biografía de la Federación Médica de Cuba, 36.
18. Zulawski and Palmer address the importance of this issue for Bolivian and Costa Rican medicine. See Zulawski, Unequal Cures, and Palmer, From Popular Medicine to Medical Populism.
19. Dechamp and Poblete Troncoso, El problema médico, 31.
20. Dechamp and Poblete Troncoso, El problema médico, 24–31.
21. "Medical Practice in Cuba."
22. "¿Y para que se hizo?," Tribuna Médica, n.d. See legajo 5, no. 103, ANC/SP, a collection of clippings related to the conflict between the FMC and the Centro Gallego, and "Comentarios," Tribuna Médica, December 20, 1927.
23. "Thousands Workless and Starving in Cuba," Daily Boston Globe, August 6, 1931.
24. Tuberculosis mortality rose from 153 annual deaths for every 100,000 residents in 1931 to 169 per 100,000 in 1933, while infant mortality rates almost tripled between 1930 and 1933 (from 51.5 per 1,000 to 144.3 per 1,000). See Buell et al., Problems of the New Cuba, 100–103.
25. Buell et al., Problems of the New Cuba, 161.
26. Buell et al., Problems of the New Cuba, 120.
27. Buell et al., Problems of the New Cuba, 117.
28. Fernández Conde, Biografía de la Federación Médica de Cuba, 48.

29. Fernández Conde, *Biografía de la Federación Médica de Cuba*, 51–52.
30. Fernández Conde, *Biografía de la Federación Médica de Cuba*, 41–43.
31. Legajo 4, no. 172, ANC/FE.
32. Whitney, *State and Revolution in Cuba*, 62.
33. García Rodríguez, *Problemas de salubridad*.
34. Hurtado Galtés, "Editorial."
35. While direct archival evidence of political patronage in medical matters is very rare, some documents attest to the continuing distribution of public health positions for political supporters and friends. See, for example, legajo 106, no. 1, ANC/SP.
36. Indeed, precisely this argument was made by four physicians who quit the FMC in protest of a 1929 tribute the organization held in honor of Machado. See legajo 63, no. 108, ANC/FE.
37. Fernández Conde, *Biografía de la Federación Médica de Cuba*, 48.
38. Fernández Conde, *Biografía de la Federación Médica de Cuba*, 46.
39. "Ala Izquierda Médica," *Tribuna Médica*, October 1934, 335.
40. "Ala Izquierda Médica," *Tribuna Médica*, October 1934, 338.
41. Pérez, *Cuba under the Platt Amendment*, 310.
42. "Disertaciones por radio: Conferencia del Doctor Luis P. Romaguera," *Tribuna Médica*, September 1933, 330.
43. Fernández Conde, *Biografía de la Federación Médica de Cuba*, 53.
44. "El decreto de la colegiación," *Tribuna Médica*, October 1933, 331.
45. Legajo 8, no. 16, ANC/SP.
46. These were the Centro Gallego, Asociación de Dependientes del Comercio de la Habana, Centro Asturiano, Asociación Canaria, and Hijas de Galicia.
47. Legajo 2, no. 117, ANC/FE.
48. J. D. Phillips, "Cuban Reds Urge Rule by Workers," *New York Times*, September 27, 1933.
49. "40,000 in Parade of Protest in Cuba," *New York Times*, September 28, 1933.
50. "Disertaciones por radio: Conferencia del Doctor Luis P. Romaguera," *Tribuna Médica*, September 1933, 333.
51. See Whitney, *State and Revolution in Cuba*, chap. 5.
52. Whitney, *State and Revolution in Cuba*, 114.
53. Russell B. Porter, "Lack of Funds Key to Crisis in Cuba," *New York Times*, September 28, 1933.
54. J. D. Phillips, "Cuban Reds Seized to End Disorders," *New York Times*, October 2, 1933.
55. "Ala Izquierda Médica," *Tribuna Médica*, October 1943, 335.
56. While in many ways physicians represented the most privileged sector of this broad medical alliance, nurses, midwives, pharmacists, and physicians shared many complaints. On the complaints of the nursing sector, see "La Asociación Nacional de Enfermeras y la Federación Médica," *Tribuna Médica*, January 1932, and "Declaraciones en torno al mutualismo," *Tribuna Médica*, June 1934, 189.
57. "Violentamente forzadas a clausurar las casas de salud de los C. regionales," *Diario de la Marina*, January 13, 1934.
58. Phillips, *Cuban Sideshow*, 269; "Violentamente forzadas a clausurar las casas de salud de los C. regionales," *Diario de la Marina*, January 13, 1934.

59. "En el registro que se realizó a las casas de salud, no ocuparon armas," *Diario de la Marina*, January 15, 1934.

60. "En el registro que se realizó a las casas de salud." *Diario de la Marina*, January 15, 1934.

61. The number is from the 1934 International Labour Office report *El problema médico y la asistencia médica mutualista en Cuba*, prepared by Cyrille Dechamp and Moisés Poblete Troncoso.

62. "El personal de sanidad abandonó las oficinas," *Diario de la Marina*, January 20, 1934.

63. "No acepta arbitraje el Colegio Médico que brindó Mendieta," *Diario de la Marina*, January 20, 1934.

64. "Numerosos cadaveres insepultados a causa de la huelga médica," *Diario de la Marina*, January 21, 1934.

65. "Huelga general," *Tribuna Médica*, January 1934, 5.

66. "Un teniente de policia agoniza por falta de asistencia médica," *Diario de la Marina*, January 20, 1934.

67. "No han sida aceptadas las proposiciones del C. Medico," *Diario de la Marina*, January 22.

68. "Hail Recognition in Havana as Boon," *New York Times*, January 23, 1934.

69. "No han sida aceptadas las proposiciones del C. Medico," *Diario de la Marina*, January 22.

70. "Un teniente de policia agoniza por falta de asistencia médica," *Diario de la Marina*, January 20, 1934.

71. "Fallecen sin asistencia médica los enfermos en los hospitales," *Diario de la Marina*, January 21, 1934.

72. "Fallecen sin asistencia médica los enfermos en los hospitales," *Diario de la Marina*, January 21, 1934; "Terminó ayer noche la huelga médica en toda la república," *Diario de la Marina*, January 24, 1934.

73. "Una hermosa iniciativa del Centro Asturiano," *Diario de la Marina*, January 20, 1934.

74. "Impresiones," *Diario de la Marina*, January 20, 1934.

75. "No han sida aceptadas las proposiciones del C. Medico," *Diario de la Marina*, January 22, 1934.

76. "No han sida aceptadas las proposiciones del C. Medico," *Diario de la Marina*, January 22, 1934.

77. Letter from G. R. Martoreli to President Carlos Mendieta, January 22, 1934, legajo 10, no. 62, ANC/SP.

78. "En un tiroteo frente a una botica murió el Doctor Borges," *Diario de la Marina*, January 21, 1934; "Aniversario de la muerte del Dr. Borges" *Tribuna Médica*, January, 1935, 8. In 1927, Borges, then a member of the Ala Izquierda Estudiantil, was expelled from the University of Havana for his revolutionary activity. Later, he was forced into exile. After the overthrow of Machado, he returned to Cuba to devote his time to revolutionary work and helped organize the January strike as part of the Ala Izquierda Médica. After his death, he was widely hailed as Cuban medicine's first twentieth-century martyr. After the Cuban Revolution of 1959, a hospital in Pinar del Rio province would be named after Borges. See "Homenaje a la memoria del Doctor José Elias Borges," *Tribuna Médica*, January, 1935, 1.

79. "Explosión en una clinica," *Diario de la Marina*, January 22, 1934; Phillips, *Cuban Sideshow*, 298; "Terminó ayer noche la huelga médica en toda la república," *Diario de la Marina*, January 24, 1934.

80. "El pueblo pretendió quemar una botica," *Diario de la Marina*, January 23, 1934.

81. "Physicians, Nurses Strike in Cuba," *Atlanta Constitution*, January 21, 1934.

82. "Hail Recognition in Havana as Boon," *New York Times*, January 23, 1934.

83. "Los comunistas daban mueras al ABC en el sepelio de Borges," *Diario de la Marina*, January 22.

84. "Bases del arreglo médico," *Diario de la Marina*, January 24, 1934. The demanded 100-peso minimum salary was not granted, but minimum wages for medical work were established.

85. "Bombs, Shots Terrorize Cuba," *Boston Daily Globe*, February 5, 1934; "Two in Mob Killed by Cuban Soldiers," *New York Times*, February 5, 1934.

86. See "Cuba Suppresses Medical College," *New York Times*, February 17, 1934, and "Agresión Inaudita," *Tribuna Médica*, February 1934.

87. "Impresiones," *Diario de la Marina*, January 20, 1934.

88. Letter from G. R. Martoreli to President Carlos Mendieta, January 22, 1934, legajo 10, no. 62, ANC/SP.

89. "Impresiones," *Diario de la Marina*, January 20, 1934.

90. "Huelga general," *Tribuna Médica*, January 1934, 5.

91. Dechamp and Poblete Troncoso, *El problema médico*.

92. Dechamp and Poblete Troncoso, *El problema medico*, 83.

93. Dechamp and Poblete Troncoso, *El problema medico*, 86.

94. "Ala Izquierda Médica," *Tribuna Médica*, October 1934, 335.

95. "Ala Izquierda Médica," *Tribuna Médica*, October 1934, 335.

96. Dechamp and Poblete Troncoso, *El problema médico*, 3.

97. "Ala Izquierda Médica," *Tribuna Médica*, October 1934, 338.

98. Odio Pérez, "Socialización," 363. Cuban physician Eduardo Odio Pérez was one of the four physicians who had quit the FMC in protest of its honoring President Machado at a 1928 event. See legajo 4, no. 172 and no. 173, and legajo 63, no. 108, ANC/FE.

99. Odio Pérez, "Socialización," 363.

100. Odio Pérez, "Socialización," 363.

101. Odio Pérez, "Socialización," 364.

102. Indeed, while the Ala Izquierda organized within the FMC, the Cuban Socialist Party began a "vigorous campaign" in its journal *Vanguardia Socialista* in favor of the demands of the medical class. See "El Partido Socialista cubano," *Tribuna Médica*, July 1934, 177.

103. Odio Pérez, "Socialización," 363.

104. See Dr. Rene De la Valette's "El pasado frente al futuro," *Tribuna Médica*, December 1934, 431, and "Lucha Médica," *Tribuna Médica*, November 1934, 361.

105. Rene De la Valette, "El pasado frente al futuro," *Tribuna Médica*, December 1934, 431. For the original, see Aspinwall, "Plea for Socialized Medicine." That George Aspinwall was the pen name of a "New York surgeon who has made important contributions to the surgury [sic] of the nose, ear, and throat," and yet published articles pseudonymously, suggests that perhaps there was more room within the medical community in

Cuba than in the United States in 1934 to advocate for the radical transformation of the health system. See "The American Mercury Authors," *American Mercury*, May 1934, 128.

106. Aspinwall, "Plea for Socialized Medicine," 38.

107. The article would then be reprinted in *La Tribuna Médica*. See Alberto Inclán, "Editorial," *Tribuna Médica*, December 1934, 425. For Inclán, a better model for a country with "a bourgeoise or capitalist system" like Cuba was the U.S. Mayo Clinic or the Johns Hopkins hospital, which charged patients according to their income and provided free care to those who could not afford medical fees.

108. For a general overview of his medical and horse-breeding activities, see "Alberto Inclán, 1888–1965," *Journal of Bone and Joint Surgery*, April 1965, 646–47.

109. "Acta de la Decimatercera Asamblea Nacional," *Tribuna Médica*, January 1935, 35.

110. "Demandas de los Médicos del Sanatorio 'La Esperanza,'" *Tribuna Médica*, September 1934, 259. Indeed, according to the 1934 International Labour Office report, wages at Havana's public hospitals were "extremely low" at an average of less than $88 per month. According to Dechamp and Troncoso, these wages were particularly untenable, given the economic climate for physicians in general in the capital. Public sector doctors were increasingly unable to get a clientele outside the system and were therefore completely reliant on their wages to survive. See Dechamp and Poblete Troncoso, *El problema médico*, 24–25.

111. Fernández Conde, *Biografía de la Federación Médica de Cuba*, 65.

112. See "Protesta la Federación Médica del abandono de los hospitales," *Tribuna Médica*, July 1934, 131; "El triunfo de los médicos del Sanatorio 'La Esperanza,'" *Tribuna Médica*, October 1934, 347; and "Indiferencia Gubernamental," *Tribuna Médica*, November 1934, 397.

113. The interview was republished in *La Tribuna Médica* that month. See "Declaraciones del Doctor Bisbé," *Tribuna Médica*, January 1935, 19.

114. "Declaraciones del Doctor Bisbé," *Tribuna Médica*, January 1935, 19.

115. See the medical workers' "Manifiesto al Pueblo," legajo 72, no. 5, folio 3, Tribunal de Urgencia, ANC.

116. Fernández Conde, *Biografía de la Federación Médica de Cuba*, 66.

117. Whitney, *State and Revolution in Cuba*, 131.

118. Fernández Conde, *Biografía de la Federación Médica de Cuba*, 68.

119. Fernández Conde, *Biografía de la Federación Médica de Cuba*, 69–71.

120. "Impresiones," *Diario de la Marina*, January 20, 1934.

## CONCLUSION

1. Mencía, *La sanidad y la beneficencia en Cuba*, 4.
2. Mencía, *La sanidad y la beneficencia en Cuba*, 14.
3. Mencía, *La sanidad y la beneficencia en Cuba*, 33.
4. García Rodríguez, *Problemas de salubridad*, 16–18.
5. García Rodríguez, *Problemas de salubridad*, 15.
6. García Rodríguez, *Problemas de salubridad*, 10.
7. García Rodríguez, *Problemas de salubridad*, 11.
8. Mencía, *La sanidad y la beneficencia en Cuba*, 33.

9. This narrative is shared by those on the Right and the Left, and it structures, in different ways, the writings of Cuban exiles after 1959, as well as much of the historiography of the Cuban republic and the historiography of the Cuban Revolution published outside the island.

10. See Article 160 of the 1940 constitution.

11. García Rodríguez, *Problemas de beneficencia*, 69–70.

12. García Rodríguez, *Problemas de beneficencia*, 67.

13. García Rodríguez, *Problemas de salubridad*, 20.

14. Congreso de la República de Cuba, *Diario de sesiones del Congreso*, 7a, 92.

15. Beltrán Moreno, "Editorial," 1.

16. McGuire and Frankel, "Mortality Decline in Cuba," 84–85. On the problems with prerevolutionary and early postrevolutionary health statistics, see 99–94.

17. Roberto E. Hernández makes a similar argument, although without the statistical analysis of McGuire and Frankel, in his "La atención médica en Cuba hasta 1958."

18. While the number of scholarly works examining the revolution's health policies is extensive, recent works include Brotherton, *Revolutionary Medicine*; Andaya, *Conceiving Cuba*; Pérez, *Caring for Them from Birth to Death*; Mason et al., *Community Health Care in Cuba*; Hirschfeld, *Health, Politics, and Revolution*; Whiteford and Branch, *Primary Health Care in Cuba*; and Kath, *Social Relations and the Cuban Health Miracle*.

19. See, for example, "Discurso pronunciado por el Comandante Fidel Castro Ruz, Primer Ministro del Gobierno Revolucionario en la sesión plenaria celebrada por el Comité Conjunto de Instituciones Cívicas Cubanas, en el Salon de Actos del Colegio Médico Nacional, el 16 de Marzo de 1959," in the online database "Discursos e intervenciones del Comandante en Jefe Fidel Castro Ruz, Presidente del Consejo de Estado de la República de Cuba" (http://www.cuba.cu/gobierno/discursos/1959/esp/f160359e.html).

20. See, for example, Hirschfeld, *Health, Politics, and Revolution*; Nordlinger, "Myth of Cuban Healthcare"; and Manning, "Think the Cuban Healthcare System Is Ideal?"

# BIBLIOGRAPHY

### ARCHIVES CONSULTED

Charlottesville, Va.
    Library of the University of Virginia, Special Collections Library
        Papers of Jefferson Randolph Kean
College Park, Md.
    National Archives of the United States of America
        Records of the Military Government of Cuba, 1898–1903
        Records of the Provisional Government of Cuba
Havana, Cuba
    Archivo de la Oficina del Historiador de la Ciudad de la Habana
        Actas Capitulares del Ayuntamiento de la Habana, Libro de Borradores
    Archivo Nacional de Cuba, La Habana
        Audencia de la Habana
        Fondo Especial
        Registro de Asociaciones
        Secretaría de la Presidencia
        Tribunal de Urgencia
    Biblioteca Nacional de Cuba José Martí
New York, N.Y.
    Columbia University Archives
        Homer Folks Papers
Philadelphia, Pa.
    Historical Society of Pennsylvania
        John R. Brooke Papers
        Citizens' Permanent Relief Committee Records
Washington, D.C.
    Library of Congress, Manuscripts Division
        Papers of Clara Barton
        Papers of William Crawford Gorgas
        Papers of Edwin Greble
        Papers of Leonard Wood

## PERIODICALS, CUBA

Anales de la Academia de Ciencias Médicas, Físicas, y Naturales de La Habana
Anales de la Oftalmología (Havana)
Arquitectura (Havana)
Boletín Médico Municipal de la Habana
Boletín Mensual de la Liga Contra la Tuberculosis de Cuba (Havana)
Boletín Oficial de la Secretaría de Sanidad y Beneficencia de la Isla de Cuba (Havana)
Boletín Oficial del Departamento de Beneficencia de la Isla de Cuba (Havana)
Crónica Médico-Quirúrgica de la Habana (Havana)
Cuba Contemporánea: Revista Mensual (Havana)
Diario de la Marina (Havana)
El Diario Español (Havana)
La Discusión (Havana)
El Figaro (Havana)
Gaceta Oficial de la República de Cuba
La Habana Médica (Havana)
Havana Post (Havana)
La Higiene (Havana)
La Lucha (Havana)
Medicina de Hoy (Havana)
El Mundo (Havana)
La Política Cómica (Havana)
El Progreso Médico (Havana)
Revista de Ciencias Médicas (Havana)
Revista de Humanidades Médicas (Camagüey)
Tribuna Médica (Havana)
El Triunfo (Havana)
La Union (Güines)
Vida Nueva (Havana)

## PERIODICALS, UNITED STATES

American Medical Association Bulletin
American Journal of Nursing
Boston Daily Advertiser
Boston Daily Globe
Boston Medical and Surgical Journal
California and Western Medicine
Chicago Daily Tribune
Harper's Weekly
Idaho Daily Statesman
Journal of the American Medical Association
Journal of the Association of Military Surgeons of the United States
Medical News
Medical Record
Minneapolis Journal
New York Times
Omaha World Herald
Outlook
San Francisco Chronicle
Springfield Republican
The Sun (Baltimore)
Washington Post

## PUBLISHED AND UNPUBLISHED SOURCES

Actas de la Octava Conferencia de Beneficencia y Corrección de la Isla de Cuba. Havana: La Moderna Poesía, 1910.
Actas de la Primera Conferencia Panamericana de Eugenesia y Homicultura de las Repúblicas Americanas. Havana: El Gobierno de la República de Cuba, 1928.
Actas de la Segunda Conferencia Panamericana de Eugenesia y Homicultura de las Repúblicas Americanas. Buenos Aires: Frascoli y Bindi, 1934.
Actas y Trabajos del Segundo Congreso Médico Nacional, Habana, Febrero 24–28 de 1911. Havana: El Universal, 1911.

Adair, Jennifer. *In Search of the "Lost Decade": Everyday Rights in Post-Dictatorship Argentina*. Berkeley: University of California Press, 2020.

Adamovsky, Ezequiel. *Historia de la clase media Argentina: Apogeo y decadencia de una ilusión, 1919–2003*. Buenos Aires: Planeta, 2009.

Adelman, Jeremy. *Colonial Legacies: The Problem of Persistence in Latin American History*. New York: Routledge, 1999.

Aguilar, Luis E. *Cuba 1933: Prologue to Revolution*. Ithaca, N.Y.: Cornell University Press, 1972.

Ahlman, Jeffrey S. *Living with Nkrumahism: Nation, State, and Pan-Africanism in Ghana*. Columbus: Ohio State University Press, 2017.

Ahmed, Faiz. *Afghanistan Rising: Islamic Law and Statecraft between the Ottoman and British Empires*. Cambridge: Harvard University Press, 2017.

Aldereguía, Gustavo. "La tuberculosis en la raza negra: Réplica al Señor Gustavo E. Urrutia." *Diario de la Marina*, September 15, 1929.

Aleman, José. "Consideraciones sobre 444 enfermos examinados bajo el punto de vista de tuberculosis pulmonar." *Actas del Segundo Congreso Médico Nacional*. In *Actas y Trabajos del Segundo Congreso Médico Nacional, Habana, Febrero 24–28 de 1911*, 24–29. Havana: El Universal, 1911.

Alfonso, Manuel F. "La beneficencia en Cuba." *Boletín Oficial de la Secretaría de Sanidad y Beneficencia de la Isla de Cuba*, March 1915.

Alfonso y García, Ramón María. *La prostitución en Cuba y especialmente en La Habana: Memoria de la comisión de higiene especial de la Isla de Cuba elevada al Secretario de Gobernación cumpliendo un precepto reglamentario*. Havana: Imprenta Fernández, 1902.

Alonso García, Alicia. "Diego Tamayo Figueredo: Médico y patriota cubano." *Revista de Humanidades Médicas* 15, no. 1 (2015): 196–205.

Ames, David W. "Negro Family Types in a Cuban Solar." *Phylon* 11, no. 2 (1950): 159–63.

Andaya, Elise. *Conceiving Cuba: Reproduction, Women, and the State in the Post-Soviet Era*. New Brunswick, N.J.: Rutgers University Press, 2014.

Anderson, Warwick. *Colonial Pathologies: American Tropical Medicine, Race, and Hygiene in the Philippines*. Durham: Duke University Press, 2006.

———. "Where Is the Postcolonial History of Medicine?" *Bulletin of the History of Medicine* 7, no. 23 (1998): 522–30.

Aragón, Ernesto. "El Concurso Nacional de Maternidad de 1918." *Boletín Oficial de la Secretaría de Sanidad y Beneficencia de la Isla de Cuba*, February 1918, 149–77.

Argote-Freyre, Frank. *Fulgencio Batista: From Revolutionary to Strongman*. New Brunswick, N.J.: Rutgers University Press, 2006.

Armus, Diego. *The Ailing City: Health, Tuberculosis, and Culture in Buenos Aires, 1870–1950*. Durham: Duke University Press, 2011.

———, ed. *Disease in the History of Modern Latin America: From Malaria to AIDS*. Durham: Duke University Press, 2003.

Arvey, Sarah R. "Sex and the Ordinary Cuban: Cuban Physicians, Eugenics, and Marital Sexuality, 1933–1958." *Journal of the History of Sexuality* 21, no. 1 (2012): 93–120.

Aspinwall, George W. "A Plea for Socialized Medicine." *American Mercury*, September 1934, 34–40.

Bangs, John Kendrick. *Uncle Sam Trustee.* New York: Riggs Publishing, 1902.
Barcia Zequeira, María del Carmen. *Una sociedad en crisis: La Habana a finales del siglo XIX.* Havana: Editorial Ciencias Sociales, 2000.
Barnet, Enrique. *Concepto actual de la medicina: Trabajo leído en la sesión solemne del 15 de Mayo de 1902.* Havana: La Prueba, 1905.
———. *Conversaciones del doctor.* Havana: Secretaría de Sanidad y Beneficencia, 1914.
———. *La peste bubónica.* Havana: Junta Superior de Sanidad de la Isla de Cuba, 1903.
———. *La sanidad en Cuba.* Havana: Imprenta Mercantil, 1905.
Barney, Sandra Lee. "Maternalism and the Promotion of Scientific Mothering during the Industrial Transformation of Appalachia, 1880–1930." *NWSA Journal* 11, no. 3 (Autumn 1999): 68–92.
Barton, Clara. *The Red Cross in Peace and War.* Washington, D.C.: American Historical Press, 1899.
Bay y Sevilla, Luis. *La vivienda del pobre: Sus peligros en el orden moral y de la salud.* Havana: Impresa Montalvo, Cárdenas, y Ca., 1924.
Bell, Morag. "'The Pestilence That Walketh in Darkness': Imperial Health, Gender and Images of South Africa c. 1880–1910." *Transactions of the Institute of British Geographers* 18, no. 3. (1993): 327–41.
Beltrán Moreno, Sebastián. "Editorial: La miseria, causa del fracaso de toda política sanitaria." *Medicina de Hoy* 2, no. 1 (January 1937): 1–2.
Bender, Thomas. *A Nation among Nations: America's Place in World History.* New York: FSG/Hill & Wang, 2006.
Birn, Anne-Emanuelle. *Marriage of Convenience: Rockefeller International Health and Revolutionary Mexico.* Rochester, N.Y.: University of Rochester Press, 2006
Bivins, Roberta. "Coming 'Home' to (post)Colonial Medicine: Treating Tropical Bodies in Post-War Britain." *Social History of Medicine* 26, no. 1 (February 2013): 1–20.
Bliss, Katherine. *Compromised Positions: Prostitution, Public Health, and Gender Politics in Revolutionary Mexico.* University Park: Pennsylvania State University Press, 2001.
Blum, Ann S. *Domestic Economies: Family, Work, and Welfare in Mexico City, 1884–1943.* Lincoln: University of Nebraska Press, 2009.
Bronfman, Alejandra. *Measures of Equality: Social Science, Citizenship, and Race in Cuba, 1902–1940.* Chapel Hill: University of North Carolina Press, 2004.
Brotherton, P. Sean. *Revolutionary Medicine: Health and the Body in Post-Soviet Cuba.* Durham: Duke University Press, 2012.
Buell, Raymond Leslie, et al. *Problems of the New Cuba: Report of the Commission on Cuban Affairs.* New York: Foreign Policy Association, 1935.
Burton, Antoinette, ed. *Archive Stories: Facts, Fictions, and the Writing of History.* Durham: Duke University Press, 2005.
Cabrera, Raimundo. *La Casa de Beneficencia y la Sociedad Económica: Sus relaciones con los gobiernos de Cuba.* Havana: Imprenta La Universal, 1914.
Calvo Peña, Beatriz. "Prensa, política y prostitución en la Habana finisecular: El caso de La Cebolla y la 'polémica de las meretrices.'" *Cuban Studies/Estudios Cubanos* 36 (2005): 23–49.

Cañizares, Dulcila. *San Isidro, 1910: Alberto Yarini y su época*. Havana: Editorial Letras Cubanas, 2001.

Cañizares Esguerra, Jorge. "New World, New Stars: Patriotic Astrology and the Invention of Indian and Creole Bodies in Colonial Spanish America, 1600–1650." *American Historical Review* 104, no. 1 (1999): 33–68.

Cantero, Trinidad. "La enfermera: Los derechos y consideraciones que se le deben dispensar." In *Memoria Oficial. Tercera Conferencia Nacional de Beneficencia y Corrección de la Isla de Cuba. Celebrada en Matanzas del 2 al 4 de Abril de 1904*, 301–3. Havana: La Moderna Poesía, 1904.

———. "Escuela de enfermeras." In *Primera Conferencia Nacional de Beneficencia y Corrección de la Isla de Cuba. Celebrada en La Habana del 19 al 22 de Marzo de 1902*, 383–85. Havana: La Moderna Poesía, 1902.

Carassai, Sebastián. *The Argentine Silent Majority: Middle Classes, Politics, Violence, and Memory in the Seventies*. Durham: Duke University Press, 2014.

Casavantes Bradford, Anita. *The Revolution Is for the Children: The Politics of Childhood in Havana and Miami, 1959–1962*. Chapel Hill: University of North Carolina Press, 2014.

Casey, Matthew. *Empire's Guestworkers: Haitian Migrants in Cuba during the Age of US Occupation*. Cambridge: Cambridge University Press, 2017.

Caulfield, Sueann. *In Defense of Honor: Sexual Morality, Modernity, and Nation in Early Twentieth-Century Brazil*. Durham: Duke University Press, 2000.

Caulfield, Sueann, Sarah C. Chambers, and Lara Putnam. *Honor, Status, and Law in Modern Latin America*. Durham: Duke University Press, 2005.

Cepeda, Rafael. *Eusebio Hernández: Ciencia y patria*. Havana: Editorial de Ciencias Sociales, 1991.

Céspedes, Benjamín de. *La prostitución en la ciudad de la Habana*. Havana: Establecimiento Tipográfico O'Reilly, 1888.

Chailloux Cardona, Juan Manuel. *Síntesis histórica de la vivienda popular: Los horrores del solar habanero*. 1945. Havana: Editorial de Ciencias Sociales, 2008.

Chambers, Sarah C. *From Subjects to Citizens: Honor, Gender, and Politics in Arequipa, Peru, 1780–1854*. University Park: Pennsylvania State University Press, 1999.

Chapman, Charles E. *A History of the Cuban Republic: A Study in Hispanic American Politics*. New York: Macmillan, 1927.

Chazkel, Amy. *Laws of Chance: Brazil's Clandestine Lottery and the Making of Urban Public Life*. Durham: Duke University Press, 2011.

Childs, Matt D. *The 1812 Aponte Rebellion in Cuba and the Struggle against Atlantic Slavery*. Chapel Hill: University of North Carolina Press, 2006.

Coll y Nuñez, Paula. *Memoria de los trabajos realizados por el Comité Antituberculoso de las Damas Isabelinas*. Havana: Imprenta del Ejército, 1932.

Congreso de la República de Cuba. Cámara de Representantes, Sesión Ordinaria. *Diario de sesiones del Congreso de la República de Cuba*, tercera legislatura 3, no. 8 (April 27, 28, 1903): 89–103.

*Constitution and By-laws of the Professional Club Oscar Primelles*. New York: n.p., n.d.

*Contra la tísis: Cartilla dedicada a las clases populares Habana, Cuba*. Havana: Departamento de Sanidad, 1902.

Cook, Mercer. "Urrutia." *Phylon* 4, no. 3 (1943): 220–32.
*Core Curriculum on Tuberculosis: What the Clinician Should Know.* 6th ed. Atlanta: CDC, 2013.
Cosculluela, José A. *La salubridad urbana: Con especial referencia a la ciudad de La Habana.* Havana: Compostela y Chacón, 1925.
Cosse, Isabella. "Mafalda: Middle Class, Everyday Life, and Politics in Argentina, 1964–1973." *Hispanic American Historical Review* 94, no. 1 (2014): 35–75.
Cuadrado, Gaston. "Necesidad de higiene pública." *Crónica Médico-Quirúrgica de la Habana* 28 (1902): 254–60.
Cuba. Departamento de Beneficencia. *El Nuevo Departamento de Beneficencia: Sus fines y sus métodos.* Havana: Departamento de Beneficencia, 1900.
Cuba. Dirección Nacional del Censo. *Census of the Republic of Cuba: 1919.* Havana: Maza, Arroyo, y Caso, 1922.
Cuba. Oficina Nacional del Censo. *Censo de la República de Cuba, 1907.* Washington, D.C.: Oficina del Censo de los Estados Unidos, 1908.
Cuba. Secretaría de Sanidad y Beneficencia. *Servicio de Higiene Infantil: A manera de divulgación científica, con motivo del reparto de premios en el Concurso Nacional de Maternidad, Habana, 6 de enero de 1919.* Havana: n.p., 1919.
Danielson, Ross. *Cuban Medicine.* New Brunswick, N.J.: Transaction, 1979.
De Barros, Juanita. *Reproducing the British Caribbean: Sex, Gender, and Population Politics after Slavery.* Chapel Hill: University of North Carolina Press, 2014.
De Barros, Juanita, Steven Paul Palmer, and David Wright, eds. *Health and Medicine in the Circum-Caribbean, 1800–1968.* New York: Routledge, 2009.
Dechamp, Cyrille, and Moises Poblete Troncoso. *El problema médico y la asistencia médica mutualista en Cuba.* Translated by Rafael de la Torre. Havana: n.p., 1934.
Dehogues, Jorge L. "Condiciones que deben exigirse a los enfermos para ser admitidos en hospitales y dispensaries." In *Memoria Oficial. Primera Conferencia Nacional de Beneficencia y Corrección de la Isla de Cuba. Celebrada en La Habana del 19 al 22 de Marzo de 1902,* 407–9. Havana: La Moderna Poesía, 1902.
de la Cruz y Ugarte, Carlos. *Obligaciones del estado en relación con la beneficencia infantil.* Havana: n.p., 1927.
de la Fuente, Alejandro. *Havana and the Atlantic in the Sixteenth Century.* Chapel Hill: University of North Carolina Press, 2008.
———. *A Nation for All: Race, Inequality, and Politics in Twentieth-Century Cuba.* Chapel Hill: University of North Carolina Press, 2001.
———. "Two Dangers, One Solution: Immigration, Race, and Labor in Cuba, 1900–1930." *International Labor and Working-Class History,* no. 51 (1997): 30–49.
de la Guardia, Vicente. *Higiene pública: Algunas consideraciones relativas á la ciudad de la Habana.* Havana: Imprenta J.A. Casanova, 1901.
de la Portilla, Florencio. "Contribución al estudio y tratamiento de las gastroenteritis en los niños." In *Actas y Trabajos del Segundo Congreso Médico Nacional, Habana, Febrero 24–28 de 1911,* 233–35. Havana: El Universal, 1911.
Delfín, Manuel. *La Casa del Pobre, institución benéfica genuinamente cubana.* Havana: La Propagandista, 1914.
———. *Nociones de higiene.* Havana: La Propagandista, 1901.
———. *Treinta años de médico.* Havana: La Propagandista, 1909.

Delgado García, Gregorio. "Dr. Enrique Núñez de Villavicencio y Palomino, gran figura de la cirugía cubana en la guerra y en la paz." *Cuadernos de la Historia de la Salud Pública* 84 (1998): 39–55.

Departamento de Sanidad de la Habana. *Manual de práctica sanitaria. Para uso de jefes e inspectores de sanidad, médicos, funcionarios, etc., de la república de Cuba.* Havana: n.p., 1905.

De Quesada y Miranda, Gonzalo. *Anecdotario martiano.* Havana: Ediciones Patria, 1948.

Deulofeu, Emma. "Aire puro en el tratamiento de la tuberculosis." *Vida Nueva*, February 1912, 130–31.

Dirección General del Censo. *Census of the Republic of Cuba, 1919.* Havana: Maza, Arroyo y Caso, 1920.

Dore, Elizabeth, and Maxine Molyneux, eds. *Hidden Histories of Gender and the State in Latin America.* Durham: Duke University Press, 2000.

Duque, Matías. "Al 'Medical Record': 'La Amenaza Cubana.'" *Boletín Oficial de la Secretaría de Sanidad y Beneficencia de la Isla de Cuba*, June 1909, 341–44.

———. "Sanidad y beneficencia." *Boletín Oficial de la Secretaría de Sanidad y Beneficencia de la Isla de Cuba*, April 1909, 5–6.

Echenberg, Myron. "Pestis Redux: The Initial Years of the Third Bubonic Plague Pandemic, 1894–1901." *Journal of World History* 13, no. 2 (Fall 2002): 429–49.

———. *Plague Ports: The Global Urban Impact of Bubonic Plague, 1894–1901.* New York: New York University Press, 2007.

Edelmann, Ernesto. "Desinfección urbana." *Anales de la Academia de Ciencias Médicas, Físicas, y Naturales de la Habana* 36 (May 1900): 339–43.

"Escuela de enfermeras de la République de Cuba: Discursos de los Doctores C. E. Finlay y Enrique Nuñez." *Boletín Oficial del Departamento de Beneficencia de la Isla de Cuba* 2, no. 13 (November 1902): 285–91.

Espinosa, Mariola. *Epidemic Invasions: Yellow Fever and the Limits of Cuban Independence, 1878–1930.* Chicago: University of Chicago Press, 2009.

Farber, Samuel. *Revolution and Reaction in Cuba, 1933–1960: A Political Sociology from Machado to Castro.* Middletown, Conn.: Wesleyan University Press, 1976.

Fariñas Borrego, Maikel. *Sociabilidad y cultura del ocio : La élites habaneras y sus clubes de recreo, 1902–1930.* Havana: Fundación Fernando Ortiz, 2009.

Fernández, Edelmira. "Escuela central de enfermeras cubanas." In *Memoria Oficial. Séptima Conferencia Nacional de Beneficencia y Corrección de la Isla de Cuba*, 281–85. Havana: La Moderna Poesía, 1908.

Fernández Conde, Augusto. *Biografía de la Federación Médica de Cuba.* Havana: Colegio Médico de la Habana, 1945.

Ferreira, Roquinaldo. *Cross Cultural Exchange in the Atlantic World: Angola and Brazil during the Era of the Slave Trade.* Cambridge: Cambridge University Press, 2012.

Ferrer, Ada. *Freedom's Mirror: Cuba and Haiti in the Age of Revolution.* New York: Cambridge University Press, 2014.

———. *Insurgent Cuba: Race, Nation, and Revolution, 1868–1898.* Chapel Hill: University of North Carolina Press, 1999.

*Fiebre amarilla: Instrucciones populares para evitar su contagio y propagación.* Havana: Junta Superior de Sanidad, 1906.

Finch, Aisha K. *Rethinking Slave Rebellion in Cuba: La Escalera and the Insurgencies of 1841–1844*. Chapel Hill: University of North Carolina Press, 2015.

*Fines y reglamento de la "Liga de Higiene Social" fundada a iniciativas del Director de Sanidad Dr. J. A. López del Valle*. Havana: n.p., 1924.

Finlay, Carlos E. "Algunos problemas respecto a las escuelas de enfermeras." In *Memoria Oficial. Tercera Conferencia Nacional de Beneficencia y Corrección de la Isla de Cuba. Celebrada en Matanzas del 2 al 4 de Abril de 1904*, 79–83. Havana: La Moderna Poesía, 1904.

———. "Escuelas de enfermeras." In *Memoria Oficial. Primera Conferencia Nacional de Beneficencia y Corrección de la Isla de Cuba. Celebrada en La Habana del 19 al 22 de Marzo de 1902*, 356–61. Havana: La Moderna Poesía, 1902.

Fischer, Brodwyn. *A Poverty of Rights: Citizenship and Inequality in Twentieth-Century Rio de Janeiro*. Stanford, Calif.: Stanford University Press, 2008.

Fischer, Sibylle. *Modernity Disavowed: Haiti and the Cultures of Slavery in the Age of Revolution*. Durham: Duke University Press, 2004.

Fosalba, Rafael E. "La mortinatalidad y mortalidad infantil en la República de Cuba." *Anales de la Academia de Ciencias Médicas, Físicas, y Naturales de la Habana* 51 (1914): 88–444.

Foucault, Michel. *The Birth of the Clinic: An Archaeology of Medical Perception*. New York: Vintage Books, 1975.

French, John D. "The Laboring and Middle-Class Peoples of Latin America and the Caribbean: Historical Trajectories and New Research Directions." In *Global Labour History: A State of the Art*, edited by Jan Lucassen, 289–333. Bern, Switzerland: Peter Lang, 2006.

Fuentes, Juan B. "Casas de vecindad, dispensario especial." In Departamento de Sanidad de la Habana, *Manual de Práctica Sanitaria. Para uso de Jefes e Inspectores de Sanidad, Médicos, Funcionarios, etc., de la República de Cuba*, 839–57. Havana: n.p., 1905.

———. "Como puede intervenir el estado en el axilio a las familias pobres?" In *Actas y trabajos de la Septima Conferencia Nacional de Beneficencia y Corrección de la Isla de Cuba*, 354–363. Havana: La Moderna Poesía, 1908.

Funes Monzote, Reinaldo. *El despertar del asociacionismo científico en Cuba, 1876–1920*. Havana: Centro de Investigación y Desarrollo de la Cultura Cubana Juan Marinello, 2005.

Galarreta, Luís Adam. "La inmigración haitiana, jamaiquina y china: Influencia desfaborable en nuestro estado sanitario." *Crónica Médico-Quirúrgica de la Habana* 47 (March 1921): 94–97.

Gandarilla, Julio César. *Contra el yanqui: Obra de protesta contra la Enmienda Platt y contra la absorción y el maquiavelismo norteamericanos*. Havana: Rambla, Bouza, y ca., 1913.

García Mendoza, Alberto. "Las viviendas de los pobres y la tuberculosis." In *Memoria Oficial. Segunda Conferencia Nacional de Beneficencia y Corrección de la Isla de Cuba. Celebrada en Santa Clara del 24 al 26 de Mayo de 1903*, 329–34. Havana: La Moderna Poesía, 1904.

García, Angel, and Piotr Mironchuk. *Los soviets obreros y campesinos en Cuba*. Havana: Editorial de Ciencias Sociales, 1987.

García, Guadalupe. *Beyond the Walled City: Colonial Exclusion in Havana*. Berkeley: University of California Press, 2016.

García González, Armando. "El desarrollo de la eugenesia en Cuba." *Asclepio* 51 (1999): 85–100.

García González, Armando, and Raquel Álvarez Peláez. *En busca de la raza perfecta: Eugenesia e higiene en Cuba (1898–1958)*. Madrid: Consejo Superior de Investigaciones Científicas, 1999.

García Rodríguez, Félix. *Problemas de beneficencia: Lo poco que se ha hecho, lo mucho que puede hacerse*. Havana: Imprenta Librería Nueva, 1937.

———. *Problemas de salubridad*. Havana: Imprenta Librería Nueva, 1940.

Gillette, Howard. "The Military Occupation of Cuba, 1899–1902: Workshop for American Progressivism." *American Quarterly* 25, no. 4 (1973): 410–25.

Gómez, Edualdo. *Compilación sanitaria de Cuba*. Havana: Sindicato de Artes Gráficas, 1929.

González Pagés, Julio César. *En busca de un espacio: Historia de las mujeres en Cuba*. Havana: Editorial de Ciencias Sociales, 2005.

Gorgas, William Crawford. "The Conquest of the Tropics for the White Race." *Boston Medical and Surgical Journal* 160, no. 24 (June 17, 1909): 765–67.

———. "A Short Account of the Results of Mosquito Work in Havana, Cuba." *Journal of the Association of Military Surgeons of the United States* 7 (1903): 133–39.

———. *The Work of the Sanitary Department of Havana, with Special Reference to the Repression of Yellow Fever*. New York: William Wood, 1901.

Grandin, Greg. *The Last Colonial Massacre: Latin America in the Cold War*. Chicago: University of Chicago Press, 2004.

Guiteras, Juan. "La inmigración china." *Anales de la Academia de Ciencias Médicas, Físicas, y Naturales de La Habana* 50 (1913): 248–99.

———. "Mortalidad de niños en la república." *Boletín Oficial de la Secretaría de Sanidad y Beneficencia de la Isla de Cuba*, December 1913, 664–74.

———. "An Open Letter." *Boletín Oficial de la Secretaría de Sanidad y Beneficencia de la Isla de Cuba*, June 1912, 679–80.

———. "La peste bubónica en Cuba." *Boletín Oficial de la Secretaría de Sanidad y Beneficencia de la Isla de Cuba*, September 1914, 313–47.

———. "La sanidad cubana y la opinión extranjera." *Boletín Oficial de la Secretaría de Sanidad y Beneficencia de la Isla de Cuba*, June 1909, 1–4.

Gutiérrez, John A. "Disease, Empire, and Modernity in the Caribbean: Tuberculosis in Cuba, 1899–1909." Ph.D. diss., City College of New York, 2013.

———. "'An Earnest Pledge to Fight Tuberculosis': Tuberculosis, Nation, and Modernity in Cuba, 1899–1908." *Cuban Studies* 45 (January 2017): 280–96.

Helg, Aline. *Our Rightful Share: The Afro-Cuban Struggle for Equality, 1886–1912*. Chapel Hill: University of North Carolina Press, 1995.

Hernández, Eusebio, and Rafael Cepeda. *Ciencia y patria*. Havana: Editorial de Ciencias Sociales, 1991.

Hernández, Eusebio, and Domingo F. Ramos. *Homicultura*. Havana: Secretaría de Sanidad y Beneficencia, 1911.

Hernández, Roberto E. "La atención médica en Cuba hasta 1958." *Journal of Inter-American Studies* 11, no. 4 (1969): 533–57.

Hibbard, Eugenia. "Como viven nuestros pobres." *El Mundo* (Havana), January 31, 1912.

———. "Trabajos sobre la tuberculosis en Cuba." In *Memoria Oficial. Octava Conferencia Nacional de Beneficencia y Corrección de la Isla de Cuba. Celebrada En Sagua la Grande los Días 8, 9 y 10 de Enero de 1910*, 281–93. Havana: La Moderna Poesía, 1911.

Hibbard, M. Eugénie. "Cuba: A Sketch." *American Journal of Nursing* 4, no. 9. (1904): 696–702.

———. "The Establishment of Schools for Nurses in Cuba." *American Journal of Nursing* 2, no. 12 (1902): 985–91.

Hicks, Anasa. "Hierarchies at Home: A History of Domestic Service in Cuba from Abolition to Revolution." Ph.D. diss., New York University, 2017.

Hill, Robert Thomas. *Cuba and Porto Rico, with the Other Islands of the West Indies: Their Topography, Climate, Flora, Products, Industries, Cities, People, Political Conditions, etc.* London: T. Fisher Unwin, 1898.

Hirschfeld, Katherine. *Health, Politics, and Revolution in Cuba since 1898.* New Brunswick, N.J.: Transaction, 2008.

Hoganson, Kristin L. *Fighting for American Manhood: How Gender Politics Provoked the Spanish-American and Philippine-American Wars.* New Haven: Yale University Press, 1998.

Horst, Jesse. "Sleeping on the Ashes: Slum Clearance in Havana in an Age of Revolution, 1930–65." Ph.D. diss., University of Pittsburgh, 2016.

Hunt, Nancy Rose. *A Colonial Lexicon: Of Birth Ritual, Medicalization, and Mobility in the Congo.* Durham: Duke University Press, 1999.

Hurtado Galtés, Félix. "Editorial: El problema económico de la clase médica." *Tribuna Médica*, June 15, 1930, 3–4.

Ibarra, Jorge. *Prologue to Revolution: Cuba, 1898–1958.* Boulder, Colo.: Lynne Rienner, 1998.

Iglesias Utset, Marial. *Las metáforas del cambio en la vida cotidiana: Cuba, 1898–1902.* Havana: Ediciones Union, 2003.

*Instrucciones populares para evitar el contagio y la propagación de la escarlatina.* Havana: Junta Superior de Sanidad, 1903.

Iturria, Miguel. *Españoles en la cultura cubana.* Sevilla: Editorial Renacimiento, 2004.

Jacobsen, Joaquín L. "The Problem of Tuberculosis in Cuba." *Transactions of the Sixth International Congress on Tuberculosis*, 113–25. Washington, D.C.: William Fell, 1908.

Joseph, Gilbert, and Daniel Nugent, eds. *Everyday Forms of State Formation: Revolution and the Negotiation of Rule in Modern Mexico.* Durham: Duke University Press, 1994.

Jover, Verena. "La institución de la enfermera cubana y la caridad." In *Memoria Oficial. Primera Conferencia Nacional de Beneficencia y Corrección de la Isla de Cuba. Celebrada en La Habana del 19 al 22 de Marzo de 1902*, 386–88. Havana: La Moderna Poesía, 1902.

Kath, Elizabeth. *Social Relations and the Cuban Health Miracle.* Brunswick, N.J.: Transaction, 2010.

Katz, Michael B. *In the Shadow of the Poorhouse: A Social History of Welfare in the United States.* New York: Basic Books, 1986.

Kean, Jefferson Randolph. "Hospitals and Charities in Cuba." *Journal of the Association of Military Surgeons of the United States* 12 (1903): 140–49.

———. "Needs of the Department of Charities of Cuba." In *Memoria Oficial. Primera Conferencia Nacional de Beneficencia y Corrección de la Isla de Cuba. Celebrada en La Habana del 19 al 22 de Marzo de 1902*, 537–42. Havana: La Moderna Poesía, 1902.

———. *Report of Major J. R. Kean, Major and Surgeon, U.S.A., Superintendent, Department of Charities*. In U.S. War Department, *Civil Report of Brigadier General Leonard Wood, Military Governor of Cuba*, 1901, vol. 5. Washington, D.C.: Government Printing Office, 1901.

Klein, Naomi. *The Shock Doctrine: The Rise of Disaster Capitalism*. Toronto: Knopf Canada, 2007.

Kraut, Alan M. *Silent Travelers: Germs, Genes, and the "Immigrant Menace."* Baltimore: Johns Hopkins University Press, 1994.

Kuhn, Thomas. *The Structure of Scientific Revolutions*. Chicago: University of Chicago Press, 1962.

Lambe, Jennifer L. *Madhouse: Psychiatry and Politics in Cuban History*. Chapel Hill: University of North Carolina Press, 2017.

Lasso, Marixa. *Myths of Harmony: Race and Republicanism during the Age of Revolution, Colombia, 1795–1831*. Pittsburgh: University of Pittsburgh Press, 2007.

Laveaga, Gabriela Soto. *Jungle Laboratories: Mexican Peasants, National Projects, and the Making of The Pill*. Durham: Duke University Press, 2009.

Laveaga, Gabriela Soto, and Claudia Agostoni. "Science and Public Health in the Century of Revolution." In *A Companion to Mexican History and Culture*, edited by William H. Beezley, 561–74. Malden, Mass.: Blackwell, 2011.

Lawlor, Clark. *Consumption and Literature: The Making of the Romantic Disease*. New York: Palgrave Macmillan, 2006.

Lebredo, Mario G. "La mortalidad infantil y medidas que deben ponerse en práctica a fin de disminuirla." *Boletín Oficial de la Secretaría de Sanidad y Beneficencia de la Isla de Cuba*, August 1917, 208–33.

Le-Roy y Cassá, Jorge. *Inmigración anti-sanitaria*. Havana: Dorrbecker, 1929.

———. *La mortalidad infantil en Cuba: Notas demográficas*. Havana: Impresa y Librería de Lloredo y Ca., 1914.

———. "La sanidad en Cuba: Sus progresos." *Cuba contemporánea: Revista mensual* 3, no. 1 (September 1913): 43–63.

*El libro del Centro Asturiano de la Habana, 1889–1927*. Havana: n.p., 1928.

López, A. Ricardo, and Barbara Weinstein, eds. *The Making of the Middle Class: Toward a Transnational History*. Durham: Duke University Press, 2012.

López, Enrique. "Ambliopía por desnutrición." *Anales de la oftalmología* 2, no. 9 (March 1900): 85–87.

López, Kathleen M. *Chinese Cubans: A Transnational History*. Chapel Hill: University of North Carolina Press, 2013.

López del Valle, José Antonio. *Los adelantos sanitarios de la república de Cuba*. Havana: Imprenta La Propagandista, 1924.

———. "Casas de vecindad." *Boletín Oficial de la Secretaría de Sanidad y Beneficencia de la Isla de Cuba*, August 1917, 264–72.

———. *Los certificados médicos pre-nupciales: Historia, consideraciones médico-sanitarias, ventajas y aplicación práctica de esa medida*. Havana: Secretaría de Sanidad y Beneficencia, 1927.

———. *El Departamento de Sanidad de la Habana: Su organización, procedimientos y marcha*. Havana: n.p., 1905.

———. "Desenvolvimiento de la sanidad y de la beneficencia en Cuba, durante los últimos diez y seis años." *Boletín Oficial de la Secretaría de Sanidad y Beneficencia de la Isla de Cuba*, December 1914, 702–766.

———. *Lecciones populares sobre la tuberculosis*. Havana: Secretaría de Sanidad y Beneficencia, 1911.

———. "The Nationalization of Sanitary Services. Address Read Before the Special Session of the Board, Havana, Cuba, March 7, 1908." Havana: n.p., 1908.

López Denis, Adrian. "Disease and Society in Colonial Cuba, 1790–1840." Ph.D. diss., University of California, Los Angeles, 2007.

Mallon, Florencia. *Peasant and Nation: The Making of Postcolonial Mexico and Peru*. Berkeley: University of California Press, 1995.

Maluquer de Motes Bernet, Jordi. *Nación e inmigración: Los españoles en Cuba (ss. XIX y XX)*. Havana: Ediciones Júcar, 1992.

Manning, Hadley Heath. "Think the Cuban Healthcare System Is Ideal? No Cigar. Not Even Close." *Washington Examiner*, November 29, 2016.

Markel, Howard. *Quarantine! East European Jews and the New York City Epidemics of 1892*. Baltimore: Johns Hopkins University Press, 1999.

Martínez, Emilio. "La asistencia médica a domicilio: Su organización—No debe ser función del Estado." In *Memoria Oficial. Segunda Conferencia Nacional de Beneficencia y Corrección de la Isla de Cuba. Celebrada en Santa Clara del 24 al 26 de Mayo de 1903*, 123–30. Havana: La Moderna Poesía, 1904.

Martinez-Alier, Verena. *Marriage, Class, and Colour in Nineteenth-Century Cuba*. Cambridge: Cambridge University Press, 1974.

Martínez Moreno, José. "Algunas consideraciones sobre la manera de ser de nuestros hospitales." *Memoria Oficial. Tercera Conferencia Nacional de Beneficencia y Corrección de la Isla de Cuba. Celebrada en Matanzas del 2 al 4 de Abril de 1904*, 53–60. Havana: La Moderna Poesía, 1904.

Mason, Susan E., et al., eds. *Community Health Care in Cuba: An Enduring Model*. Chicago: Lyceum Press, 2009.

Matthews, Franklin. *The New-Born Cuba*. New York: Harper & Brothers, 1899.

McCoy, Alfred W., and Francisco A. Scarano, eds. *Colonial Crucible: Empire in the Making of the Modern American State*. Madison: University of Wisconsin Press, 2009.

McDonald, Daniel. "Peripheral Citizenship: The Popular Politics of Rights, Welfare, and Health in São Paulo, 1960–1993." Ph.D. diss., Brown University, forthcoming.

McGuire, James W., and Laura B. Frankel. "Mortality Decline in Cuba, 1900–1959: Patterns, Comparisons, and Causes." *Latin American Research Review* 40, no. 2 (2005): 83–116.

McKiernan-González, John. *Fevered Measures: Public Health and Race at the Texas-Mexico Border, 1848–1942*. Durham: Duke University Press, 2012.

McLeod, Marc. "'Sin Dejar de Ser Cubanos': Cuban Blacks and the Challenges of Garveyism in Cuba." *Caribbean Studies* 31, no. 1 (January–June 2003): 75–105.

———. "'We Cubans Are Obligated Like Cats to Have a Clean Face': Malaria, Quarantine, and Race in Neocolonial Cuba, 1898–1940." *The Americas* 67, no. 1 (2010): 57–81.

McNeill, J. R. *Mosquito Empires: Ecology and War in the Greater Caribbean, 1620–1914*. Cambridge: Cambridge University Press, 2010.

Meade, Teresa A. *Civilizing Rio: Reform and Resistance in a Brazilian City, 1889–1930*. University Park: Pennsylvania State University Press, 1997.

Meckel, Richard A. *Save the Babies: American Public Health Reform and the Prevention of Infant Mortality, 1850–1929*. Rochester, N.Y.: University of Rochester Press, 1990.

Mederos de Fernández, Rafaela. *La mujer en el frente social de Cuba: Recopilación de 44 años de labor, 1894–1938*. Havana: Impresa Editora de Publicaciones, 1939.

———. "Protección a la niñez: Tema oficial del Congreso Nacional de Madres." *Memoria del Primer Congreso Nacional de Mujeres Organizado por la Federación Nacional de Asociaciones Femeninas*, 315–21. Havana: La Universal, 1923.

"Medical Practice in Cuba: Address of Dr. J. M. Penichet, Delegate of the Cuban Federation of Physicians to the House of Delegates of the American Medical Association." *Journal of the American Medical Association*, June 11, 1927, 1890–91.

*Memoria del Primer Congreso Nacional de Mujeres Organizado por la Federación Nacional de Asociaciones Femeninas*. Havana: La Universal, 1923.

*Memoria del Segundo Congreso Nacional de Mujeres*. Havana: La Universal, 1927.

*Memoria Oficial. Primera Conferencia Nacional de Beneficencia y Corrección de la Isla de Cuba. Celebrada en La Habana del 19 al 22 de Marzo de 1902*. Havana: La Moderna Poesía, 1902.

*Memoria Oficial. Segunda Conferencia Nacional de Beneficencia y Corrección de la Isla de Cuba. Celebrada en Santa Clara del 24 al 26 de Mayo de 1903*. Havana: La Moderna Poesía, 1904.

*Memoria Oficial. Tercera Conferencia Nacional de Beneficencia y Corrección de la Isla de Cuba. Celebrada en Matanzas del 2 al 4 de Abril de 1904*. Havana: La Moderna Poesía, 1904.

*Memoria Oficial. Sexta Conferencia Nacional de Beneficencia y Corrección de la Isla de Cuba. Celebrada en Cienfuegos del 30 de Marzo al 2 de Abril de 1907*. Havana: La Moderna Poesía, 1907.

*Memoria Oficial. Séptima Conferencia Nacional de Beneficencia y Corrección de la Isla de Cuba. Celebrada en Cárdenas del 18 al 20 de Abril de 1908*. Havana: La Moderna Poesía, 1908.

*Memoria Oficial. Octava Conferencia Nacional de Beneficencia y Corrección de la Isla de Cuba. Celebrada en Sagua la Grande los Días 8, 9 y 10 de Enero de 1910*. Havana: La Moderna Poesía, 1911.

Mencía, Manuel. *La sanidad y la beneficencia en Cuba: Informe presentado al Sr. Presidente de la República y al Consejo de Secretarios*. Havana: Molina y Cia., 1936.

Merelles, Mariá. "Reposo." *Vida Nueva*, February 1912, 128–30.

Meza, Ramon. "Nuestra inmigración util debe ser protegida." In *Memoria Oficial de la Quinta Conferencia Nacional de Beneficencia y Corrección de la Isla de Cuba*. Havana: La Moderna Poesía, 1906.

Milanich, Nara B. *Children of Fate: Childhood, Class, and the State in Chile, 1850–1930*. Durham: Duke University Press, 2009.

Mitchell, Timothy. *Rule of Experts: Egypt, Techno-Politics, Modernity*. Berkeley: University of California Press, 2002.

Moore, Robin D. *Nationalizing Blackness: Afrocubanismo and Artistic Revolution in Havana, 1920–1940*. Pittsburgh: University of Pittsburgh Press, 1997.

Motes Bernet, Jordi Maluquer de. *Nación e inmigración: Los Españoles en Cuba (ss. XIX y XX)*. Havana: Ediciones Júcar, 1992.

Mulhall, Michael G. *The Dictionary of Statistics*. London: Routledge and Sons, 1903.

Naranjo Orovio, Consuelo, and Armando García González. *Medicina y racismo en Cuba: La ciencia ante la inmigración canaria en el siglo XX*. Canary Islands: Centro de la Cultura Popular Canaria, 1996.

Neptune, Harvey. *Caliban and the Yankees: Trinidad and the United States Occupation*. Chapel Hill: University of North Carolina Press, 2007.

New York State Medical Association. *Medical Directory of New York, New Jersey, and Connecticut*. New York: New York State Medical Association, 1902.

Nordlinger, Jay. "The Myth of Cuban Healthcare." *National Review*, July 11, 2007, https://www.nationalreview.com/2007/07/myth-cuban-health-care/.

Nuñez, Emiliano. "Asistencia hospitalaria y asistencia a domicilio." In *Memoria Oficial. Primera Conferencia Nacional de Beneficencia y Corrección de la Isla de Cuba. Celebrada en La Habana del 19 al 22 de Marzo de 1902*, 266–75. Havana: La Moderna Poesía, 1902.

Odio Pérez, Eduardo. "Socialización de los servicios médicos y afines." *Tribuna Médica*, November 1934, 363–64.

O'Donnell, Mary Agnes. "Dificultades con que se tropieza en las escuelas de enfermeras." In *Memoria Oficial. Primera Conferencia Nacional de Beneficencia y Corrección de la Isla de Cuba. Celebrada en La Habana del 19 al 22 de Marzo de 1902*, 373–76. Havana: La Moderna Poesía, 1902.

Offner, Amy. *Sorting Out the Mixed Economy: The Rise and Fall of Welfare and Developmental States in the Americas*. Princeton: Princeton University Press, 2019.

Ortiz, Fernándo. "Consideraciones criminológicas acerca de la inmigración en Cuba." In *Memoria Oficial de la Quinta Conferencia Nacional de Beneficencia y Corrección de la Isla de Cuba*, 343–55. Havana: La Moderna Poesía, 1906.

Ortiz y Coffigny, Julio, "Algunas consideraciones sobre las escuelas de enfermeras en relación con el reglamento general." In *Memoria Oficial. Tercera Conferencia Nacional de Beneficencia y Corrección de la Isla de Cuba. Celebrada en Matanzas del 2 al 4 de Abril de 1904*, 84–89. Havana: La Moderna Poesía, 1904.

Palmer, Steven. "Beginnings of Cuban Bacteriology: Juan Santos Fernández, Medical Research, and the Search for Scientific Sovereignty, 1880–1920." *Hispanic American Historical Review* 91, no. 3 (2012): 445–68.

———. *From Popular Medicine to Medical Populism: Doctors, Healers, and Public Power in Costa Rica, 1800–1940*. Durham: Duke University Press, 2003.

———. *Launching Global Health: The Caribbean Odyssey of the Rockefeller Foundation*. Ann Arbor: University of Michigan Press, 2010.

Palmer, Steven, José Antonio Piqueras, and Amparo Sánchez Cobos, eds. *State of Ambiguity: Civic Life and Culture in Cuba's First Republic*. Durham: Duke University Press, 2014.

Pappademos, Melina. *Black Political Activism and the Cuban Republic.* Chapel Hill: University of North Carolina Press, 2011.
Parker, D. S. *The Idea of the Middle Class: White-Collar Workers and Peruvian Society, 1910–1950.* University Park: Pennsylvania State University Press, 1998.
Parker, William Belmont. *Cubans of To-day.* New York: Putnam's, 1919.
Patterson, K. D. "Yellow Fever Epidemics and Mortality in the United States, 1693–1905." *Social Science and Medicine,* April 1992, 855–65.
Peard, Julyan G. "Tropical Disorders and the Forging of a Brazilian Medical Identity, 1860–1890." *Hispanic American Historical Review* 77, no. 1 (February 1997): 1–44.
Pérez, Cristina. *Caring for Them from Birth to Death: The Practice of Community-based Cuban Medicine.* Lanham, Md.: Lexington Books, 2008.
Pérez, Louis A., Jr. *Cuba between Empires, 1878–1902.* Pittsburgh: University of Pittsburgh Press, 1983.
———. *Cuba under the Platt Amendment, 1902–1934.* Pittsburgh: University of Pittsburgh Press, 1986.
———. *On Becoming Cuban: Identity, Nationality, and Culture.* Chapel Hill: University of North Carolina Press, 1999.
Pérez, Pelayo. "La vivienda de nuestra clase pobre." *Arquitectura* 2, no. 2 (August 1918): 11–16.
Phillips, Ruby Hart. *Cuban Sideshow.* Havana: Cuban Press, 1935.
Plasiencia, Leonel. "La leche que se consume en la Habana, por su composición es buena: Es sucia bacteriológicamente por malas manipulaciones." *Boletín Oficial de la Secretaría de Sanidad y Beneficencia de la Isla de Cuba,* March 1914, 241.
Pons, Juan B. "La tuberculosis en el porvenir." In *Actas y Trabajos del Segundo Congreso Médico Nacional, Habana, Febrero 24–28 de 1911,* 29–32, Havana: El Universal, 1911.
Porter, Roy. "What Is Disease?" In *The Cambridge Illustrated History of Medicine,* edited by Roy Porter, 82–117. Cambridge: Cambridge University Press, 1996.
*Proceedings of the Twenty-Eighth National Conference of Charities and Correction.* Boston: George H. Ellis, 1901.
*Programa. Convención Nacional de Sociedades Cubanas de la Raza de Color.* Havana: Molina y Cia., 1936.
Pruna, Pedro M. "National Science in a Colonial Context: The Royal Academy of Sciences of Havana, 1861–1898." *Isis* 85, no. 3 (September 1994): 412–26.
Pruna Goodgall, Pedro M. *La Real Academia de Ciencias de la Habana, 1861–1898.* Madrid: CESIC, 2002.
Putnam, Lara. *Radical Moves: Caribbean Migrants and the Politics of Race in the Jazz Age.* Chapel Hill: University of North Carolina Press, 2013.
Quintard, Lucy W. "Nursing in Cuba." *Third International Conference of Nurses: Pan-American Exposition, Buffalo.* Cleveland: Press of J. B. Savage, 1901.
Quiza Moreno, Ricardo. *Imaginarios al ruedo: Cuba y los Estados Unidos en las exposiciones internacionales (1876–1904).* Havana: Ediciones Unión, 2010.
Ramírez Ros, Primitivo. "Sobre el mismo tema de la tuberculosis: Aclaración a la Señora Consuelo de Govantes." *Diario de la Marina,* September 8, 1929.
———. "La tuberculosis en la raza negra." *Diario de la Marina,* August 18, 1929.

Ramos, Domingo F. "Servicio de Higiene Infantil: Informe." *Boletín Oficial de la Secretaría de Sanidad y Beneficencia de la Isla de Cuba*, August 1914, 229–41.
Renda, Mary A. *Taking Haiti: Military Occupation and the Culture of U.S. Imperialism, 1915–1940*. Chapel Hill: University of North Carolina Press, 2001.
Reverby, Susan, and David Rosner. "'Beyond the Great Doctors' Revisited: A Generation of the 'New' Social History of Medicine." In *Locating Medical History*, edited by Frank Huisman and John Warner, 167–93. Baltimore: Johns Hopkins University Press, 2004.
Riaño San Marful, Pablo. *Gallos y toros en Cuba*. Havana: Editorial Fundación Fernando Ortiz, 2002.
Robaina, Tomás Fernández. *El Negro en Cuba, 1902–1958: Apuntes para la historia de la lucha contra la discriminación racial*. Havana: Editorial de Ciencias Sociales, 1995.
Roberts, Samuel Kelton, Jr. *Infectious Fear: Politics, Disease, and the Health Effects of Segregation*. Chapel Hill: University of North Carolina Press, 2009.
Rodgers, Daniel. *Atlantic Crossings: Social Politics in a Progressive Age*. Cambridge: Harvard University Press, 2000.
Rodríguez de Tío, Lola. "Asilo huérfanos de la patria." In *Memoria Oficial. Segunda Conferencia Nacional de Beneficencia y Corrección de la Isla de Cuba. Celebrada en Santa Clara del 24 al 26 de Mayo de 1903*, 57–65. Havana: La Moderna Poesía, 1904.
Rodríguez Expósito, César. *Carlos J. Finlay: 1833–1915*. Havana: Ministerio de Salud Pública, Consejo Científico, 1965.
———. *Dr. Juan N. Dávalos: El sabio que sueña con las bacterias*. Havana: Ministerio de Salud Pública, 1967.
———. "La Primera Secretaría de Sanidad del Mundo se Creó en Cuba." *Cuadernos de la Historia de la Salud Pública*, no. 25 (1964): 7–34.
Rogaski, Ruth. *Hygienic Modernity: Meanings of Health and Disease in Treaty-Port China*. Berkeley: University of California Press, 2004.
Romero Sanchez, Susana. *The Building State: Urbanization, Rural Modernization, and the Reinvention of History in Colombia, 1920–1957*. Forthcoming.
Rosenberg, Charles E. *The Care of Strangers: The Rise of America's Hospital System*. New York: Basic Books, 1987.
Rosenberg, Charles, and Jeanne Golden, eds. *Framing Disease: Studies in Cultural History*. New Brunswick, N.J.: Rutgers University Press, 1992.
Rosner, David. *A Once Charitable Enterprise: Hospitals and Health Care in Brooklyn and New York, 1885–1915*. Cambridge: Cambridge University Press, 1982.
Rothstein, William G. "Trends in Mortality in the Twentieth Century." In *Readings in American Health Care: Current Issues in Socio-Historical Perspective*, edited by William G. Rothstein, 71–86. Madison: University of Wisconsin Press, 1995.
Rubens, Horatio S. *Liberty: The Story of Cuba*. New York: Brewer, Warren, and Putnam, 1932.
Ruiz, Ramón Eduardo. *Cuba: The Making of a Revolution*. Amherst: University of Massachusetts Press, 1968.
Sánchez de Fuentes, Alberto. "Profilaxis de la tuberculosis en Cuba." *Boletín Oficial de la Secretaría de Sanidad y Beneficencia de la Isla de Cuba*, July–December 1927, 539–49.
Sánchez Martínez, Luis. *Guía del policía cubano*. 2nd ed. Havana: Comas y López, 1914.

Sanders, James E. *The Vanguard of the Atlantic World: Creating Modernity, Nation, and Democracy in Nineteenth-Century Latin America*. Durham: Duke University Press, 2014.

Santos Fernández, Juan. "Discurso leído en la sesión solemne celebrada el día 15 de Mayo de 1902." *Anales de la Academia de Ciencias Médicas, Físicas, y Naturales de la Habana* 39 (1902–3): 4–10.

———. "La inmigración." *Anales de la Academia de Ciencias Médicas, Físicas, y Naturales de la Habana* 43, no. 7 (1907): 4–25.

Scarpaci, Joseph L., Roberto Segre, and Mario Coyula. *Havana: Two Faces of the Antillean Metropolis*. Chapel Hill: University of North Carolina Press, 2002.

Schurz, Carl. "The Philanthropic Policy." *Harper's Weekly*, April 9, 1898, 339.

Scott, Julius. *The Common Wind: Afro-American Currents in the Age of the Haitian Revolution*. New York: Verso, 2018.

Sippial, Tiffany A. *Prostitution, Modernity, and the Making of the Cuban Republic, 1840–1920*. Chapel Hill: University of North Carolina Press, 2013.

Sixth International Congress on Tuberculosis. *Transactions of the Sixth International Congress on Tuberculosis, Washington, D.C., September 28 to October 5, 1908*. Philadelphia: W. F. Fell Company, 1908.

Starr, Paul. *The Social Transformation of American Medicine: The Rise of a Sovereign Profession and the Making of a Vast Industry*. New York: Basic Books, 1982.

"Starvation of Reconcentrados in Cuba." *Boston Medical and Surgical Journal* 137, no. 14 (November 4, 1897): 478.

"Statistics of Physicians of Paris since the Thirteenth Century." *Woman's Medical Journal*, June 1904, 132.

Stepan, Nancy. *The Hour of Eugenics: Race, Gender, and Nation in Latin America*. Ithaca, N.Y.: Cornell University Press, 1991.

———. "The Interplay between Socio-Economic Factors and Medical Science: Yellow Fever Research, Cuba, and the United States." *Social Studies of Science* 8, no. 4 (1978): 397—423.

———. *Picturing Tropical Nature*. Ithaca, N.Y.: Cornell University Press, 2001.

Stern, Alexandra Minna. "Making Better Babies: Public Health and Race Betterment in Indiana, 1920–1935." *American Journal of Public Health* 92, no. 5 (2002): 742–52.

———. "Responsible Mothers and Normal Children: Eugenics, Nationalism, and Welfare in Postrevolutionary Mexico, 1920–1940." *Journal of Historical Sociology* 12, no. 4 (December 1999): 369–97.

Stoler, Ann Laura. *Along the Archival Grain: Epistemic Anxieties and Colonial Common Sense*. Princeton: Princeton University Press, 2010.

———, ed. *Haunted by Empire: Geographies of Intimacy in North American History*. Durham: Duke University Press, 2006.

Stoner, K. Lynn. *From the House to the Streets: The Cuban Women's Movement for Legal Reform, 1898–1940*. Durham: Duke University Press, 1991.

Stubbs, Jean. "Gender Constructs of Labour in Prerevolutionary Cuban Tobacco." *Social and Economic Studies* 37, no. 1/2 (1988): 241–69.

Suárez, Miguel R. "Notes from Cuban Relief Department." In *Proceedings of the Twenty-Seventh National Conference on Charities and Correction*, 374–79. Boston: George H. Ellis, 1900.

———. "Partial Review of Charitable Work Done by the Government of Intervention in Cuba." In *Addresses before the First National Conference of Charities and Corrections of the Island of Cuba*, 3–29. Havana: Rambla & Bouza, 1902.
Suárez Findlay, Eileen. *Imposing Decency: The Politics of Sexuality and Race in Puerto Rico, 1870–1920*. Durham: Duke University Press, 1999.
Suchlicki, Jaime. *Cuba, from Columbus to Castro*. New York: Scribner, 1974.
Sullivan, Frances Peace. "Radical Solidarities: U.S. Capitalism, Community Building, and Popular Internationalism in Cuba's Eastern Sugar Zone, 1919–1939." Ph.D. diss., New York University, 2012. ProQuest (AAT 3546477).
Sussman, George D. "The End of the Wet-Nursing Business in France, 1874–1914." *Journal of Family History* 2, no. 3 (1977): 237–58.
Tabares del Real, José A. *La Revolución del 30: Sus dos últimos años*. Havana: Editorial de Ciencias Sociales, 1973.
Taboadela, J. A. *Report of the Work Done by the Department in Favor of the Protection of Infancy*. Havana: La Moderna Poesía, 1914.
Tamayo y Figueredo, Diego. *Discurso leído en la aperture del curso académico de 1905 a 1906*. Havana: M. Ruiz, 1905.
———. "Necesidad de asociaciones particulares de carácter filantrópico que protejan a determinados inmigrantes." In *Memoria Oficial de la Quinta Conferencia Nacional de Beneficencia y Corrección de la Isla de Cuba*, 335–42. Havana: La Moderna Poesía, 1906.
———. "La vivienda en procomún." In *Memoria Oficial de la Sexta Conferencia Nacional de Beneficencia y Corrección de la Isla de Cuba*, 236–40. Havana: La Moderna Poesía, 1907.
Teuma, Emilio. *La secretaría de sanidad y beneficencia: Su origen, el fundador, apuntes para el estudio del progreso patrio*. Havana: La Prueba, 1917.
Thomas, Hugh. *Cuba, or, the Pursuit of Freedom*. New York: Da Capo Press, 1998.
Thurner, Mark. *From Two Republics to One Divided: Contradictions of Postcolonial Nationmaking in Andean Peru*. Durham: Duke University Press, 1997.
Thurner, Mark, and Andrés Guerrero, eds. *After Spanish Rule: Postcolonial Predicaments of the Americas*. Durham: Duke University Press, 2003.
Tomes, Nancy. *The Gospel of Germs: Men, Women, and the Microbe in American Life*. Cambridge: Harvard University Press, 1998.
Tone, John Lawrence. *War and Genocide in Cuba, 1895–1898*. Chapel Hill: University of North Carolina Press, 2006.
Trouillot, Michel-Rolph. *Silencing the Past: Power and the Production of History*. Boston: Beacon Press, 1995.
Tupper, Henry Allen. *Columbia's War for Cuba: A Story of the Early Struggles of the Cuban Patriots, and of All the Important Events Leading up to the Present War Between the United States and Spain for Cuba Libre, 1898*. New York: P. B. Bromfield & Co., 1898.
Turda, Marius, and Aaron Gillette. *Latin Eugenics in Comparative Perspective*. London: Bloomsbury, 2014.
Tyrrell, Ian. *Reforming the World: The Creation of America's Moral Empire*. Princeton: Princeton University Press, 2010.
Ubieta, Enrique. *Efemérides de la revolución cubana*. Vol. 2. Havana: La Moderna Poesía, 1911.

Urban, Kelly. "The 'Black Plague' in a Racial Democracy: Tuberculosis, Race, and Citizenship in Republican Cuba, 1925–1945." *Cuban Studies* 45 (January 2017): 319–39.

———. "The Sick Republic: Tuberculosis, Public Health, and Politics in Cuba, 1925–1965." Ph.D. diss., University of Pittsburgh, 2016.

U.S. Agency for International Development. *Nutrition and Tuberculosis: A Review of the Literature and Considerations for TB Control Programs*. USAID, 2010.

U.S. Census Office. *Census Reports*. Vol. 3, *Twelfth Census of the United States, Taken in the Year 1900, Vital Statistics*. Pt. 1, *Analysis and Ratio Tables*, ccxlv. Washington, D.C.: United States Census Office, 1902.

U.S. War Department. *Annual Reports of the War Department for the Fiscal Year Ended June 30, 1899, Report of the Major-General Commanding the Army*. Washington, D.C.: Government Printing Office, 1899.

———. *Annual Reports of the War Department for the Fiscal Year Ended June 30, 1900*. Washington, D.C.: Government Printing Office, 1900.

———. *Civil Report of Brigadier General Leonard Wood, Military Governor of Cuba, 1901*. Washington, D.C.: Government Printing Office, 1901.

———. Office of the Census of Cuba. *Report on the Census of Cuba, 1899*. Washington, D.C.: Government Printing Office, 1899.

Valdés, Juan B. "Mortalidad Infantil: Sus Causas, Medios Para Prevenirlas y Combatirlas." In *Septima Conferencia de Beneficencia y Corrección de la Isla de Cuba*, 99–115. Havana: La Moderna Poesía, 1908.

Varona Suárez, Manuel. "Homicultura: Notas sobre los trabajos de los Dres. E. Hernández y D. F. Ramos." *Boletín Oficial de la Secretaría de Sanidad y Beneficencia de la Isla de Cuba*, December 1910, 1–3.

Vaughan, Mary Kay. *Cultural Politics in Revolution: Teachers, Peasants, and Schools in Mexico, 1930–1940*. Tucson: University of Arizona Press, 1997.

Vaughan, Megan. "Healing and Curing: Issues in the Social History and Anthropology of Medicine in Africa." *Social History of Medicine* 7, no. 2 (September 1994): 283–95.

Veeser, Cyrus. *A World Safe for Capitalism: Dollar Diplomacy and America's Rise to Global Power*. New York: Columbia University Press, 2002.

Vidal Rodríguez, José Antonio. *La emigración gallega a Cuba: Trayectos migratorios, inserción y movilidad laboral, 1898–1968*. Madrid: Centro Superior de Investigaciones Científicas, 2005.

Vogel, Morris J. *The Invention of the Modern Hospital: Boston, 1870–1930*. Chicago: University of Chicago Press, 1980.

Wade, Peter. *Race and Ethnicity in Latin America*. London: Pluto Press, 1997.

Wailoo, Keith. *Dying in the City of the Blues: Sickle Cell Anemia and the Politics of Race and Health*. Chapel Hill: University of North Carolina Press, 2001.

Walker, Louise E. *Waking from the Dream: Mexico's Middle Classes after 1968*. Stanford, Calif.: Stanford University Press, 2013.

Wangensteen, Owen H., and Sarah D. Wangensteen. *The Rise of Surgery: From Empiric Craft to Scientific Discipline*. Folkestone: Dawson, 1978.

Warren, Adam. *Medicine and Politics in Colonial Peru: Population Growth and the Bourbon Reforms*. Pittsburgh: University of Pittsburgh Press, 2010.

Weinstein, Barbara. *For Social Peace in Brazil: Industrialists and the Remaking of the Working Class in São Paulo, 1920–1964*. Chapel Hill: University of North Carolina Press, 1997.

Whiteford, Linda M., and Laurence G. Branch. *Primary Health Care in Cuba: The Other Revolution*. Lanham: Rowman and Littlefield, 2007.

Whitney, Robert. *State and Revolution in Cuba: Mass Mobilization and Political Change, 1920–1940*. Chapel Hill: University of North Carolina Press, 2001.

Wilson, Erastus. *El problema urgente: El saneamiento de la Habana y su puerto*. Havana: La Prueba, 1898.

Wood, Leonard. "The Military Government of Cuba." *Annals of the American Academy of Political and Social Science* 21 (1903): 1–30.

Worboys, Michael. *Spreading Germs: Disease Theories and Medical Practice in Britain, 1865–1900*. Cambridge: Cambridge University Press, 2000.

Wright, Irene Aloha. *Cuba*. Macmillan: New York, 1910.

Zulawski, Ann. "Environment, Urbanization, and Public Health: The Bubonic Plague Epidemic of 1912 in San Juan, Puerto Rico." *Latin American Research Review* 53, no. 3 (2018), 500–516.

———. *Unequal Cures: Public Health and Political Change in Bolivia, 1900–1950*. Durham: Duke University Press, 2007.

# INDEX

Aballí, Ángel Arturo, 142, 185
advertising, and health campaigns, 53, 62, 95, 135–36
Agramonte, Aristedes, 100
air, and disease, 160–62
Ala Izquierda Estudiantil, 164
Ala Izquierda Médica, 172, 178–79, 185–86, 190, 194–99
Albarrán Domínguez, Pedro, 1–2, 83, 206
Aldereguía, Gustavo Adolfo, 163–64, 170
Alfonso y García, Ramon María, 58
American Medical Association, 182
American Red Cross, 28–32, 37–38
antibiotics, 62, 118, 158, 161, 173
Antillean. See West Indians
archives, 11–12, 14–15, 37, 39–40
August Revolution, 84

bacteriology, 2–4, 53, 56, 63, 72–73, 87, 91, 100–101, 108–9, 218n44
Bandera, Quintín, 151
Bando de Piedad, 157, 248n84
Bangs, John Kendrick, 45
Baracoa, 1, 19
Barnet, Enrique, 48–49, 57, 93, 103–4, 131–34
Barton, Clara, 30, 38
Batista, Fulgencio, 190, 193, 198–200, 208
Bay y Sevilla, Luis, 161, 168
*beneficencia*: colonial, 26–27, 47; U.S. Military Government reorganization of, 34–36; funding and state support, 41–46; and a right to welfare, 205–6
black fraternal societies, 164, 171

bodegas, 105, 117, 187
Borges, José Elias, 192, 237n78
breastfeeding, 17, 61, 119, 129–38, 144
Brooke, John R., 31
Brotherton, P. Sean, 15
bubonic plague, 7, 9–10, 13, 56; symptoms, 87, 93; third pandemic of, 90, 92–93, 115; mitigation measures, 94–95; public declaration of, 95–98, 100, 102; economic effects, 97–98, 102, 110–14; and debates over provenance, 99–100, 109–11

Canary Islands, 9, 10, 99–100, 103, 109, 111, 180
Cantero, Trinidad, 71–72, 77, 79–80
Casa de Beneficencia y Maternidad, 26, 42, 211–12nn28–29
Castro, Fidel, 208
Catholic Church, charities, 19, 26; opposition to professional nursing, 50, 72, 76–78; and health education, 61; and disease outbreaks, 95, 219n60
Central Cuban Relief Committee, 28
Centro Asturiano, 86, 93, 180, 193, 235n14, 236n46
Centro Gallego, 180, 190, 236n46
*centros regionales*. See Spanish immigrant mutual aid societies
Céspedes, Carlos Manuel de, 4, 204
Chailloux, Juan Manuel, 151–53, 155, 157
Chelala Aguilera, José, 198
children, 8, 14, 151, 203; and the reconcentration, 19–22, 24–25, 27, 30, 120; and the U.S. Military Government in

Cuba, 31, 33, 35, 37–40; as laborers, 61; and Chinese immigration, 92; and poverty, 107, 120–23, 151, 156–57, 162; and tuberculosis, 146, 148. See also crèches; Industrial School for Girls; infant mortality; mothering; orphans
Children's Health Service, 24, 128–30, 135, 137, 139–40, 144
China, 92–93, 103, 105
Chinese immigrants, 9, 60, 92, 105, 115
cholera, 56, 92
circum-Caribbean, as space of exchange, 9, 51, 66, 69, 92–93
cleanliness, 49, 54, 73, 94, 103, 129
Club Adelante, 171
Club Profesional Oscar Primelles, 218n35
Confederación Nacional Obrera de Cuba (CNOC), 186, 190, 193
Conservative Party, 98, 99, 165
Constitution of 1901, 69–70
Constitution of 1940, 14, 153, 200, 204–7
Conversaciones del doctor, 104–5, 132, 134
Cosculluela, José A., 160, 168, 174
Covadonga Hospital, 86, 87, 107, 180, 235n14
COVID-19, 18
crèches, 126–27, 129–30, 133, 137, 138–40, 143, 145, 166, 168, 170
Cuban Academy of Science, 7, 48, 55–56, 59, 68, 92, 123, 131, 151, 154
Cuban Anti-Tuberculosis League, 61–62, 79, 146, 162, 164, 167–68
Cuban Communist Party, 164, 186
Cuban Medical College, 176–77, 187–94, 197–98
Cuban Medical Federation, 166, 172, 175–200
Cuban Orphan Society, 34

Damas Isabelinas, 146, 162, 167
Davenport, Charles, 141
Department of Public Charities, 34–37, 40–40, 42–44, 46, 64, 73, 81–82, 205
Deulofeu, Emma, 160

Diario de la Marina (newspaper), 78–79, 115, 146, 165, 168, 191–92, 194–95, 197, 200
Diario Español (newspaper), 99–102, 110–13
Directorio Social Revolucionario "Renacimiento," 171
dispensaries, 7, 41, 42, 59, 64, 128, 133, 149, 162, 169, 177, 185, 198, 205, 214n81. See also Dispensario Furbush; Dispensario La Caridad
Dispensario Furbush, 68, 158, 168, 198
Dispensario La Caridad, 19–20, 26, 60, 78, 121
doctors: participation in Cuban independence struggle, 5, 56–58, 124–25; education, 19, 57, 62, 125, 171, 179, 199, 217n32; class origin, 19, 179–80; doctor-patient ratio in Cuba, 55, 195–96, 217n26; political affiliations, 56–60, 178–79, 184–87. See also Cuban Medical Federation; hospitals; patronage
domestic workers, 86, 122, 137
Duque, Matías, 70, 84, 85,

education. See doctors; education; health education; nursing schools
El Mundo (newspaper), 102, 117–18, 136
El Triunfo (newspaper), 95, 98, 100–101, 108–9, 112
enteritis, 3, 26, 66, 117–19, 130
Espinosa, Mariola, 5, 68
Estrada Palma, Tomás, 48, 71, 84
eugenics, 127, 140–42

Féderación Médica de Cuba. See Cuban Medical Federation
Fernández, Edelmira, 79–80
Ferrer, Ada, 4, 32, 154
Finlay, Carlos E., 46–47, 76, 78, 187, 217n6
Finlay, Carlos Juan, 3–4, 53, 56, 67, 84, 201
Folks, Homer, 34–36, 38–40
food: cost of, 6, 23, 122, 169; imports, 10, 24, 122, 189; contaminated, 26, 60, 118; donations, 27–33, 37–39, 46, 119–21, 124, 129, 134, 137–39, 143, 145; subsidized, 169–70, 174

France, influence on Cuban medicine, 2, 125, 127–28, 140, 228n29
Fuente, Alejandro de la, 153, 154, 164
fumigation, 88, 95, 105–6, 108, 110–13

Gandarilla, Julio César, 70
gender, 6–9, 11, 15, 22, 27, 30, 33; and poverty, 19, 37–41, 119–23; and medical nationalism, 50, 60–63, 71–76; and mortality, 161–62; and hospital admission, 222n110
General Wood Laboratory, 71
Gillette, Howard, Jr., 36
glanders, 65, 67–68, 220n58
Gómez, José Miguel, 128
Gómez, Juan Gualberto, 154, 165
Gómez, Miguel Mariano, 201
Gorgas, William Crawford, 52, 54, 68, 90
Grau San Martín, Ramón, 176–77, 187–90
Great Britain, 67, 93, 108, 133
Great Depression, 182–83; and mortality in Cuba, 235n24
Greble, Edwin St. John, 123, 124, 214n89
Guanabacoa, 29–30, 107–8
Guardia, Vicente de la, 65, 66
Guerra Chiquita, 57, 125, 211n3
Guiteras, Antonio, 187
Guiteras, Juan, 28, 87, 92, 96–97, 99, 101, 103, 106, 108, 111, 202

Haiti, 14, 96, 115,
Havana, growth and demographics, 9–11, 91, 149; racialized/gendered labor market, 32–33, 91, 119, 122, 153. *See also* housing; real estate speculation; tenements; unemployment
Havana Department of Public Health, 53–54, 64–65, 67, 87, 89, 84, 94–114, 129, 132, 136, 169,
Havana Relief Department, 32
health education, 7–8, 58–62; and mothers, 63, 80, 126, 128, 130, 132–34, 136, 137; nurses and, 72–73; as basis of antituberculosis campaign, 150, 158–62, 167–68. *See also* infant mortality: state responses to; nursing: home visits; tuberculosis
Hernandez, Eusebio, 57, 124–29, 138, 140–41, 144, 163, 218n32
Hibbard, Eugenie, 15, 75, 160, 169
Hicks, Anasa, 122
Hoganson, Kristin, 27
homiculture, 126–28, 138, 140–42
Honduras, 125
hospitals, public: conditions in, 20, 26, 53, 73, 74, 183, 198–99, 201; and the U.S. occupation, 31, 34–36, 53; administrative reform, 35–36, 41–42, 73; state funding, 41–43, 183, 198–99, 201; admittance, 43–44, 78, 82, 185, 205; and nursing, 73–75, 78; as gendered spaces, 74–75, 222n110; corruption and patronage, 82, 183; and doctors, 185, 194, 196, 197, 198, 200
housing: conditions, 15, 64, 66, 119, 142, 203; costs, 8, 11, 122, 147, 149, 152–53, 163, 203; and race, 151, 153, 156, 158, 173–74. *See also* real estate speculation; tenements
Hurtado Galtés, Félix, 179, 180, 184
Hyatt, George W., 29–30
hygiene, 4, 7, 13, 14, 48–50, 56, 58–61, 63, 72, 90, 94, 98, 103, 202. *See also* cleanliness; health education; medical nationalism; mothering; tuberculosis

"Ideales de una raza," 146, 149, 164–67, 170
Iglesias Utset, Marial, 54, 62
immigration: and infant mortality, 120; policy, 90–93, 114–15, 172; and whitening, 58, 60. *See also* Chinese immigrants; Spanish immigrants; West Indians
Industrial School for Girls, 33, 38
infant mortality, 7, 8, 11, 15, 22, 60, 160, 207; as national indicator, 15, 120, 144; causes of, 118–19, 131; and poverty, 121–22, 183; and race, 122–23, 140–44; state responses to, 128–30, 137–38,

INDEX 263

140–41, 144, 204. *See also* breastfeeding; crèches; homiculture; milk; mothering; National Motherhood Competitions
International Labour Office, 181, 193–96, 199

Jacobsen, Joaquín, 61, 68, 155, 163, 167–69, 202
Jover, Verena, 77, 80

Kean, Jefferson Randolph, 25, 35, 37, 42–44, 76, 78, 82–84
Koch, Robert, 4, 56
Kraut, Alan, 115

labor movement, 186, 187, 190–91, 192–94, 200. *See also* Confederación Nacional Obrera de Cuba
La Casa del Pobre, 121, 123–24, 168
*La Discusión* (newspaper), 95, 97–98, 100, 107–10
La Esperanza Sanitorium, 158, 169, 198; patient demographics, 161–62;
*La Higiene* (journal), 14, 19, 63, 121, 133
*La Lucha* (newspaper), 72, 102–3, 109, 113
Lebredo, Mario G., 87, 137
Le-Roy y Cassá, Jorge, 60, 202, 216n3
Ley de Colegiación Médica Obligatoria, 187–90, 193
Liberal Party, 84, 95–96, 98–100
Liga Contra la Tuberculosis. *See* Cuban Anti-Tuberculosis League
López del Valle, José Antonio, 15, 82, 94, 103, 136–37, 140, 149, 160, 219n52
*Los Cubanos en Campaña* (newspaper), 66, 74
Los Fosos (shelter), 24–25, 37, 39–40

Machado, Gerardo, 12, 163–64, 171, 176, 178–79, 182–87, 189–90, 236n36
Magoon, Charles, 81, 84, 123
malaria, 7, 66–67, 97, 115, 201, 227n93
Malberty, José Ángel, 1–2, 4, 11, 57, 83–84
malnutrition, 11, 15, 19, 26, 31, 117, 126, 142, 144

Martí, José, 57, 150, 154
Matanzas, 23, 192
maternal health, 17, 126–29, 140
Mazorra Hospital, 26, 36, 198, 200
McKinley, William, 28
medical nationalism, 3–8, 10–11, 14, 103, 114, 149–50, 202–3, 208; and state responsibility for the health of citizens, 2–3, 8–9, 41–43, 169–74; as cultural revolution, 16, 50, 60–64, 70; and U.S. empire, 69–70, 83–85, 89, 96–97, 187; and nursing, 71–80; and infant mortality, 119–20, 133, 137; and raceless nationalism, 165–73
*Medical Record* (journal), 96
Méndez Capote, Domingo, 108, 154, 155
Mendieta, Carlos, 190–94, 198–200
Menocal, Mario G., 98–100, 128, 135, 138
Menocal, Raimundo, 57, 75
Mercedes Hospital, 57, 72, 75, 76, 127, 142, 191, 198
Merelles, Maria, 162
*mestizaje*, 142
Mexico, 9, 57, 62, 93, 133, 205
Miami, 191
milk: cost of, 23, 26; and infant mortality, 118–19, 126, 138, 144, 219n60; milk inspection, 129–32
Ministry of Health and Public Charities. *See* Secretaría de Sanidad y Beneficencia
Montalvo, Rafael, 59
mosquitoes: extermination of, 5, 67–68, 82–83, 94, 118, 201, 220n81; role in causing yellow fever, 53, 56, 67, 217n17
mothering, 16, 63, 119–20, 133, 133, 142. *See also* scientific motherhood; women

National Conferences on *Beneficencia* and Corrections, 46–47, 77, 79, 155
National Congress of Cuban Mothers, 137–39, 230n79
National Congress of Mothers (U.S.), 155
National Convention of Cuban Societies of the Race of Color, 171–72

National Laboratory for Scientific Investigation, 87, 93, 95, 101,
National Medical College, 176–77, 187–94, 197–98
National Motherhood Competition (Concurso Nacional de Maternidad), 135–36, 143
National Women's Congresses (Cuba), 230n89
New Orleans, 9, 68, 216nn10–11
New York City, 34, 36, 41, 57, 62, 72, 75, 97, 126, 141
New York State Charities Aid Association, 35
Nuñez, Emiliano, 57, 73
Nuñez de Villavicenio, Enrique, 57, 74, 120
Nuñez Portuondo, Ricardo, 183, 187
nursing: and nationalism, 71–72, 77–80; opposition to, 75–80; and race, 76–77; and education, 129–30; home visits, 133, 135, 149, 158, 160–62, 173
nursing schools, 7, 36, 43, 46, 49–50; creation of, 73–75; conflicts over, 75–77; and the 1934 medical strike, 190–91

obstetrics, 124–28
Odio Pérez, Eduardo, 196–98
O'Donnell, Mary Agnes, 72, 76
orphanages, 26, 34, 38, 40–41, 43; and institutionalization, 35, 37
orphans: and the reconcentration, 20, 26, 28, 37, 38; and adoption, 35; as nursing students, 76, 206; and prostitution, 211n23. *See also* Department of Public Charities; orphanages

Pan-American Conference on Eugenics and Homiculture, 160
Pappademos, Melina, 171
Partido Independiente de Color, 153, 164
Pasteur, Louis, 4, 56, 217n32
patronage, 82–84, 124, 161, 174, 184, 201, 203, 235n35
pauperism, 22, 31–33, 35, 39, 46, 169
Penichet, J. M., 182

Pérez, Louis A., Jr., 32, 62, 114, 186
pharmacies, 95, 177, 191–92, 197
pharmacists, 171, 177, 187, 190, 191–92, 236n56
Philadelphia, 28, 41, 57
Pinard, Adolphe, 125–26, 128, 140, 218n32
Platt Amendment, 7, 49, 51, 64, 69–70, 83–84, 89, 102, 114, 187, 202
Politica Cómica, 97
Pozo Gato, Catalina, 153
*Progreso Médico* (journal), 66
prostitution, 25, 78, 138, 151, 153, 211n23
puericulture, 125–28, 228n29, 230n89
Puerto Rico, 9, 97

quarantine, 10, 13, 16, 64, 88, 97, 100, 105–16
Quinta de Dependientes, 52, 190, 193
Quintard, Lucy, 73, 76, 77

race: and the labor market, 8, 15, 91–92, 119, 122, 153; and the reconcentration, 21; and access to medical care, 21, 74–75, 161–62; and U.S. relief efforts, 27–28, 32; and U.S. views of Cuban health conditions and capacities, 51, 54, 70, 96–97; and immigration, 58, 60, 89–93, 114–16; and health disparities, 123, 142–43, 148–49, 162; and housing, 150–58; and health demands of Cubans of color, 163–73
raceless nationalism, 4, 11, 17, 150, 154, 164–66, 170
racial segregation: of colonial *beneficencia* institutions, 27; of Spanish-immigrant hospitals, 27, 163, 165–66; and housing, 152–53
Ramírez Ros, Primitivo, 146–47, 164–67, 170–71
Ramos, Domingo F., 118, 120, 124, 126–29, 134, 141–42
rats, as disease vectors, 9–10, 88, 94–95, 98, 103–6, 113, 118
real estate speculation, 11, 149
reconcentration, 5, 16, 21–29, 31–33, 37–41, 43, 58, 72–73, 76, 215n96, 221n103;

INDEX 265

mortality, 5, 20, 24–25, 211n5; as counterinsurgency strategy, 19–20; Cuban relief efforts, 19–20, 25–27; economic effects, 23–24; and race, 27, 212n34; U.S. relief efforts, 27–31. *See also* American Red Cross; United States: relief work; U.S. Military Government in Cuba: relief work of
Red Cross. *See* American Red Cross
Reed, Walter, 67
Regla, 107–8
regulations: and fines, 53, 54, 67, 81, 94, 111, 157; health, 65, 81, 129, 131, 137, 158–60; flouting of, 159–60, 174
rents. *See* housing costs
rights, health, 2–4, 8, 13–14, 43–46, 150, 163–75, 202–8
Roberts, Samuel K., 149
rural health, 140, 172, 181, 201, 207–8

Sabas Alomá, Maríblanca, 154, 170
Sánchez de Fuentes, Alberto, 168
sanitation, 45, 52–54, 67, 69, 70, 94–95, 98–99, 105, 108, 113
Santiago de Cuba, 31–32, 76–77, 105
Santos Fernández, Juan, 48–49, 61, 68, 91
scientific charity, 34–42, 46–47
scientific motherhood, 130–37
Secretaría de Sanidad y Beneficencia: creation of, 1–3, 80–85; and corruption, 12, 174, 184, 201, 203; official *boletín* of, 15, 139, 148. *See also* medical nationalism; nursing; patronage; Platt Amendment
sewage system, 51, 64–65, 201, 220n75
Sisters of Charity, 73–78, 138–39
slavery, 4, 125, 170
smallpox, 68, 75, 92, 97, 115, 220n72
Social Hygiene League, 142
socialized medicine, 196–200, 207–8
*solares*. *See* tenements
Spain: source of desired immigration, 6, 90–91, 115–16; and counterinsurgency, 19–20; and "backwardness," 51, 70, 114; as a disease threat, 89, 91, 99–100, 114–15. *See also* Canary Islands; Guerra Chiquita; reconcentration; "Spanish-American War"; Spanish immigrants; Ten Years War; War of Independence, final
"Spanish-American War," 5, 22, 28–29, 31, 38 and U.S. naval blockade, 26, 27, 29, 73
Spanish immigrant mutual aid societies: medical benefits, 10–11, 92, 180–81, 207, 235n15; as racially exclusive, 27, 163, 165–66; conflict with Cuban Medical Federation, 177–78, 182–83, 188–90, 193–95, 197, 200; class composition, 180, 235n13. *See also* Centro Asturiano; Centro Gallego.
Spanish immigrants, 8, 9, 10, 27, 52, 74, 86, 89–91; role in Cuban and urban economy, 10, 91, 98–99, 113, 153, 176, 189; associationalism, 80, 92, 180, 193; relationship with Cuban public health authorities, 100–104, 106, 108–9, 111–14. *See also* Spanish immigrant mutual aid societies
starvation, 5, 20, 23–31, 71, 198, 208
Stepan, Nancy, 5, 127
stigma, 78–79, 92, 115
strikes: medical, 11, 177–78, 181, 183, 186, 189–95, 197–200; general labor, 186, 189, 193, 197, 199–200
Suárez, Miguel R., 30, 32–33, 39–40
sugar industry, 4, 23, 91,

Tamayo Figueredo, Diego, 57, 71, 151, 154–55, 157, 217n19, 218n32, 218n35
tenements, 8, 11, 107, 147, 162–63; as racially coded black spaces, 105, 147, 150–54, 163; and disease, 147, 154–56, 166–70; state regulation of, 159–60, 174. *See also* housing conditions; racial segregation; real estate speculation
Ten Years War, 56–57, 125, 204, 211n3
tetanus, 2
Teuma, Emilio, 85
tobacco factories, 122, 163,
tourism, 97–98

Tribuna Medica, 179, 182–83, 195–98
Triscornia quarantine station, 106, 107, 129
tropical environment, 48–49, 62, 90–91, 216n3
tuberculosis: and race, 8, 11, 16, 92, 148, 151, 161–67, 170–72; research, 56, 142; transmission, 56, 147–48; and alcohol, 61; popular education, 61–62, 80, 81, 127, 159, 162–63; and the U.S. Military Government in Cuba, 66–67, 68–69; state efforts to control, 80, 158–61, 173, 205; and poverty, 121, 122, 123, 147–48, 155–57, 183, 206; mortality, 146–47, 231n5; symptoms, 147–48; treatment and prevention, 150, 162; state vs. private responsibility, 168–72, 174; private antituberculosis efforts (see Casa del Pobre, La; Cuban Anti-Tuberculosis League; Damas Isabelinas). See also Koch, Robert; La Esperanza Sanitorium; tenements
typhoid, 56, 66, 97, 201, 220n72

unemployment, 11, 91, 142, 147–48, 163, 171, 182–83, 185, 195, 204
United States: interventionism, 20–21, 27–28, 49, 69–70, 83–84, 89; relief work, 20–21, 27–30; views on Cuban poor, 31–32, 45–46; accusations of Cuban sanitary backwardness, 53–54, 96–97. See also American Red Cross; Platt Amendment; U.S. Military Government in Cuba; U.S. Provisional Government in Cuba
University of Havana, 125, 142, 151–53, 171, 179, 187, 199
Urban, Kelly, 161
Urrutia, Gustavo, 164–67, 170–71
U.S. Military Government in Cuba (1899–1902), 5–6, 20, 80; relief work of, 30–33; support for private charities, 37–38; and hospitals, 41–44, 73–78; sanitary campaign, 51–55, 59; yellow fever campaign, 51–55, 67–68; relationship with Cuban physicians, 64–66, 68–70. See also Department of Public Charities; Folks, Homer; Los Fosos; Wood, Leonard; yellow fever; Yellow Fever Commission
U.S. Provisional Government in Cuba (1906–1909), 84, 123

vaccines, 56, 68, 129, 199, 218n32
Valdés, Juan, 133, 134
Varona Suárez, Miguel, 128
Vida Nueva (journal), 85, 112, 154

War of Independence, final (1895–1898), 3, 5, 16, 20, 22, 31, 57–58, 73, 75–76, 109, 125, 127, 206
West Indian, 9, 60, 92, 114–15
wet nurses, 17, 63, 129, 133
Weyler, Valeriano, 19, 23–26, 29, 110
Whitney, Robert, 184
women: and wages, 11, 32, 119, 122–23, 143, 148; employment, 11, 33, 37–39, 72–73, 79, 142, 148; effects of the reconcentration on, 20–22, 25, 27–28; and relief, 28, 30–33, 37–41; reformers, 137–40. See also gender; infant mortality; mothering; nursing
Women's Committee for the Protection of Children in Habana Nueva, 137–40
Wood, Leonard, 34–39, 48, 68–69, 71

yellow fever, 2–3, 5–7, 9, 49–56, 94, 96, 101, 118, 120, 126, 133, 174; acquired immunity, 3, 52; outbreaks in the U.S., 51; symptoms, 51–52; U.S. efforts to control, 51–54, 66–69; Carlos J. Finlay's mosquito theory, 56; and the Platt Amendment, 69–70, 83–84; and immigration, 90–91; campaign as a model for other health campaigns, 126, 144, 163, 169
Yellow Fever Commission, 64, 66–67

INDEX 267

## ENVISIONING CUBA

Daniel A. Rodríguez, *The Right to Live In Health: Medical Politics in Postindependence Havana* (2020).

Tiffany A. Sippial, *Celia Sánchez Manduley: The Life and Legacy of a Cuban Revolutionary* (2020).

Ariel Mae Lambe, *No Barrier Can Contain It: Cuban Antifascism and the Spanish Civil War* (2019).

Henry B. Lovejoy, *Prieto: Yorùbá Kingship in Colonial Cuba during the Age of Revolutions* (2018).

A. Javier Treviño, *C. Wright Mills and the Cuban Revolution: An Exercise in the Art of Sociological Imagination* (2017).

Antonia Dalia Muller, *Cuban Émigrés and Independence in the Nineteenth-Century Gulf World* (2017).

Jennifer L. Lambe, *Madhouse: Psychiatry and Politics in Cuban History* (2017).

Devyn Spence Benson, *Antiracism in Cuba: The Unfinished Revolution* (2016).

Michelle Chase, *Revolution within the Revolution: Women and Gender Politics in Cuba, 1952–1962* (2015).

Aisha K. Finch, *Rethinking Slave Rebellion in Cuba: La Escalera and the Insurgencies of 1841–1844* (2015).

Christina D. Abreu, *Rhythms of Race: Cuban Musicians and the Making of Latino New York City and Miami, 1940–1960* (2015).

Anita Casavantes Bradford, *The Revolution Is for the Children: The Politics of Childhood in Havana and Miami, 1959–1962* (2014).

Tiffany A. Sippial, *Prostitution, Modernity, and the Making of the Cuban Republic, 1840–1920* (2013).

Kathleen López, *Chinese Cubans: A Transnational History* (2013).

Lillian Guerra, *Visions of Power in Cuba: Revolution, Redemption, and Resistance, 1959–1971* (2012).

Carrie Hamilton, *Sexual Revolutions in Cuba: Passion, Politics, and Memory* (2012).

Sherry Johnson, *Climate and Catastrophe in Cuba and the Atlantic World during the Age of Revolution* (2011).

Melina Pappademos, *Black Political Activism and the Cuban Republic* (2011).

Frank Andre Guridy, *Forging Diaspora: Afro-Cubans and African Americans in a World of Empire and Jim Crow* (2010).

Ann Marie Stock, *On Location in Cuba: Street Filmmaking during Times of Transition* (2009).

Alejandro de la Fuente, *Havana and the Atlantic in the Sixteenth Century* (2008).

Reinaldo Funes Monzote, *From Rainforest to Cane Field in Cuba: An Environmental History since 1492* (2008).

Matt D. Childs, *The 1812 Aponte Rebellion in Cuba and the Struggle against Atlantic Slavery* (2006).

Eduardo González, *Cuba and the Tempest: Literature and Cinema in the Time of Diaspora* (2006).

John Lawrence Tone, *War and Genocide in Cuba, 1895–1898* (2006).

Samuel Farber, *The Origins of the Cuban Revolution Reconsidered* (2006).

Lillian Guerra, *The Myth of José Martí: Conflicting Nationalisms in Early Twentieth-Century Cuba* (2005).

Rodrigo Lazo, *Writing to Cuba: Filibustering and Cuban Exiles in the United States* (2005).

Alejandra Bronfman, *Measures of Equality: Social Science, Citizenship, and Race in Cuba, 1902–1940* (2004).

Edna M. Rodríguez-Mangual, *Lydia Cabrera and the Construction of an Afro-Cuban Cultural Identity* (2004).

Gabino La Rosa Corzo, *Runaway Slave Settlements in Cuba: Resistance and Repression* (2003).

Piero Gleijeses, *Conflicting Missions: Havana, Washington, and Africa, 1959–1976* (2002).

Robert Whitney, *State and Revolution in Cuba: Mass Mobilization and Political Change, 1920–1940* (2001).

Alejandro de la Fuente, *A Nation for All: Race, Inequality, and Politics in Twentieth-Century Cuba* (2001).

www.ingramcontent.com/pod-product-compliance
Lightning Source LLC
Chambersburg PA
CBHW032033300426
44117CB00009B/1044